Into Our Own Hands

Into Our Own Hands

The Women's Health Movement in the United States, 1969–1990

Sandra Morgen

Rutgers University Press
New Brunswick, New Jersey, and London

8-30-2005
LAN
 # 24

Library of Congress Cataloging-in-Publication Data

Morgen, Sandra.
    Into our own hands : the women's health movement in the United States,
1969–1990 / Sandra Morgen.
      p. cm.
    Includes bibliographical references and index.
    ISBN 0-8135-3070-9 (cloth: alk. paper) — ISBN 0-8135-3071-7 (pbk. : alk. paper)
    1. Women's health services—United States. 2. Women's health services—
Political aspects—United States. 3. Feminism—United States. I. Title.

RG103 .M67 2002
362.1'98'0973—dc21

                       2001048614

British Cataloging-in-Publication data for this book is available from the British
Library

For permissions to previously published material see Preface and Acknowledg-
ments.

Manufactured in the United States of America

To the many women across the world who have struggled for affordable, dignified and quality health care for themselves and their families; and

in memory of

*my mother, Sadye Block Morgan (1927–1991),
whose struggle with cancer demonstrated wisdom, courage and strength;*

*in the hope
that women will continue to work individually and collectively for a healthier, more equitable and just world.*

Contents

Afterword: The Movement in the 1990s: Accomplishments
and Continuing Challenges

Preface and Acknowledgments

In January 1973 the Supreme Court decision in *Roe* vs. *Wade* legalized abortion. Several months later my mother, age forty-six, was diagnosed with breast cancer. That fall, I entered the doctoral program in anthropology at the University of North Carolina. I did not know it then, but groups of women in communities across the United States were enacting feminism by forming women's health clinics and reclaiming their right to greater control over their bodies and their health care.

These were heady times. During the 1960s and 1970s, women, communities of color, welfare recipients, students, and antiwar activists organized powerful social movements that were reshaping North American society. Anthropologists, some of them anyhow, were reflecting on the legacy of colonialism in our disciplinary theory and practice. To me, the prospect of fieldwork in some faraway place felt wrong, even imperialistic. Instead, I wanted to weave my political, personal, and scholarly passions together, to study the process of social transformation all around me. So I rejected the time-tested theory that we learn about *us* by studying the *other* and decided to study not just the *us* of the United States, but the *us* of feminist activism.

In early 1977, when the women's health movement was fresh, radical, and rich with promise, I began what became more than two years of ethnographic research in one of those health clinics, one located on the East Coast. Women's health was never just a scholarly interest for me, a trained medical anthropologist. When I worked at the women's health collective, my daily work—pregnancy testing; birth control, abortion, and pregnancy counseling; routine gynecological health services; working with women struggling to survive poverty or to escape domestic violence; health care advocacy; being a member of a collectively run clinic—was simultaneously fieldwork and an expression of my personal and political commitments. My work there ended in 1979, when my mother's cancer recurred and I went home to live with my parents during her second course of chemotherapy. I wrote my dissertation while I was helping care for my mother.

In the past quarter century a revolution has transformed women's health care. That revolution was sparked not primarily by technological advances, white-coated physicians, or managers of HMOs. Rather, ordinary women conceived and reinvented history in the late 1960s when they demanded knowledge about their bodies, sought greater control over their own health care, and forced their way into medical schools and the rooms where health policy decisions are made. From seeds of activism, women organized health collectives, self-help groups, abortion and health information and referral services, health clinics, and organizations that advocated for change in many aspects of women's health care. Ironically, few people today realize this was a grassroots revolution organized by white middle-class and working-class women, by middle-class and working-class women of color, by lesbians and heterosexuals.

During the time I worked at the feminist clinic, I learned what it meant for women to work together without bosses or professional or male authority figures to act, to create change. I felt buoyed and elated as I helped write grants for the organization, provided lay health care very different from what women received in mainstream medical practices, participated in the collective process of sustaining the organization and using it as a base from which to advocate for change. The rigors of efforts to build consensus also taught me about political divisions, conflicts between high ideals and daily realities, burnout. After I completed a dissertation and several articles based on my research in the movement, I moved away from the work for many years, in part because my own engagement complicated interpretation in ways that I did not yet have the tools to understand. I knew that the movement had become a painful place to be, and I did not yet understand how the lessons I was learning—about the extraordinary difficulties of collective structure, about dilemmas of class and racial difference, about the potentially co-opting power of the state and assaults by the New Right—could illuminate either social theory or social change efforts.

What I didn't know then was that the same difficulties and dangers presided over other social movements, too, and that I would discover them again in the collective *we* that works from a variety of (mostly allied) locations in higher education (women's studies and women's research centers, black and ethnic studies, cultural and postcolonial studies) to transform the academy. I remember vividly the moment when I began to understand that endless turmoil within the women's health movement echoed what had happened in many other progressive movements. Charles Payne (1995) made that connection for me in *I've Got the Light of Freedom: The Organizing Tradition and the Mississippi Freedom Struggle*. Payne tracks the growth and diversification of the Student Non-Violent Coordinating Committee (SNCC) from its early days as the "Beloved Community" of local people who found the movement "an oasis of personal trust" (1995, 366) into its later incarnation as a forum for militant analysis and "contentious and dogmatic behavior . . . that would never have been tolerated" by its first members, for whom "nothing was more important than relationships with concrete individuals" (1995, 373). Contention is inevitable in organizations that aim to change the way people think and act, Payne reminded me.

I came back to research on the women's health movement in the early 1990s when I saw how little attention was being paid to the role of grassroots activism in the dramatic changes in women's health care over the two previous decades. I noticed (how could I not?) that the heroic and innovative campaigns against AIDS and breast cancer were presented as if they were spontaneous and unprecedented, as if they had no connection with and owed none of their successes to the women's health movement. I heard countless debates about health care reform that rarely, and then barely, mentioned the work of activists from the women's and the community health and civil rights movements, who had fought for change for many years. I drove past office buildings that advertised women's health care, but the names on all the signs had the initials M.D. after them. I saw bookstore shelves literally overflowing with books about women's health, books that themselves provided evidence of enormous changes in the amount and kind of information available to women about our bodies, and that often failed to acknowledge the role of the women's health movement as catalyst to that flood of information. I have taught scores of courses on women's health, political activism, and feminist theory to bright, energetic students of women's studies, anthropology, and sociology over the years. They may have heard of, and some may have read, *Our Bodies, Ourselves*. Otherwise they know very little about the women's health movement, even though many consider themselves feminists.

And so in this book I have told the stories of some of the tens of thousands of activists who worked so hard and effectively for change, and of the organizations they built and sustained to promote knowledge, choice, and health care reform. The research on which this book is based depends on the voices of women. It includes interviews with forty-five women's health activists; fieldwork from 1977 to 1979 in one feminist health clinic; and hundreds of primary documents from the movement (collected over twenty-five years, including many given to me by the women I interviewed); a survey conducted in 1990 of fifty women's health organizations; and scholarly and popular articles about the movement. The forty-five women I interviewed include leaders and staff of key women's health advocacy organizations: the National Women's Health Network, the National Black Women's Health Project, the National Latina Health Organization, the Federation of Feminist Women's Health Centers, the Boston Women's Health Book Collective, DES Action, Advocates for Medical Information, the Coalition for the Medical Rights of Women, HealthRight, and the Committee to End Sterilization Abuse. I also interviewed current or past directors or staff of eleven different feminist clinics located across the United States.

Their memories of the movement are social. Of course, they speak as individuals, in the words of Ana Maria Alonso, turning "action into text"(1988, 34). But as they recall how they formed, staffed, retreated from, stayed in, critiqued, and defended their organizations, they identify themselves within a group or groups and create narratives about how the group began and sometimes about how it ended. They articulate collective experience and through it create social meaning that constitutes now, as it always did, political discourse. In their stories, the women's health movement surges back out of memory and into focus. From the voices and experiences of women who have built the women's health movement, I have endeavored to forge a coherent historical study of a movement that was almost always experienced locally but that quickly achieved national and then international scope.

In the following chapters I move between two conventions—the anthropological convention of not identifying people or organizations by name and the historical convention of naming names and locations and attributing particular statements to particular people. This approach may be confusing (and perhaps irritating) to some readers, but my work demanded compromise between the methods and insights of the two disciplines. Some women who agreed to let me use their names, and indeed, wanted me to do so, will find that I ended up inventing pseudonyms for them because I am concerned about violating the confidentiality I promised to others whose identities may be closely related to theirs. In general, when I am constructing a historical picture of the movement, I tend to use the names of individuals and organizations. When I am analyzing the dynamics of change in the movement, especially changes that involve internal organizational dynamics, I often do not reveal the identity of individuals or organizations. I hope the reader can move relatively easily through the book and adapt to these shifting conventions.

This book builds on the scholarship and insights of those who have studied the movement before me. Scholarship such as Sheryl Ruzek's now classic book on the women's health movement (1978) and Rosalind Petchesky's work on abortion and reproductive rights (1984) have been influential in my evolving understanding of the movement, as has been the work of many others whose work is cited in the book. And I hope this book will inspire and help others study this important but too-little known movement, including key aspects of the movement not comprehensively addressed in this book. I focus on the period from 1969 through the very early 1990s and on women's reproductive health care, the focus of much feminist health activism in the 1970s and 1980s. I do not include extensive discussion of the broader pro-choice movement, and I have limited my research so that activism on birthing, home birth and midwifery; breast cancer; and AIDS are addressed only briefly. Whether it makes sense to talk about separate women's health, home birth/midwifery, breast cancer, and AIDS movements is debatable. But for the purposes of this book I have restricted my coverage of the broader women's health movement to efforts to change routine gynecological health care.

I wrote this book because it is important to know that political activism makes a difference. Most of us understand how thoroughly politics infuses the abortion issue, but politics saturate other aspects of women's health care as well: struggles over birth control, most recently over Norplant and Depo-Provera; pregnancy and birthing; breast cancer; AIDS; differential rates of morbidity and mortality for poor women and women of color; the safety of hormone replacement therapies; the morning-after pill; environmental causes of cancer and other chronic illnesses; medical experimentation; the cost and accessibility of primary health care. I wrote this book to show that it is not just highly paid lobbyists, physicians, professional associations, and politicians who influence health policy and practices, but also women from diverse social locations who have worked individually and collectively to produce accessible information; develop alternatives to mainstream medical care; question the safety and efficacy of medical and pharmaceutical treatments; and organize demonstrations and other protest activities; as well as those who have made their voices heard in myriad other ways.

I first began to do research about the women's health movement in the mid 1970s. One can accumulate many debts of gratitude over a quarter century. I certainly have. Countless women devoted valuable commitment, time, and energy to build and sustain the women's health movement. I have talked personally to, worked with, or read the work of more than one hundred of these women. To them, many of whom will be unnamed here because of reasons of confidentiality, I owe my deepest gratitude for trusting me with your experiences and memories. I expect some of you may disagree with aspects of my conclusions or wish my emphases in the book had been different. But I hope that readers who were or are involved in the movement will be able to discern the deep respect I have for their collective work and accomplishments and will understand that my intent in writing this book is to help, perhaps in some small way, strengthen social justice movements. I hope they will also forgive whatever errors there may be in the details of stories pieced together from interviews, movement documents, and my own fieldwork.

Over the past several years a number of people have played crucial roles in helping this manuscript become a book. I can never thank them enough. Joan Zirker is a consummate writer/editor who helped me strengthen and clarify my prose and turn chapters into engaging stories. Barbara Sutton, a graduate student in sociology at the University of Oregon, was the ultimate research assistant: she combined careful attention to detail and accuracy with dedication and good humor. Other research assistants—Thembisa Waetjen, Nancy Leeper, Alice Julier, and Holly Langan—each helped enormously by collecting, organizing, and summarizing data and/or references.

Four of my colleagues and friends read and commented on drafts of this book. To them I am eternally grateful. The list of the ways they helped me is too long to print here, but it comes under the multiple headings of wise counsel, suggestions for snappy titles, pep talks, and, most of all, sustaining friendship. Thank you, Carol Stack, Nancy Tuana, Joan Acker, and Karen Brodkin, for everything.

I am blessed by the friendship and support of other friends and colleagues who helped this book happen mainly by being there and being supportive and for teaching me so much by word and deed. Thanks especially to Joan Bayliss, Lynn Bolles, Ann Bookman, Bonnie Thornton Dill, Linda Fuller, Eileen and Anthony Giardina, Angela Ginorio, Margaret Hallock, Elizabeth Higginbotham, Dorothy Holland, Greg McLaughlan, Irwin Noparstak, Rob Proudfoot, Bill and Lynne Rossi, and Lynn Stephen.

My women's group—we have been together almost a decade—has heard far more about this book than most nonacademics would have endured. Thanks for that and for everything else: Pearl Chang, Bev Holman, Mary Hinman, Cindy Manning, and Margie Miska. Lynn Berg and Lesli Morrison helped me remember that one needs a body to write and thrive.

Thanks to everyone at Rutgers University Press for the many different ways they helped make this book happen in the world, and especially to Helen Hsu and Marlie Wasserman, who served as midwives, welcoming the book to the press and ushering it through its many stages of production. I also thank Monica Phillips for her copyediting.

For the past ten years I have worked in a wonderful community of scholars and staff at the Center for the Study of Women in Society at the University of

Oregon. I cannot thank all of you by name, but each of you, through your many contributions to CSWS, have made my work over the past decade worthwhile and fun. Thanks, especially, to Lynne Fessenden, Marie Harvey, Terri Heath, Shirley Marc, Judith Musick, Beth Hege Piatote, Lin Reilly, and Diana Taylor for ways you helped, day to day, so that I was able, sometimes, to focus on my research.

My family has been and is bedrock for me. Thanks for believing in me and the worth of what I do, thanks for your generosity, thanks for being the first place in which I learned the importance of community. My father, Dr. Robert Morgen, has taught me by the way he lives the importance of high quality health care and challenges me intellectually. My mother, to whom this book is dedicated, was and is inspiration in so many ways. My sisters, Barbara Morgen and Betsy Glen, have given me unfailing support over the years, and my brother, Richard Morgen, also lent encouragement along the way.

I met the man who later became my husband, Robert Hill Long, at about the midpoint in my two years of fieldwork in a feminist health clinic in the late 1970s. He moved from North Carolina to join me there, and we have moved several times since, like many other couples, struggling to find a way to balance the demands of two careers. Robert, I thank you for the solid foundation that our partnership is, for the poetry you write and live, for the sacrifices, and for the many joys of family.

My children, Seth Morgen Long and Sarah Morgen Long, have been the source of the greatest happiness I have known in life. There were certainly times when working on this book and my other work came at the expense of spending precious time with them. Seth and Sarah, thanks for your patience and understanding, and most of all, for being just who you are and are becoming.

I gratefully acknowledge the following for the use of material previously published in other versions: Sage Publications, for permission to use material previously published in "Class Experience and Conflict in a Feminist Workplace: A Case Study," in *Women and Work: Race, Ethnicity and Class* (1997), ed. Elizabeth Higginbotham and Mary Romero; Temple University Press, for permission to use material previously published in "It Was the Best of Times, It Was the Worst of Times: Emotional Discourse in the Work Cultures of Feminist Health Clinics," in *Feminist Organizations: Harvest of the New Women's Movement* (1995), ed. Myra M. Ferree and Patricia Yancey Martin; Elsevier Science, for permission to use material previously published in "The Dynamics of Cooptation in a Feminist Health Clinic," *Social Science and Medicine* 23, no. 2 (1986): 201–210; *Human Relations Journal,* for permission to use material previously published in "Personalizing Personnel Decisions in Feminist Organizational Theory and Practice," *Human Relations* 47, no. 6 (1994): 665–684.

Into Our Own Hands

Part I
In the Beginning

Chapter 1

Conceiving History

In 1969 a few dozen women met in Boston, Chicago, and Los Angeles and forged alliances that would revolutionize women's health care in the United States. In New York and Ann Arbor that year, two other women were working independently to identify and understand the effects of commonly prescribed estrogens. They didn't know each other at first; but they had in common a need for information about how their bodies worked, about how the health care women received affected both their health and their view of themselves. In different sites, through different means, across the country, women began to take their health care into their own hands, to wrest back some control over their sexuality, their reproductive lives, and their health from their doctors, and particularly their obstetrician-gynecologists. They imagined change and they made it happen.

The moment was right. By 1969 radical activism was transforming the political landscape of the United States. The civil rights, along with women's, antiwar, student, and welfare rights movements had mobilized hundreds of thousands of women and men whose political visions, while varying, contributed to an evolving critique of racism, sexism, capitalism, and imperialism. Radical rhetoric, huge demonstrations, an alphabet soup of new organizations and intensive grassroots organizing resulted in hard-won victories such as the Equal Pay Act (1963), the Civil Rights Act (1964), Executive Order 11246 (initiating affirmative action in 1965), and widespread acts of resistance to the draft, segregation, the humiliation of women in welfare offices, and more.

Within the broadly defined Left, ideological and organizational change was incessant. From the roots of the civil rights movement grew Black Power, La Raza, the United Farm Workers (UFW), the American Indian Movement, and women's liberation. Women's groups formed within and outside of radical organizations such as Student Nonviolent Coordinating Committee (SNCC) and Students for Democratic Society (SDS). In 1966, as the National Organization for Women (NOW) was formed in Washington, D.C., the Association to Repeal Abortion Laws (later to become the National Association for Repeal of Abortion Laws, or NARAL) was founded in California. The following year abortion reform bills were introduced in at least twenty-five state legislatures (Solinger 1998, xii) and progressive clergy in New York constituted a formal (illegal) abortion referral network.

In 1968 "C-R" (consciousness-raising) emerged as a symbol and tactic of a growing women's liberation movement. In the spring of 1968 Martin Luther King Jr. was assassinated in Memphis. Two months later Robert Kennedy met with the same fate. Political rage grew, culminating on the streets of Chicago at the Democratic convention. Chaos in Chicago and the national turmoil over Vietnam overwhelmed the candidacy of Democratic nominee Hubert Humphrey, and Richard Nixon triumphed in the November election.

Four months after Nixon's inauguration, during one of the first women's liberation conferences in Boston, eight middle-class white women gathered in a room on the campus of Emmanuel College for a workshop on women and their bodies. Nancy Hawley, the workshop leader, just had a daughter two weeks before. The women talked about childbirth, sexuality, relationships, birth control, and abortion (it was illegal); and they talked about their doctors, who were depicted by women in the workshop as "condescending, paternalistic, judgmental, and non-informative" (Boston Women's Health Book Collective [BWHBC] 1973, 1). Christening themselves "the doctor's group," the eight women hoped to find medical professionals willing to share expertise in constructive ways. But as they gathered around Jane Pincus's kitchen table in the next few weeks, "we realized just how much we had to learn about our bodies" (1). So they decided on a summer project: together, they would mend their lack of knowledge.

Over the next few months, each of them researched one of the topics that had occupied them at their first meeting. To that list, they added women's anatomy and physiology, venereal disease, pregnancy, menopause, and nutrition. Then they taught each other what they had learned, and in the autumn, meeting in a student lounge at MIT and using mimeographed copies of their research papers as a text, they publicly offered their first course on women and their bodies. At the end of a dozen or so sessions, many participants "felt both eager and competent to get together in small groups and share what they had learned with other women" (1). The women of the collective hoped that the process would replicate itself. It did. Demand for the research papers grew.

In December 1970, the nonprofit New England Free Press printed 5,000 copies of *Women and Their Bodies*. The book sold well; 15,000 copies were in print by April 1971, and by December that number had quadrupled. By 1973, when the collective incorporated and contracted with Simon and Schuster to publish the book, the New England Free Press had printed 350,000 copies of the retitled *Our Bodies, Ourselves*. Millions of copies later, this book has changed the landscape of women's health care in the United States and throughout the world.

When Heather Booth, SNCC volunteer and veteran of the Mississippi Freedom Summer, took the floor at the February 1969 meeting of the Chicago-based organization, Voters Committed to Change, she told her audience that "it was essential to frame the problem of abortion in terms of . . . women having the right to control their reproduction" (Kaplan 1995, 5). A twenty-six-year-old mother of two toddlers who heard Booth's talk understood that reproductive control could be a matter of life and death. Jenny (a pseudonym chosen by Kaplan 1995) had just had a legal abortion. She had fought hard for it. Diagnosed with Hodgkin's disease two years before, during her second pregnancy, she had become pregnant again very quickly after giving birth to her younger child. Three doctors—a gynecologist, a radiologist, and an oncologist—recommended termination of the pregnancy, but the hospital board refused permission, only relenting after Jenny convinced two psychiatrists that she would kill herself if she could not secure an abortion. Listening to Heather Booth, Jenny knew that she must join the Abortion Counseling Service of Women's Liberation. In spring 1969, following months of discussion and study, the Abortion Counseling Service of Women's Liberation created an organization called Jane. Its members, all "Jane," helped women secure safe, illegal abortions.

If you dialed 643–3844 in Chicago, you'd hear her voice: "This is Jane from women's liberation. If you need assistance, leave your name and phone number and someone will call you back." From 1969 to 1973, one Jane or another returned the calls of almost eleven thousand women. At first, the twenty or so members of the collective (almost all of them white and middle class) acted only as intermediaries between clients and abortion providers, counseling women about what to expect during the procedure and settling the price. They could rely on only a few doctors. Jane members researched each provider carefully to ensure safety.

The collective's members quickly became frustrated with the cost of the abortions (about five hundred dollars) and with their inability to control the procedures. Finding one practitioner willing to negotiate fees, they began to refer many women to him. As they accompanied clients to their abortions, they discovered how simple the procedure was. When they learned that their principal provider was not an M.D., that he had been trained through an apprenticeship with a doctor, some members of Jane decided that if he could do the procedure, then so could they. The discovery that the provider had not been an M.D. and the decision to do abortions themselves caused a crisis within Jane. Some members of the collective left. But others stayed on and began to assist at abortions. Through apprenticeship they learned to do the procedure. By the summer of 1971, Janes (especially Jenny) were doing half the abortions themselves. They lowered the price. Many women paid no more than fifty dollars, and, at last, Jane was able to offer free abortions as well.

Soon the Janes were performing all the procedures. That's how they thought abortions ought to be done: by women, for women, as acts of liberation and empowerment. Janes held the hands of their clients, rubbed their legs, made them cups of tea, explained post-procedure medications to suppress bleeding and prevent infection, performed Pap smears, handed out copies of *Our Bodies, Ourselves,* and provided birth control information and supplies. And they telephoned each woman after her abortion to make sure her recovery was uncomplicated. They also counseled clients about conditions that required medical intervention at a hospital. In four years, Jane had not a single fatality.

Only once did the Chicago police interfere with the operation of the service, which appeared to enjoy tacit protection from area law enforcement agencies. On the afternoon of May 3, 1972, seven Janes were arrested at a high-rise apartment building on South Shore Drive, where that day's abortions were to take place. By the time their case was scheduled for trial, the Supreme Court's decision in *Roe* vs. *Wade* (January 22, 1973) had overturned restrictions on abortion during the first two trimesters of pregnancy, and charges against the women were dropped. Although abortion was legal now in Illinois, many Janes were reluctant to close the service, which had been good for them as well as for the women they helped: "Everyone . . . was encouraged to go beyond what they thought they could do in terms of competence, taking responsibility, leadership because of the necessity of our work," one of the Janes recalled (Jane 1990, 6).

On May 20, 1973, more than one hundred of those new women celebrated the end of Jane—in public, finally—at the Oak Park home of one of the members. Nick, the practitioner who had worked with Jane longest and trained women to do abortions, came to the party. For the first and only time, he saw all the Janes together: "He had half expected wild-eyed revolutionaries dressed in motorcycle jackets and combat boots. Instead, gathered on . . . [the] brick-walled terrace in the sunshine, was a group of ordinary women in sundresses and shorts, eating and talking. They did not fit the image he had in his mind. They looked too normal, too straight" (Kaplan 1995, 280). And that they were. But these women had been moved by the times and the challenges they faced, "challenges [that] transformed us individually. We were pushed through some kind of hidden, invisible wall. We became women we didn't expect to become, who we loved becoming" (Jane 1990, 6).

Carol Downer attended her first meeting of the Los Angeles chapter of the National Organization of Women in 1969. The white, working-class house-wife and mother of six threw herself into the struggle to liberalize California's abortion laws, but she quickly tired of legal maneuvers. "We needed different power relations," she thought. "Things had to be done differently" (Downer 1990). Downer wanted women to start clinics and perform abortions themselves. With five other white housewives "who had 24 children among us and a combined medical experience of over a hundred years," she found an abortion provider who agreed to teach them the procedure, and one day, as she watched him insert an IUD into a woman's uterus, Downer had a kind of conversion experience (FFWHC 1981b, 17).

> There she was up in the stirrups, with a speculum in, and there, voila, was a cervix. I think the reason it had such a momentous impact on me is that I was going out and doing all this public speaking and looking at it [the need for abortion] so intellectually, so politically. And then to see how beautiful and simple and accessible a cervix was overwhelmed me with the significance of it . . . I immediately ran out and told every woman friend I had, this is going to change everything. (Downer 1990)

Downer had been pregnant seven times (she had one illegal abortion); she had had more gynecological examinations than she could begin to remember. But she had never seen a cervix before. That privilege had been reserved for the doctor, who wielded his speculum beneath a sheet that shielded women from the sight of their own bodies. Suddenly, Downer understood how easy it would be to learn what the doctor knew. Arming herself with a plastic speculum, a flashlight, and a mirror, she figured out how to examine her own cervix. On April 7, 1971, during a meeting at Everywoman's Bookstore in Los Angeles, she invited the thirty or so women who had come to talk about taking control of their reproductive lives to watch as she lay on a desk, placed a clear plastic speculum into her vagina, and demonstrated the process of cervical self-examination. The effect was electrifying. "The energy that is unleashed by doing self-examination was a moving force in everything we did," said

Downer (1990).

And they did a lot. The women practiced cervical self-examination together weekly, and they began to demonstrate the procedure for others in the community. Lorraine Rothman developed a menstrual extraction kit that she called the Del-Em, which gave women unprecedented control over their monthly periods. Downer and Rothman traveled to the 1971 national conference of the National Organization for Women, where they demonstrated cervical self-examination and menstrual extraction. With the help of other women at the conference, they planned a twenty-three-city tour to spread the ideas and techniques of self-help. Beginning in November 1971, they crossed the country, teaching what they had learned about their bodies. One of their stops was Chicago. After that demonstration some members of Jane bought mirrors, determined to offer every woman who came to them for an abortion to see, as Carol Downer had, how simple and accessible her cervix was. "In the beginning, we would ask women whether they wanted to see their cervixes," one Jane reported. "After a time, we just said, 'Here, look at your cervix.' We tried to share knowledge because knowledge is strength" (Jane 1990, 4).

When Downer and Rothman returned from their tour, they were given the use of two rooms in the Los Angeles Women's Center for a phone, a desk, and a table on which to demonstrate self-examination. The rooms also housed the Women's Abortion Referral Service (WARS), which contracted with a local hospital for blocks of time during which women could receive abortions "from our hand-picked physicians" (by now, abortion laws had been liberalized in California). Members of WARS "accompanied women and counseled them every step of the way, making sure that they received abortions in a respectful atmosphere." The women had become "aggressive medical consumers" (FFWHC 1981b, 18). Soon they would be health care providers as well. In 1972 they opened the Los Angeles Feminist Women's Health Center (LAFWHC), one of the first women-controlled health and abortion clinics in the country.

In 1969 Barbara Seaman burst the bubble of public complacency about oral contraceptives with her pioneering study, *The Doctors' Case against the Pill.* Nine years earlier, oral contraceptives had been approved by the Food and Drug Administration (FDA). Now eight million women in the United States (and four to seven million more throughout the world) used the medication, which was widely regarded as safe and effective. Demand was strong, physicians were comfortable prescribing the pill, and pharmaceutical companies looked forward to increasing sales. But Seaman, a health columnist for such mainstream magazines as *Ladies Home Journal, Good Housekeeping,* and *Brides* kept hearing from readers who described alarming side effects from oral contraceptives—depression, loss of libido, weight gain, blood clots, heart attack, and stroke. Inundated by questions, Seaman began to gather information about the pill.

Her commitment to women's health issues had begun a dozen years before, immediately after the birth of her first child. Like the other women in the maternity ward, Seaman was given pills to take every four hours. When she asked about the pills, nurses refused to identify them. The medication (laxatives, she discovered later), made her son, whom she was breastfeeding, ill. Hospital personnel didn't foresee the problem. All new mothers were given laxatives because it was taken for granted that they would use formula to feed their babies. After the birth of her daughter in 1960, Seaman says, "I found my vocation when I sold my first article on how to subvert the breastfeeding practices in hospitals to a magazine called *Mother's Manual* for $50" (Bloom and Parsons 1994, 1). Barbara Seaman liked to know what medication she was taking. As a columnist to whom other women turned for advice, she felt obligated to learn about the medication they were taking, too.

Seaman interviewed women who used oral contraceptives, uncovered studies of cerebrovascular, cardiovascular, and other classes of complications in subspecialty medical journals, talked with doctors, and reviewed meetings of medical associations and groups such as the World Health Organization, which held conferences on the pill's safety in 1965 and 1967. With the support of some doctors who shared her concern—the director of the contraceptive clinic at Johns Hopkins University School of Medicine wrote the introduction to *The Doctors' Case against the Pill*—Seaman produced a coherent and devastating critique of physicians, pharmaceutical companies, and the Food and Drug Administration for failing to protect women from drugs that had potentially serious side effects, and for failing to inform them of those dangers.

The Doctors' Case against the Pill ignited a firestorm of controversy that led Senator Gaylord Nelson to convene hearings on the pill in 1970. The Senate hearings generated even more controversy about the dangers of oral contraceptives, the silence of manufacturers and population control experts about those dangers, and the FDA's complicity in that silence. The outcome of the hearings was a new requirement that drug companies include a package insert detailing possible side effects with every prescription of the pill. Barbara Seaman lost her columns with the women's magazines, probably because of pressure from pharmaceutical industry executives. But her career as a women's health activist and advocate continued. Editions of *The Doctors' Case against the Pill* were published in Germany, Holland, and England, and twenty-five years after its first appearance, a new edition was released in this country. Seaman's work helped establish the principle of informed consent—the right to full disclosure of the possible effects of a medication or a medical procedure—that most Americans now take for granted.

Belita Cowan started tracking another story about estrogens in 1969. Working part time at University Hospital in Ann Arbor while finishing a master's degree in English, Cowan worried about the effects of diethylstilbestrol (DES), the "morning-after pill," which was routinely prescribed to students as a contraceptive after unprotected intercourse. In recently completed trials at University Hospital (the results would appear in the *Journal of the American Medical Association* [JAMA]), not one of one thousand women who had been given DES reported a pregnancy. Nor did any participants report serious reactions to the drug.

But Belita Cowan had heard from friends and students who had taken the morning-after pill about short-term side effects, including severe nausea. She had also heard of pregnancies among participants in the study. And she knew that research linked maternal ingestion of DES with cancers in daughters. With a group of local women who had been patients at the University of Michigan's student health center, Cowan organized Advocates for Medical Information (AMI) to educate women about DES and to oppose the use of the morning-after pill at University Hospital and at other student health centers in the United States. In 1971, with a grant from student government, AMI undertook an independent survey of women who had taken DES as a contraceptive. Sixty-nine women responded to the AMI survey. Only one-quarter of them had ever been contacted by health service doctors after their treatment with DES. The JAMA study was flawed and the DES emergency was spreading.

Recognizing that local campaigners needed a national strategy, Cowan consulted with Ralph Nader and feminist activists to prepare for a press conference in Washington, D.C., in December 1972. After the press conference, the dangers of DES leapt from the pages of *herself,* a women's newspaper Cowan had helped establish several months before (it was sold in Ann Arbor grocery stores along with *Time, Newsweek, Seventeen,* and the tabloids), into the national media spotlight.

Belita Cowan and Barbara Seaman were bound to meet, destined to become friends. During their late-night, long-distance telephone calls, they talked about an idea: a Washington-based lobbying group devoted to women's health issues. In 1974, Seaman and Cowan joined with three other feminists—psychologist Phyllis Chesler, physician Mary Howell, and activist and later attorney Alice Wolfson—to found the National Women's Health Network.

Conceiving History

The Boston Women's Health Book Collective, Jane, Carol Downer, Lorraine Rothman, the Los Angeles Feminist Women's Health Center, Barbara Seaman, and Belita Cowan conceived history. They imagined, as did countless others, new ways of thinking about their bodies and taking control of their reproductive lives. Then they acted. Working from their own kitchens or from borrowed rooms in schools, churches, and community centers, they presided over the multiple births of the women's health movement. This movement was never monolithic, flourished in many different sites at once, and was the midwife for many different organizations and organizational forms over the next three decades.

I embrace the metaphor of conception not just because it is obvious for a movement whose heart was women's reproductive experience and health, but because I want to underline the process by which this national social movement was imagined and enacted. I use the phrase *conceiving history* for its double meaning: it compares the generative dynamics of movement making with the creation of narratives that describe those dynamics. Almost thirty years after the multiple beginnings of the women's health movement, I, too, have conceived history as I form ideas about the movement and the women who mothered it, as I represent thoughts, feelings, and actions through which they served as agents of change. I have sifted through hundreds of historical documents and hundreds of hours of conversations with activists, and I remember what it was like to be a fieldworker and member of a feminist health clinic for more than two years in the late 1970s. From these materials, I have selected particular events and organizations and the words of individual women and I have built a narrative necessarily partial and evocative that tries to capture what it felt like to be part of the women's health movement, what it felt like to make the movement grow.

The need for such a narrative is clear. In 1969, a woman who placed herself under a doctor's care had the duty to do what she was told. Now she has the right to gather information and resources to make her own decisions about her sexuality, her reproductive life and health, even her treatment for breast cancer. Not all women want to exercise that right. But the commitment of the women's health movement to autonomy and informed consent has transformed health care in this country for women (and for men). Despite the movement's impact and the centrality of movement participation in the lives and memories of so many women in so many communities, the story of the women's health movement is not widely known.

In this book I want to tell that story, to unfurl the political meaning of the movement, to recognize the crucial roles grassroots organizing and local feminist health organizations played in changing women's health care and policy at the national level. But I'm chastened by contemporary social theory that warns against telling too neat, too unified, too coherent and single a story (Foucault 1980; Touraine 1981; Nicholson 1990; Butler and Scott 1992). Critical historiography and critical social theory remind us that historical representation is always conceived, experienced, and interpreted by individuals (including scholars) whose vision and understanding is shaped by their own social location within a complex system of power relations. Histories are not innocent. They filter, emphasize, de-emphasize, and expurgate as they (re)conceive the past.

This is a book about how modern social movements are experienced and structured as political forces. I aim to show how individuals and organizations spread out across the country came to conceive of and identify themselves as contributors to a national social movement. I explore the mechanisms by which the women's health movement transcended the grassroots groups and local activism that constituted the movement experience for most of its participants and represent the *nationalness* of the effort. But the challenge I faced, like other social movement scholars, comes from the fact that while the phenomenon I am writing about—the women's health movement—was and is national, indeed international, in reach, my research data came from individuals and mostly locally situated organizations. As I moved back and forth between the experiences of individuals, the histories of organizations and the national scope and impact of the movement, I recognized that my problem—the need to "solder a multiplicity of personal, local, and regional historicities" into a national story, to borrow Ana Alonso's words—mirrored the experience movement participants undergo as they construct a sense of themselves as part of a larger historical process (Alonso 1988, 40).

Most contemporary social movements burn their way into the popular imagination as pictures of foundational events or leaders. So, as the stories are popularly told, the civil rights movement begins in 1955 with Rosa Parks and Martin Luther King Jr. and the Montgomery bus boycott. The gay liberation movement begins in 1969 with the explosive events at the Stonewall bar in New York City. The antiwar movement begins with the disputes over free speech that erupt at the University of California at Berkeley in 1964, when administrators forbade students to set up informational tables, solicit memberships, or collect funds for political causes in Sproul Plaza. The farmworker movement begins when Cesar Chavez emerges to lead agricultural workers on protest marches through the fields of the Salinas valley. Although participants know that the origins of these movements are deeply rooted, broader, and more complex than emblematic leaders or big events suggest, such representations nevertheless powerfully shape our common understandings of social change.

Women's health organizations (with a few exceptions) resisted hero making. The movement always hewed to its local beginnings. Not often or primarily did it represent itself through national demonstrations or in the persons of nationally recognized leaders. Indeed, the larger women's health advocacy organizations of the mid–1970s and 1980s do not and cannot account for the movement's existence as a national phenomenon. Instead, its nationalness depended on its multiple points of emergence, the dense interconnections among individuals and organizations that developed over time, and its visibility. "The parameters of the local and global [here read national] are often indefinable or indistinct," Grewal and Kaplan argue. "They are permeable constructs. How one separates the local from the global is difficult to decide when each thoroughly infiltrates the other" (1994, 11). As they reinvented their health care more than thirty years ago, women faced this challenge: to create a national or movement-wide coherence from many local beginnings and continuances.

This account of the women's health movement differs not just from the stories favored by the power structures it challenged, but also from narratives of what Charles Payne calls *normative history*, historiography "premised on the assumption that national institutions work more or less as advertised, that shared values are the key to understanding change" (1995, 420). Normative history focuses on the actions of a few visible leaders, on transformations that start at the top and move downward. It depicts a system that incorporates—as it disempowers—critique. The foundational stories of the women's health movement turn normative history on its head. The excitement, the passion, the power of its collective vision and action grew on many different root stocks, out of the experience of individual women in many different locations—experience that was nevertheless common enough that women recognized their own feelings in others as they talked together about their interactions with the health care system, especially around reproductive issues.

A movement's beginnings constitute reference points, not only for the historian or the social scientist, but also for activists within the movement, as they look back to the past to understand the present and chart the future. Foundational stories create shared history and sustain collective identity, the core of the lived experience of belonging to a social movement. Paul Ricoeur has argued that social groups "form images of themselves in relation to a set of founding events and re-enact this shared link to a collective past in public life as well as in everyday life" (1978, 45). Here, Ricoeur echoes what Bellah et al. (1985) call *community of memory*. Those who are encompassed in a community of memory need not have lived together the remembered events. But knowing the events, knowing their meanings for a social group, and feeling part of that group through the sharing of memory—these are ways communities of memory constitute themselves. John Gillis suggests the "core meaning of any individual or group identity, namely, as sense of sameness over time or space, is sustained by remembering; and what is remembered is defined by the assumed identity." Too often, Gillis says, "we refer to both as if they had the status of material objects—memory as something to be retrieved; identity as something that can be lost as well as found. We need to be reminded that memories and identities are not fixed things, but representations or constructions of reality" (1994, 3).

So also are the foundational stories that drive a movement's evolving self-consciousness. These stories signal the moment of rupture between tacit acceptance of things as they are and resistance, mobilization toward the new. They explain and inspire. They aim to create a sense of shared history and to make possible a sense of shared identity. They commemorate moments, individuals, ideas, and actions, but they flow toward a larger story, a story of change. Foundational stories are told in social movements for the same reasons that families and nations tell stories about themselves—to construct a history with roots to a present that is shared and hopes for a future in which individuals have a common stake.

I don't claim that these four are the only stories that could be told about the origins of the women's health movement. In chapter 3 I will look at others. But each of these four stories begins in 1969 with a moment that signaled rupture with the past; each marks the passions, the creativity, the differing strategies, and the variety of meanings of the politics of the women's health movement; and each shows the irreducible indebtedness of social movements to local histories, embodied practices, and collective memory. I have tried to retell these stories as I have found them reported within the movement. But foundational stories are not best understood as receptacles for history. Rather, they frame history, draw lines of demarcation within which we create historical meaning as we make connections between past and present.

At some moment in its history, after ideas and actions have begun to create a sense of it, a social movement is named, declared to be. Then the process of historical construction can begin, a future can be envisioned in which the movement is a significant actor. Of course, foundational stories begin before that moment. But once a movement is declared to be, they function as scaffolds for remembered history and for the articulation of shared goals. They are not free-floating text; their telling and retelling, by particular people in the context of particular political purposes or agendas, embody the discursive process of movement making.

By focusing on the concepts of social memory and collective identity as ways of examining what it means to talk about a national social movement, I emphasize the discursive dimension of social movements. As Jane Mansbridge has argued, "The entity—'women's movement' or 'feminist movement'—to which they [politically active feminists] feel accountable is neither an aggregation of organizations nor an aggregation of individual members but a discourse. It is a set of changing, contested aspirations and understandings that provide conscious goals, cognitive backing, and emotional support for each individual's evolving feminist identity" (1995, 27). In the next chapter, I explore how the foundational stories of the women's health movement contributed to the making of the movement, first in the imaginations of participants, next in the real world of social movement organizations: how the women-and-their-bodies workshop at Emmanuel College evolved into the Boston Women's Health Book Collective; how public demonstrations of cervical self-examination evolved into the elaborated politics of self-help and women-controlled clinics of the Feminist Women's Health Centers; how Jane created itself in open secrecy and transformed the rhetoric of autonomy into safe, deprofessionalized abortions; how Barbara Seaman and Belita Cowan harnessed the power of media to expose the complicity of physicians, drug companies, and the FDA in concealing the effects of medications prescribed to women.

Chapter 2

Foundational Stories and Movement Making

In this chapter I examine the importance of foundational stories in the process of movement making, using narrative history to foreground the critical process of conceiving of the movement as a movement, extra-organizational in scope, as a political force. This kind of narrative weaves together many threads of movement making: the founding and building of organizations, conferences, protests, networks, and coalitions; the development of manifestos, pamphlets, handbooks, and other print and nonprint materials to explain and advocate for movement goals; action plans that capture the attention of the media, public officials, and policy makers who control resources and procedures the movement wants to change; enlistment of active and passive members in a base of support, and more. I (re)construct the narratives of the four foundational stories introduced in chapter 1 based on interviews with activists and organizational documents about the projects and strategies of the women's health movement. Documentary sources include my own and other published interviews with key actors, archival material from organizations, and movement publications. The retellings rely on the words, images, themes, and tones of the women who first shared these stories among themselves and their friends.

"A Good Story": Our Bodies, Ourselves

The bold inventiveness and stunning success of the work of the Boston Women's Health Book Collective (BWHBC) make this the most widely known foundational story of the women's health movement. In the past thirty years the BWHBC has sold millions of copies of multiple editions of the book in the United States and globally. Savvy negotiations with their publisher have resulted in many thousands of discounted copies sold or donated to clients of feminist health clinics and abortion referral services in the United States and abroad.

In the 1973 edition of *Our Bodies, Ourselves,* and in editions since, the collective tells its own history, called "A Good Story," as the book's preface. They began with the facts: how "it all began at a small discussion group on 'women and their bodies'" (1) at the Boston conference in 1969, followed by the summer of research and the development of the fall course on women and their bodies. They then use their own story of learning and sharing to inspire others to do the same and to legitimize the knowledge in the book."

"As we developed the course we realized more and more that we were really capable of collecting, understanding, and evaluating medical information . . . We were equally struck by how important it was for us to be able to open up with one another and share our feelings about our bodies. The process of talking was as crucial as the facts themselves" (BWHBC 1973, 1).

They described themselves as individuals and as a group, and in this edition, like the others, they included a photograph of themselves.

> You may want to know who we are. We are white, our ages range from 24 to 40, most of us are from middle-class backgrounds and have had at least some college education, and some of us have professional degrees. Some of us are married, some of us are separated, and some of us are single . . . We are white middle class women, and as such can describe only what life has been for us . . . The group has been on-going for three years and some of us have been together since the beginning. (1973, 1–2)

They were clear that their book differs from most of the medical information available, that their goal was to present information that would be liberating,

> Our book contains real material about our bodies and ourselves that isn't available elsewhere, and we have tried to present it in a new way—an honest, humane, and powerful way of thinking about ourselves and our lives. We want to share the knowledge and power that comes with this way of thinking and we want to share the feelings we have for each other . . . In trying to figure out why this has had such a life-changing effect on us, we have come up with several important ways in which this kind of body education has been liberating for us and may be a starting point for the liberation of many other women. (1973, 2)

Like the Janes who were "pushed through an invisible wall" by the demands of their work and became women they "loved becoming," like Carol Downer and Lorraine Rothman, who unleashed tremendous excitement when they demonstrated the techniques of cervical self-examination and menstrual extraction, the women of BWHBC loved their transformation. And they believed that women who read *Our Bodies, Ourselves* could share the same exhilaration, tap the same energy, and change their own lives. Moreover, they emphatically define their collective experience as political: "The experience of learning just how little control we had over our lives and bodies, the coming together out of isolation to learn from each other in order to define what we needed, and the experience of supporting one another in demanding the changes that grew out of our developing critique—all were crucial and formative political experiences for us. We have felt our potential power as a force for political and social change" (1973, 3). The political message of the book continues throughout the book, culminating in the final chapter, which is a strong indictment of capitalist and sexist health care.

Empowerment was good, but power caused complications. BWHBC sought to make all its decisions through building consensus. In an unpublished document, also called "A Good Story" (presumably written in 1975 based on its reference to the collective being together six years), members discuss their struggles over power. As they prepared their research papers for publication by the New England Free Press, one woman was doing much of the work single-handedly. "Taking a leadership role felt both natural to her and met some personal needs. The group, in turn, needed her energy and perseverance . . . So far, so good: in our developing fluid leadership model it was natural that one or two people would emerge as initiators or leaders in a certain area of our work. Yet over the months she grew to hold an increasing influence in all aspects of what we did" (BWHBC 1975, 11). The "fluid leadership model," so characteristic of organizations within the women's health movement, always produced issues of dominance, and issues of dominance always produce tensions. BWHBC defused that tension slowly, carefully, and with respect, first by defining it as "a whole group issue."

> During the year or more that it took to work it out, the key was our ability to use the model of personal sharing that was such a central part of our teaching and our being together. . . . It means a lot to us that our support comes as much from our respect and caring for her as a friend as it does from our need to be rid of such dominance (BWHBC 1975, 12).

Their model of personal sharing helped BWHBC members break out of the familiar pattern of hierarchical leadership into which they were slipping and redefine power. "Gradually a stronger sense of self-respect and equality has settled among us, and we have found ourselves with a changed notion of what power itself can be . . . As we emerged from the struggle with more self-understanding, our group intact and our friendships deepened, we realized that there can be power without dominance, that power can also be 'power-with'" (BWHBC 1975, 13). While the version of "A Good Story" that prefaced editions of the book until the early 1990s did not explicitly detail the group's internal conflicts, beginning in the second edition there is a brief reference to "some conflict between our work load as authors of a widely selling book and our desire to be a close personal support group" (1979, 14).

Scholarly sobriety constrains against superlatives, but it would be difficult to exaggerate the impact of *Our Bodies, Ourselves*. "At first, the book was not so much read as it was absorbed. It was an antidote to the horror stories of medical indignities and insensitivity that many women harbored without sharing. For many common physical problems, it was as good as a visit to a clinician—or better, because it was full of respect for women's desire to know about themselves and full of the personal voices of women who had been there and been through it" (Robb 1979, 21). Erupting into the void (there were few popular books about women's health before it), *Our Bodies, Ourselves* created its own niche market. Women everywhere read the book and talked about it. Before long, "sensitive doctors began using it as a thorough reference for undramatic complaints that professional textbooks neglected" (Robb 1979, 21).

By the end of 1973, the year of its first commercial publication, many colleges, universities, and even medical schools had adopted *Our Bodies, Ourselves* as a text, and more would follow in the years to come. The collective was famous now, and there was more work to do than ever before: negotiations through Simon and Schuster with European and Japanese publishers; efforts to translate *Our Bodies, Ourselves* into Spanish; decisions about how to allocate royalties; discussions of future projects (BWHBC would eventually publish *Ourselves and Our Children* [1978] and *Ourselves Growing Older* [1987]), including future revisions of *Our Bodies, Ourselves*; and appearances as workshop leaders and speakers on women's health care issues and sexuality.

In 1984 the BWHBC published *The New Our Bodies, Ourselves.* They wrote a new preface, although it was followed by the version of "A Good Story" that had been part of the book since 1973. In the new preface they once again revealed to readers much about the process of writing the book, sharing their decisions about what chapters and material to include and exclude, their heavier reliance on the burgeoning new literature on women's health, and their attempts to include more material about women internationally and women of color. They caught up their readers on changes in their personal lives: new children, divorces, marriages and new relationships, the onset of "hot flashes," illnesses and deaths in their families, changes of residence. They emphasized that the medical establishment is "tied more closely than ever to other businesses in this profit-oriented economy" (1984, xiii). And they concluded that the process of sustaining their collective has not been easy:

> Yet our efforts (along with so many others) to form a community of women are still evolving and, despite their strengths, are quite fragile. A competitive society like ours makes it difficult to work collectively, to be open, to trust one another. It is more difficult to be a feminist these days than it was in the optimistic climate of the early seventies. And when the many women with backgrounds and experiences different from our own speak up and tell the truth about their lives, they make clear just how diverse this huge community is. Sometimes the great differences between us—race, class, ethnicity sexual preference, values and strategies—turn us against each other. (1984, xiv)

In the process of sharing their own story along with the information that millions of women worldwide had come to depend on, the BWHBC kept alive the spark and the political vision that defined their work as more than just a best-selling book, but, additionally, as a part of movement making. In the 1979 edition, the BWHBC identified itself with the work of many other women's health groups as part of a women's health movement. The description of the movement grows from several pages in the 1979 edition to an entire thirteen-page chapter in the 1984 and 1992 editions. With the 1984 edition, the collective adds a new chapter, "Developing an International Awareness," that recognizes a global women's health movement and the variety of needs it must address.

Although collective members did not confront dilemmas of race or class difference among themselves, they understood that "poor women and non-white women have suffered far more from the kinds of misinformation and mistreatment that we are describing in this book. In some ways, learning about our womanhood from the inside out has allowed us to cross over the socially created barriers of race, color, income and class, and to feel a sense of identity with all women in the experience of being female" (BWHBC 1973, 2). BWHBC members honored difference in sexual preference by ceding control over the chapter on lesbianism to a group of lesbian writers, and they honored their own tradition of truthfulness by writing about the discomforts of the transaction:

> They, rightly, insisted on the same kind of final editorial control that we were struggling for with the rest of the book. Though we respected their concern, this loss of control over "our book" was exceedingly difficult for us to accept. What complicated things was that the political climate around lesbianism at that time was such that when we as straight women wanted to leave

out or to suggest changes in some section of their chapter, it seemed that we were acting out of, at best, misunderstanding, and at worst, hostility and prejudice . . . Two years later, when we came to re-revise the book, our communications with the lesbian group were easier, with far less of a sense of two opposing sides—indicating a different political atmosphere as well as more experience, age, and maturity in all of us. (BWHBC 1975, 22–23)

Because the central activity of the collective has been the distribution of feminist health education materials, most notably *Our Bodies, Ourselves*; because BWHBC always focused on process in the production of those materials; and because it has survived longer than almost any other organization associated with the first phase of the women's health movement, it is uniquely able to document and to circulate its own history. The Boston Women's Health Book Collective turned radical thought into radical text with the stacks of mimeographed papers course leaders took to their first classes on women and their bodies. Its members put their faith in the power of *words*, and learned to prevail through discourse, using the weapons of paper and ink to overcome distance. BWHBC offered health information and resources through its publications and through the specialized collection of research materials in its library, the Women's Health Information Center, in Somerville, Massachusetts; it sponsored the Women's Health and Learning Center in Massachusetts prisons to educate women about violence prevention, substance abuse, and parenting skills; it participated in political advocacy groups and in women's health coalitions and organizations; and it helped fund many feminist projects over the years.

More than a quarter century after the first Simon and Schuster printing, more than four million copies of *Our Bodies, Ourselves* have been published, in six U.S. editions and in more than fifteen different languages worldwide (BWHBC 1995). So "A Good Story" has been told four million times in print. It has also been reviewed by scholars (Mellow 1989; Yallof 1994) and by writers for the popular press (Robb 1979; Vaughn 1987; Drexler 1989). No one can estimate how often women have repeated it to each other. Part creation myth, part epic poem, part spiritual autobiography, the history of the collective recapitulates the purpose of the book itself. "What we do best," Judy Norsigian and Wendy Coppedge Sanford wrote ten years after that first meeting at Emmanuel College, "is to help women look more critically at the particulars of their health care and personal lives, to start to name the changes they want to make, and to see that they can, and in fact, have to work with others to try to effect those changes. We believe that starting at this personal level generates the motivation, energy, and skills for larger political movements; it certainly has been the source of our group's continuing and energetic public presence in the struggle for women against the organized sources of oppression" (1987, 291).

By making their process seem simple, natural, and inevitable, BWHBC sketches a hopeful activism. This is print-based consciousness raising. If we can't sit in a room with our readers, we can gather in the preface to the book, our troubles and storms resolved and judged in retrospect, to describe a vibrant and safe and respectable model for personal growth within a group. "A Good Story" is crucial because it opens up a space where women triumph together. Bracing in its frankness, admirable in its thoroughness, and mainstream in its methodology, BWHBC's discourse of education and empowerment makes straight the path for other, extra-textual discourses.

The Story of Self-Help Gynecology

The story of the origin of self-help gynecology, and specifically of cervical self-examination, is less well-known to movement outsiders. Within the women's health movement, though, Carol Downer's "discovery" of the cervix is legendary, and like all legends, it was repeated over and over again. Before she joined NOW and took up the cause of abortion rights, Downer says, "I knew very little . . . and as the mother of six children I was very tied down, very limited in my experience" (Downer 1990). But she was quick to understand that the struggle for incremental change would be long and hard, and when she first saw the cervix of another woman, she conceived a faster way to achieve new power relations. On April 7, 1971, Carol Downer demonstrated cervical self-examination in public and enacted the revolutionary rhetoric of self-help: She took her body into her own hands.

Cervical self-examination was loaded with symbolic significance. By inserting a speculum into her vagina, Downer broke two taboos—she touched her own genitals and she appropriated the tools of the medical professional to reclaim knowledge about her body. Cervical self-examination took the idea of women learning about and from their own bodies to a new level. Pursuing a baldly confrontational path, Downer and Lorraine Rothman set off on a twenty-three-city tour late in 1971 to demonstrate self-help and teach the techniques of cervical self-examination and menstrual extraction (a process similar to vacuum aspiration abortion, but using a smaller cannula and a hand pump to empty the content of the uterus, relieving menstrual cramps and regulating fertility).[1] "The reactions of women in a self-help clinic to seeing their cervixes for the first time is varied," Federation of Feminist Women Health Centers (FFWHC) members wrote later. "Almost all are delighted. Some are amazed. Some are serious. Some are awed by this experience" (FFWHC 1981b, 153). Everywhere, women bought their own plastic speculums, and new self-help groups sprang up. The idea spread like wildfire.

Downer and Rothman told their story in person, as they traveled from one community to another. They reiterated the story of the first self-help group in Los Angeles, and they added to the story the many stories from their travels. They wrote articles about gynecological self-help and developed a thirty minute black-and-white movie called *Self-Help Clinic,* which they rented and sold to groups across the country (Source Collective 1974, 178). Not content merely to know, members of the Federation of Feminist Women's Health Centers were also determined to do. In this version, movement making looked like gynecological guerilla theater, sometimes lawless and unpredictable. When police officers raided the Los Angeles Feminist Women's Health Center in September 1972, they charged Carol Downer and Colleen Wilson with a crime against the state and its health care establishment: practicing medicine without a license. Weeks before, an undercover policewoman had joined one of the center's self-help groups. Dido Hasper, health activist and later president and coordinator of FFWHC, describes what happened next: "The women got together one night a week . . . to discuss their health care. They learned how to fit diaphragms, talked about vaginal infections, prenatal care, anything that the group decided to discuss. One woman had a yeast infection and asked Carol to spoon some yogurt into her vagina" (Hasper 1981, 266).

In the fifth week of the group's meetings, police burst into the Health Center, arrested Downer and Wilson, and seized cartons of yogurt—in this instance, someone's lunch—from LAFWHC's refrigerator. Just a month earlier, in August 1972, mother and daughter Lolly and Jeanne Hirsch, of Connecticut, had invested the story of the first, public cervical self-examination with an almost sacred significance in their publication *The Monthly Extract: An Irregular Periodical.* "April 7, 1971 should be declared a holy day, a momentous holiday in the lives of all modern women . . . Just as the Equal Rights Amendment will give women access to the legal system and consciousness raising has helped us reclaim our minds and brains from psychiatry, psychology and illogical traditions, the Gynecological Self Help clinic will give us back our bodies . . . GYNECOLOGY must be taken back by WOMEN" (Hirsch and Hirsch 1972, 1).

Heroic in August, Downer was a target of oppression in September, and a symbol of resistance by October, when Lolly and Jeanne Hirsch published a special issue of *The Monthly Extract* to raise money for her defense. Colleen Wilson pleaded guilty to a reduced charge, but Downer went to trial in December 1972 and was acquitted of all counts against her (Hasper 1981, 266). The arrests and trial catapulted Downer and the LAFWHC into the headlines and made the Los Angeles Police Department the butt of jokes (and rage) throughout the emerging movement. As Downer and Rothman traveled across the country a year earlier, they inspired many instances of individual transformation and seeded or nurtured feminist health groups in many different communities. The women who had met them reacted with disbelief, anger, and determination to news of the arrests, and with joy to news of Downer's acquittal. The story explained and inspired, as Carol Downer and Lorraine Rothman had done in person. As it was told in *The Monthly Extract* and in other publications, it offered as plot points all the satisfactions of radical (and movement) triumph: oppression, resistance, victory. Moreover, the trial attracted national attention, being covered in magazines such as *Time, Newsweek,* and the *New York Times* (FFWHC 1981b, 18). According to the federation, "instead of stopping us, the medical profession had inadvertently given us a boost. We traveled even more widely and spoke at campuses and conferences about self-help" (FFWHC 1981b, 19).

Every spring, in the "season of rebirth," *The Monthly Extract* marked the anniversary of the first demonstration of cervical self-examination. Clearly, Lolly and Jeanne Hirsch meant to make Downer a hero. When a reader complained that the publication was "objectifying Carol, first as a body, second as a superstar, and to be indulging in heroine worship," the editor replied, "Yes, I want to create women heroes for the 20th century." She argued further that when the women's movement is remembered two hundred years hence, "the outstanding personalities will be Carol Downer and Lorraine Rothman, for in their heads occurred the revolutionary idea that women have the right to knowledge and the control of their own bodies" (Hirsch and Hirsch 1973, 3).

Sheryl Ruzek, who wrote one of the earliest scholarly publications on the women's health movement, agreed that the first public cervical self-examination "more than any other event transformed health and body issues into a separate movement" (1978, 53). In November 1973, the left-leaning *Ramparts* was one of the first nationally marketed magazines to notice the existence of that separate movement with the publication of "Women's Self-Help Movement, Or Is Happiness Knowing Your Own Cervix?" (Fishel 1973). Although author Elizabeth Fishel sympathized with movement goals and the value of self-help, she questioned whether the practice of cervical self-examination would lead to real change in health care policy and delivery. She also wondered whether cervical self-examination would appeal more to middle-class women who want to declare independence from their gynecologists than to poor women denied access to health care.

Carol Downer would never accept such a view. Always a controversial figure, she drew fire from many others in the women's health movement for her style of leadership and because many regarded the clinics that formed under the banner of the Federation of Feminist Women's Health Centers as unfeminist because their organizational structures deviated from the more collectivist, egalitarian models of most independent community-based feminist health clinics. Unlike the independent grassroots feminist clinics organizing across the country in the early 1970s, the clinics organized by and affiliated with the Federation of Feminist Women's Health Centers tended to have more hierarchical structures, higher fees, and a different relationship to the emerging movement because of their federated structure.

In a 1974 broadside, obviously a political response to criticisms raised within the movement, Downer explains the hard pragmatism of self-help and the FWHCs:

> Why, when some women's groups are appealing for rent money and pessimism is rampant, is Self-Help barreling along? I believe the difference lies in *class*. Self-Help comes out of a lower-class consciousness, an everyday common-sense understanding that social change is not going to be welcomed by the status-quo. We know that we will not be funded to make a revolution; we will not waste our energies applying for the proverbial foundation grant or writing the proverbial book. We will not have the support of publishers, businessmen, and certainly not doctors. We will not search for "the sympathetic woman doctor," and we're too poor to offer "free" services to anyone . . . Yes, we dare to want POWER. We want to take over women's medicine—nothing less. (Downer n.d.)

The LAFWHC collected fees for health care services, and, in general, fees at FWHCs were somewhat higher than at other feminist health clinics. Downer defends the policy:

> To survive in a male-supremacist world, we have to *compete* with male institutions (meaning we have to be efficient and businesslike) and we have to *fight* approaches and individuals that we think are incorrect. Therefore, even though we would ideally be able to provide a nurturing environment for ourselves, the best we have been able to do is strive for openness, willingness to struggle and mutual respect . . . The Self Help Clinic has been accused of being ruthless, cold and rip-offs. As one of the first feminist groups to actively engage the enemy, we often find ourselves in the thick of confrontation. To some of our sisters who have been brought up to think that all problems are "communication problems" and that being fair means taking a middle position, our insistence on taking whatever position we think is right, popular or not, is not only annoying, it's sometimes downright embarrassing . . . But no matter how annoying, how embarrassing, how unpopular it may be for us to take stands; we will continue to pursue our goal of getting

better health care for women, and will continue to take positions and oppose those whom we perceive as being either the enemy or aiding the enemy (and there *is* an enemy). (Downer 1974)

Consensus is nice if you can get it, Downer says. And so is a nurturing environment. But she proudly articulates a take-no-prisoners attitude toward conflict, and that attitude, along with FFWHC funding policies, sparked strife at several women's health movement conferences in the early and mid–1970s. Attempts to canonize Downer and to give primacy to the story of cervical self-examination were highly politicized acts. The 1973 *Circle One Self Health Handbook,* a self-help manual published and widely distributed by the Colorado Springs Women's Health clinic, pays homage to Downer and the Los Angeles Feminist Women's Health Center by crediting their work with reversing a "downhill trend in women's health care" with their "pioneering" work (Ziegler and Campbell 1973, 4). *The Monthly Extract* never stopped talking about Downer and cervical self-exam. At the same time, the Boston Women's Health Book Collective never started. No edition of *Our Bodies, Ourselves*, the most widely known document—written or otherwise—of the women's health movement, mentions Downer's procedure or the galvanizing tale of her arrest and trial. This is unlikely to be an oversight. Within the movement, which was marked with division and, often enough, tendentiousness, there was no shared origin story. Different women made different choices about how to remember the movement's birth and how to describe its development.

In 1981 the federation released a book called *A New View of a Woman's Body*, published by Touchstone Books, a division of Simon and Schuster, publisher of *Our Bodies, Ourselves*. Like *Our Bodies, Ourselves*, this book begins with a first chapter, "The Grassroots of Self-Help," that, once again, recounts the story of the invention of cervical self-examination, menstrual extraction, and the development of the Feminist Women's Health Centers. It is all there—the April 7, 1971, first self-help demonstration, the many tours, the formation of the first federation clinic, the Los Angeles Feminist Women's Health Center, and then the establishment of affiliated self-help clinics in Santa Ana and Oakland, California, and then later in Detroit, Tallahassee, Chico, and Atlanta. They share with readers the history of their previous publications, including the 1975 *Women's Health in Women's Hands*. But they boldly state their belief that this new book, *A New View of a Woman's Body,* "is the first book since the publication of *Our Bodies, Ourselves* truly to break new ground" (FFWHC 1981, 20).

Health Advocacy: From Books and Broadsides to the Capitol Steps

Barbara Seaman's warnings against oral contraceptives and Belita Cowan's findings about the dangers of DES mark the first phase in the development of the policy advocacy wing of the women's health movement. With *The Doctors' Case against the Pill* and the publication of articles about the use of diethystilbestrol (DES) as a postcoital contraceptive in herself and in other movement publications, Seaman and Cowan, among others, raised consciousness on the national level about the hazards of health care as usual and helped redefine women's health needs through a politics of engagement.

There has been no high-profile creation myth for this sector of the movement. The story of the emergence of the National Women's Health Network (NWHN) has not become the stuff of legends, nor has the importance of activist authors such as Seaman and Cowan and of advocacy organizations such as AMI in seeding the national health policy debates of the mid–1970s been well understood. The discourse of advocacy particularized the movement's challenges to the medical establishment and the state, named doctors and pharmaceutical companies and FDA administrators who failed to provide women with information about the safety and efficacy of the drugs prescribed to them, and demanded a response.

Seaman's book presented the results of highly technical medical research on oral contraceptives in language that made it accessible to women. Like *Our Bodies, Ourselves* she used the private stories and experiences of women to contest the claims and penetrate the complacency of physicians and, ultimately, a number of politicians. Her voice was strong enough to lead Senator Gaylord Nelson to organize Senate hearings in January 1970 on the safety of oral contraceptives. Although Seaman worked with Nelson's staff to prepare for the hearings, Seaman attended as an observer only. She was not invited to speak. Neither were any women who had been harmed by the Pill.

Dr. Hugh Davis, who had written the introduction to Seaman's book, was the first witness; Dr. William Spellacy, who had studied the connection between the pill and elevated triglycerides (blood fats), followed. Dr. Elizabeth Connell, who was one of several witnesses recruited by Senator Robert Dole to testify in support of the pill, warned that if women were informed of its hazards, they would stop using contraceptive methods altogether, and that the consequence would be unwanted "Nelson babies" (Bloom 1995, 1). Connell repeated the story she had told Seaman in an interview for *The Doctors' Case against the Pill.* "We asked her: 'Which risks do you mention to the patient?' She replied: 'Oh, usually the thrombophlebitis [blood clotting disorders] and not too much else. They don't understand anything else. You scare the heck out of them. We tell her that in case of anything abnormal she is to call. You don't have to outline it for them and make trouble. You don't have to plant seeds about what they're going to call about. If you tell them the symptoms they'll have them by the next day'" (Seaman 1969, 11).

Her statement embodies all the qualities members of the Boston Women's Health Book Collective had found in their doctors. It is condescending, paternalistic, judgmental, noninformative. Connell is careful not to plant seeds of doubt that her patients would call her about—the implication is wonderfully clear: She doesn't want to hear from them at all (except "in case of anything abnormal"). It was her voice, usually deeper and coming from a male physician, that women had heard so often, dismissive, disdainful, some would say contemptuous. And it was in response to that voice that women mobilized to take control of their own health care.

When Fulbright-scholar-turned-radical-activist Alice Wolfson leapt to her feet during the Senate hearings and demanded that women who had taken the pill be allowed to testify, she spoke for many other women who wanted the opportunity to talk back (Bloom 1995, 1). Wolfson, wife of a physician with the Public Health Service, was part of a group called D.C. Women's Liberation. She remembers vividly the anger and outrage that led to disrupting the hearings:

> As the testimony unfolded, we were appalled. Not a single woman was testifying, not a single pill user, not a single female researcher . . . To this day I do not remember exactly what tipped us over—what comment became too much to bear. All I remember is the outrage mounting. At first we politely raised our hands, but of course we were ignored . . . And then we were on our feet raising our hands. Still they wouldn't recognize us. That's when we began to call out our questions . . . [and] the attention of the entire room turned on us. The press rotated its cameras and microphones from the august senators to the miniskirted women. (Wolfson 1998, 271)

That day in the Senate hearing room led to intensive organizing on the issue of the safety of oral contraceptives and the demand that women be better informed about the pill's risks. Wolfson's account of that day includes her belief that this action led to the birth of the women's health movement: "I had no idea at the time that those months of intense activity and organizing would result in the birth of the women's health movement" (1998, 268). Indeed, this event did galvanize the health advocacy wing of the movement. Wolfson met Barbara Seaman for the first time that day. Later, she met Belita Cowan. They began to plan for a continuing, radical presence on Capitol Hill.

After the national press conference on the dangers of DES in Washington, D.C., in December 1972, Cowan remembers,

> I'd be sitting late at night in my kitchen talking to Barbara, who is also a night person. I told her that the lesson of Ralph Nader getting involved was not lost on me . . . I said we need to be the Ralph Naders now. We are ready.

We've got to be there. Every time something comes up the drug companies are there, the doctors are there, the reimbursement people are there, the insurance companies are there. We're not there. And they're discussing things that affect us . . . I'd have these visions and she would be so encouraging. Yes, it can be done. "Why don't you talk to Mary Howell?"[2] . . . Finally, in 1974, during one of those late night telephone conversations, we decided that we would form a women's health lobby. We would all—the whole movement—descend on Washington and we would be a key player and we would influence national health policy. We would be a force to be reckoned with. You know, it's like, "they ain't seen nothin' yet." (Cowan 1991)

Effective advocates, Cowan and Seaman knew, had to be ready to play on the political stage. Although they shared many of the goals of other women involved in the emerging women's health movement, their focus on policy demanded a different style of presentation that valued professionalism and even academic affiliation. With Phyllis Chesler (psychologist and author of *Women and Madness*), Mary Howell (physician and member of the faculty of Harvard Medical School), and Alice Wolfson, Seaman and Cowan created the National Women's Health Lobby, soon to be renamed the National Women's Health Network to "monitor Federal health agencies and ensure that the voice of a national women's health movement would be heard on Capitol Hill" (NWHN 1976, 1).

The NWHN scored its first major victory as the voice of the women's health movement in late 1975. They planned a memorial service for all the women who had died from complications related to their use of DES, birth control pills, and estrogen replacement therapy just outside the offices of the Food and Drug Administration on December 15, 1975. The FDA was meeting inside to debate the advisability of requiring package informational inserts warning women of the dangers of estrogenic drugs as a treatment for menopause. Alice Wolfson recalled the NWHN strategy that led to this high-profile action. They decided to focus on the FDA, rather than on the pharmaceutical industry that made and profited from these drugs, because the FDA "are supposed to be the watchdog, protecting us" (Wolfson quoted in Berglas 1995, 1). According to the NWHN newsletter, the protest began the process of garnering support within the FDA for package inserts for estrogenic replacement therapies. Two years later, following suits by the pharmaceutical industry and physicians associations, the FDA was able to enforce the regulation that companies inform patients of drug dangers through package inserts.

The goal of the FDA action, beyond that of better informing women about the potential dangers of estrogenic drugs, was to enhance the visibility, membership, and clout of the NWHN. And they were successful. "The demonstration was also an important step in the growth of the NWHN. For the organization to become a voice for women's health, radical steps were necessary to gather support." According to Wolfson, the protest was "never an event in itself, but a means to burst into the news and onto the world" (5).

Late in 1975, the NWHN convened meetings with more than 150 representatives of thirty different women's groups to elect the network's first board of directors, plan its activities for the following year, and discuss an organizational structure. Over the next year they moved into an office, hired Cowan as executive director, developed an information clearinghouse, continued to monitor health policy, and began to build their membership base. Within a few years they had become a highly visible, effective voice for women at some of the tables where health policy decision-making took place. Their newsletter and other publications were and are vital sources of information for women across the country about the dangers of a variety of pharmaceutical drugs (they added to their concerns about estrogenic drugs concern about medications such as tamoxifen, used in the treatment of breast cancer) and medical procedures, and about a wide variety of health research and policy issues.

The National Women's Health Network was not the only feminist health advocacy group focused on changing health policy, even in the 1970s. For more than a decade there had been groups advocating for liberalization of abortion laws, and then defending women's reproductive rights from unceasing attempts by the antiabortion movement to limit those rights in poor women, and women more generally. The Committee to End Sterilization Abuse (CESA) in New York City also took on the issue of health regulation in the early and mid–1970s, ultimately forcing the U.S. Department of Health Education and Welfare (DHEW) to issue guidelines to protect women, particularly poor women of color, from coercive sterilization abuse. On the West Coast the Coalition for the Medical Rights of Women formed in 1974, bringing together health care consumers, workers, and organizations in the Bay area to advocate for premarket testing and regulation of intrauterine devices (IUDs). They expanded their activities to include advocacy on behalf of DES daughters, women exposed to DES when their mothers took the drug during pregnancy; defense of women's reproductive rights; and other women's health issues.

In 1994, NWHN initiated a series of articles in *Network News* to commemorate "important anniversaries of the founding of the modern women's health movement in the United States" (NWHN 1994, 1). Twenty years after the NWHN's birth, the series heralded and contextualized the work of the feminist health advocates who focused their sights on national level health policy and regulation. It is clear from the choices they made about what and whom to commemorate that their perspective on the movement centers on the actions, publications, and leaders that worked at the level of public policy and health care regulation to improve women's health care and expand women's participation in health policy decision making. The series of articles includes commemoration of Frances Oldham Kelsey, a physician who as a new medical officer at the FDA blocked approval of the drug thalidomide; writer/activists Barbara Seaman, Mary Howell (who wrote a scathing critique of sexist medical education in *Why Would a "Girl" Go into Medicine*, first published under the pseudonym Margaret A. Campbell) and Doris Haire (author of *The Cultural Warping of Childbirth*, a book critical of routine hospital and physician birthing practices); Phyllis Chesler (author of *Women and Madness*); *Our Bodies, Ourselves*; the Senate pill hearings; the FDA protest of estrogenic drugs; the struggle to enact regulations to protect women from sterilization abuse; and groups and projects including the Self-Help Clinic (Downer and Rothman and the LAFWHC) and the National Black Women's Health Project.

Movement making, from the perspective of the National Women's Health Network, involved becoming a watchdog of federal health policy; an information clearinghouse that worked to assist its members to be informed health care consumers; and a forum to bring representatives from a wide variety of grassroots health organizations, health advocacy groups, medicine, nursing, and medical and health care research together on behalf of improving women's health. Over the years, women from many local, regional, or other national women's health movement organizations have served on the NWHN Board, and the network has lent its support to the development of some of these organizations, including the National Black Women's Health Project.

Jane (Doe) No More

Almost three decades have passed since *Roe* vs. *Wade* put Jane out of business. But until relatively recently the historic importance of this group as one of the founding stories of the women's health movement has not been well known. Jane, of course, operated underground, outside the law, providing abortions before abortion was legalized. Because its members faced such drastic penalties for their activities, it could tell its story only selectively, to the women who most wanted to know it. Yet its practice, developed over time and in response to the needs of women desperate for safe, low-cost abortions, offers one of the most radical instances of women taking their health care into their own hands; and although the NWHN commemoration series does not include Jane, although *Our Bodies, Ourselves* doesn't mention the organization until the 1984 edition, and then only briefly, this story, in which women band together to seize control of their reproductive lives, has emerged as a cautionary tale at times when abortion rights were heavily under threat.

The story started in code. Telephone answering machines were rare and costly in 1969, and many of the Chicago-area women who called 643–3844 had never spoken to a disembodied voice before. The protocol required something from them, an act of faith, a pledge. If you wanted help from Jane, you had to be willing to say who you were and where you could be reached, to leave a record of your voice on the tape. Like the Boston Women's Health Book Collective, Jane operated on the principles of self-reliance and mutual trust. A lot was at stake. Women who wanted abortions put their lives into Jane's hands; Janes put their lives—at the very least, their liberty—into the hands of their clients. For four years they counseled women about what to expect during the abortion; met them at "the front," the apartment or home where women gathered—often accompanied by mothers, sisters, husbands, or lovers—to await their procedures; drove them to the place the abortions were performed; and saw them home again, their control of their lives partially restored. The Janes's actions, which were extraordinary, didn't strike them as particularly brave or heroic. In fact, Jane's relatively informal and utterly pragmatic approach to its work may be its most striking legacy.

Before they inaugurated Jane, members of the Abortion Counseling Service of Women's Liberation spent several months discussing all aspects of the operation they intended to launch. First, they talked about the politics and economics of abortion. Then they took up logistical questions: "How would they handle medical emergencies, such as a woman with serious complications from an abortion? What if someone died? What would they do if one of the doctors they used was arrested, or one of them was arrested? How would they handle a police investigation?" (Kaplan 1995, 25). Finally, the group (fifteen or so women in spring 1969) started practicing counseling techniques: "They learned to describe the abortion procedure and to answer the questions women were likely to ask. They talked about ways to deal with the various emotions, like shame and self-blame, that women expressed in counseling sessions. Along with the medical information Claire [Heather Booth] wanted them to address the political dimensions and give each women a sense that her personal predicament was part of the larger socioeconomic-racial-sexual struggles that were going on at that time" (Kaplan 1995, 26–27).

With Jane, an abortion was neither sordid nor dangerous. "My very good friend got pregnant," one Jane remembers, "and went to the local free clinic and they said, 'Call 643–3844 and they can help you.' And she did. And she . . . had a wonderful experience" (Elze 1988a, 115). Many years later, another Jane recalled what the work had meant to her and to clients.

> Clearly, most of us lived fairly law-abiding lives, and had never seen ourselves in conflict with the law. When your life, your identity, and what you need to

survive is in conflict with what society dictates, it can be a real opportunity to see the world in a new way, and to understand how power works. One woman . . . had counseled a middle-aged woman from Mayor Daley's neighborhood, an Irish, Catholic working-class neighborhood. After her abortion, [the woman] said, "Well, if they are lying about this, what else are they lying about?" Those were the moments we cherished and held on to, when the commonality that all women share was illuminated. We came to understand that . . . we have always taken care of each other and can trust each other because we have the shared experience of being women in the world. (Jane 1990, 4)

Most Janes shared the experience of being white and middle class and not especially militant in appearance or manner.

I knew I wanted to do political work, women's health work . . . I came from New York, where abortions were legal. It was no big thing . . . But I moved to Chicago and my friend had her abortion and I hooked into the abortion service. It was very weird at first: here are these women doing this outrageous thing and they're all real sweet and real nice. I was very used to New York aggressive, strong, assertive women, and it was real confusing to me. How could anybody so sweet do anything so gutsy? Some had kids and husbands, and everybody had long hair. (Elze 1988a, 115)

Jane couldn't strive for visibility—except for its phone number. But monthly orientation meetings, where new members were recruited and trained, were relatively open. Many women joined Jane after they had had abortions. Some brought friends into the collective with them. The service linked up with other women's health organizations, invited Carol Downer and Lorraine Rothman to demonstrate cervical self-examination and menstrual extraction (in 1971, the concept of self-help was already very highly evolved among Janes); and information about Jane began to be available through the extensive underground abortion information and referral network across the country. Nevertheless, even after the service closed, Janes had to be careful about how they told their story and to whom. In 1975, *HealthRight* published an article on the women's health movement in Chicago that begins with the story of Jane (Chicago Women with *HealthRight* 1975, 3). Sociologist Pauline Bart presented a paper on Jane at the annual meeting of the American Sociological Association in 1977 (Bart 1987). Claudia Dreifus mentioned Jane in *Seizing Our Bodies: The Politics of Women's Health* (1977), and the service won a few paragraphs in Ruzek's important book on the movement (1978).

"What we did was an important part of the history of the women's health movement in this country, and I don't want it to go unrecognized anymore," one Jane observed. "It was real sad to me that it had faded to the point where nationally, the person most well known for speaking about Jane was not a member of Jane," another said. "And that, secondly, we had been reduced to three paragraphs in a wonderful book, *Our Bodies, Ourselves*" (Elze 1988b, 14). In the past fifteen years, as gains of the antiabortion movement made real the threat that abortion might once again be made illegal in the United States, more and more interviews with ex-Janes and brief histories of the organization have appeared (Elze 1988; Baehr 1990; Jane 1990; Podell 1990; Van Gelder 1991; King 1993). Laura Kaplan's book-length study (1995) adds detail and context to the narrative through her own recollections and interviews with many other ex-Janes.

For Jane's eleven thousand clients, the organization's foundational story was the most important legend of the women's health movement. That so many otherwise law-abiding women risked arrest, prosecution, and imprisonment in order to provide safe and affordable illegal abortions attests to the desperate need for those services and to women's commitment to meet that need, whatever the cost. That Jane members took over the procedure themselves is even more remarkable, a profound rejection of the ethos of professionalism. It wasn't very difficult to learn how to do an abortion, they told themselves. There weren't any incisions to make. By mastering a series of simple tasks, and then combining them, they reclaimed knowledge held by midwives who were the repositories of abortion skills until the procedure was criminalized in the late nineteenth century. Janes dedicated themselves to lowering the cost of abortion, thus ensuring its accessibility to poor women. Accessibility of health care was to be a contested issue in the growing grassroots clinic movement in the 1970s.

The story of Jane makes clear what is less explicit, but in fact no less critical, in the other foundational stories I have told: The struggle for safe, legal, accessible abortion was central in catalyzing women's health activism. Participants at BWHBC's "Women and Their Bodies" courses shared painful experiences of unwanted (or terminated) pregnancies. Carol Downer and Lorraine Rothman planned to open a woman-controlled abortion clinic, and their work on self-help developed as part of a strategy to circumvent restrictive abortion laws. The impulse to gain knowledge about and control over their health care always came from women's need to chart their own reproductive lives (the work of Barbara Seaman and Belita Cowan also demonstrates this simple principle).

In the days since the Supreme Court decision in Webster (1989), the story of Jane tends to be told as a form of consciousness-raising in the women's health and pro-choice movements: It promises that if abortion is recriminalized, women will gain access to the information and tools they need to bring back underground abortion—safe, inexpensive, and women controlled. Thus, even two decades after Jane dissolved, the telling of this foundational story remains part of the process of movement making, circulating stories about the past that embolden the present and promise a future in which women will not allow themselves to lose what so many individuals, organizations, and the movement that defines them fought so hard to create.

Belonging: Connections, Linkages, Identity

Foundational stories remind us that the process of movement making involves real people who acted in the (often confusing) midst of particular historical circumstances and in specific communities that influenced the nature of and the response to activism there. In the late 1960s, for example, the Chicago feminist community was deeply rooted in the New Left, the Boston feminist community less so. Historian Margaret Strobel compares the umbrella groups from which Jane (Chicago Women's Liberation Union) and the Boston Women's Health Book Collective (Bread and Roses) emerged. Although the two groups "drew members from the same segment of the population in terms of age and ideology," she observed, their organizational styles and political visions were quite different (Strobel 1995, 155). One produced books; the other performed abortions.

Local circumstances also help explain why law enforcement agencies in Chicago allowed Jane to function uninterrupted for almost four years (Jane provided abortions to the wives, girlfriends, and sisters of many police officers, and some evidence suggests that the single raid on the service in May 1972 was a mistake); and local circumstances help explain why the Los Angeles Feminist Women's Health Center was raided by police and the Board of Medical Examiners for such relatively minor infractions as fitting diaphragms and offering home remedies for yeast infections. A detailed discussion of the differences between these cities is beyond the scope of this analysis. I raise the point here only to underscore that local history always provides the soil from which particular organizations grow.

Although I agree with critics who argue that much current theory reifies the concept of social movement and neglects its discursive essence, I want to explore how involvement in a social movement generates the feeling that the movement is palpable, embodied, real in nondiscursive ways, and how that feeling illuminates the process by which participants construct the experience of belonging to a national movement. In the early 1970s, concrete linkages among individuals and organizations fostered the sense of belonging to a women's health movement. Through telephone calls, letters, and other documents, visits to neighboring communities, attendance at women's health conferences, newsletters, manuals, and pamphlets, health activists nourished a sense of shared experience and collective identity.

When the group that planned to open the New Bedford Women's Center solicited advice about how to operate, women from other clinics explained the organizational structure of collectives, described the roles of different lay health workers, suggested ways to integrate volunteers, and discussed the value of incorporating as a nonprofit. They talked about problems, too. "Starting clinics is so exciting and sometimes it's easier to do than keeping one going after two years," one woman admitted in a letter to "sisters" opening the new clinic.

By the early 1970s, interorganizational support for new clinics and advocacy groups came from established organizations, principally the Boston Women's Health Book Collective and the Los Angeles Feminist Women's Health Center. For example, the first Annual Report of the new Cambridge, Massachusetts, feminist clinic, Women's Community Health Center (WCHC), includes a month-to-month chronology of such interactions:

August 1973: J.B., self-helper at large, meets . . . C.A. at a self-help presentation in Worcester, Mass. C.A. informs J.B. that there are many women in Boston who want to start a women's health center. Carol Downer [from the Los Angeles Feminist Women's Health Center] suggests a conference to bring women together for this . . .

November 1973: The First Annual Women's Health Conference is held at the Boston YWCA. Over 150 women gather. On Sunday two groups form, one to start a women-owned and controlled health center, the other to set up a women's program within an existing facility . . .

January 1974: . . . The LAFWHC begins to send $50 a week, no strings attached, hoping this will help get a woman-owned and controlled self help clinic started.

February 1974: The WCHC files for incorporation . . .

May 1974: We are becoming . . . We compile a comprehensive referral file, help women in Worcester organize a two day health conference and continue doing self help presentations . . . We receive a $5000 grant from the Boston Women's Health Book Collective . . .

July 1974: We begin our gynecological services and start our second self help group . . .

October 1974: . . . We continue to share self help throughout New England . . .

November 1974: We sponsor the Second Annual Women's Health Conference at the Boston YWCA. Gail and Beth go to the Women's Health Conference in Ames, Iowa. (WCHC 1975, 4–5)

Women's Community Health may have been unusual in the degree to which it profited from such linkages, but the pattern repeated itself over and over again: fledgling women's health organizations could count on some degree of ideological, financial, and technical support from other feminist health activists and groups.

Conferences and demonstrations also helped forge a sense of collective identity within the movement. In March 1971, more than eight hundred women gathered at a high school in New York City for what many called the first national women's health conference. Ellen Frankfort expresses amazement that so many women were drawn to the meeting. "Not a single ad or press release had announced the weekend or workshops and demonstrations. Yet women kept on arriving from places as far away as San Francisco and Seattle, having heard of the event through the genuine grassroots movement that has sprung up around women's health issues" (1972, 232). Before e-mail and the Internet, the turnout was extraordinary for a genuine grassroots movement in the earliest stages of organization. In their own communities, women who wanted to change their relationship with the health care system had already begun to meet and work together. Now they recognized that they were not alone, that their campaign—some thought of it as a crusade—was flourishing at many other sites across the country. Other national gatherings—in Iowa City in 1972, in Connecticut in 1973, in Ames, Iowa, and in Philadelphia in 1974, in Boston in 1975—offered opportunities to share information and to trade plans and tactics, and they helped develop the larger self-conception that encouraged BWHBC, for example, to imagine a national and then an international audience for *Our Bodies, Ourselves.* The sense of collective identity within the women's health movement stretched wider as a result of such national meetings, but it arose from and found justification in work that unfolded in smaller-group settings, at home.

The end of isolation marks the beginning of power. On their cross-country tour, Carol Downer and Lorraine Rothman contacted, directly or indirectly, thousands of women who hoped and planned to change the health care delivery system. Janes used mirrors to introduce thousands more to the simplicity and accessibility of their cervixes and modeled the radical spirit of self-help in their abortion protocols. The Boston Women's Health Book Collective armed millions of women with the movement's encyclopedic text, *Our Bodies, Ourselves.* Other books and manuals appeared, some shared collections of mimeographed pages, others bound and distributed by progressive or commercial presses. Through exchange of information and sharing of funding with newborn, front-line clinics (for Women's Community Health in Cambridge, fifty dollars a week, no strings attached, from LAFWHC, and a five-thousand-dollar grant from BWHBC), the separate avenues of change converged in a structure of support that had national reach.

In 1972 Ellen Frankfort, a columnist who had written a series of articles on women's health for the *Village Voice,* published *Vaginal Politics,* which articulated the movement's ideology and vision (complete with a graphic portrayal of a self-help workshop by Carol Downer and Lorraine Rothman), and fed its self-definition as a national force. The same year, Doris Haire mobilized the home birth movement against male-dominated mainstream gynecology in "The Cultural Warping of Childbirth." Phyllis Chesler's *Women and Madness,* a scarifying exploration of mental health care for women, was published in 1972. And 1972 marks the first appearance of publications that bridged the gap between the women's health movement and academic scholarship.

By the early 1970s, feminists in colleges and universities had begun to organize multidisciplinary courses in women's studies, using whatever scholarly and popular sources they could find to teach about various aspects of women's lives. Barbara Ehrenreich, who had a doctorate in biology and several years of experience in the left wing of the community health movement, teamed up with Deirdre English, a colleague at State University of New York-Old Westbury, to offer a course on women and medicine. They wrote their own teaching texts, which were published by the new Feminist Press: *Witches, Midwives, and Nurses: A History of Women Healers* and *Complaints and Disorders: The Sexual Politics of Sickness.* "We had students . . . from the Caribbean who had been midwives and then who came here and could only be practical nurses, and students from European backgrounds whose grandmothers had been able to do various herbal remedies in the old country, and we began to realize that there was this tradition of women's lay healing in many parts of the world" (Ehrenreich 1998). The story of the movement's roots had to be told.

In *Witches, Midwives, and Nurses* and *Complaints and Disorders,* Ehrenreich and English explore that tradition. The texts—pamphlets, their authors called them—were only about one hundred pages long. But their influence was profound and their distribution extraordinarily widespread. Explicitly antiracist and anticapitalist, they established a genealogy for the emerging critique of women's oppression within and by the health care industry and documented the usurpation of women's control of their own health (as healers within families and communities) by religious leaders (during the Salem witchcraft trials) and, in the mid to late nineteenth century, by medical professionals. By the mid–1970s, both mainstream and alternative presses were beginning to fill a growing popular and scholarly demand for books on women's health, and about the need for change in health care policy and in the way medical professionals treated women.[3]

I've argued that the founding of the National Women's Health Network in 1975 gave the women's health movement a unified voice and way of focusing on activities that would have a national impact, especially via the shaping of federal health policy. But that event came after the movement had achieved national scope through its activities in the service of social change, and through the conscious articulation of its politics, its goals, and its evolving collective identity. Helen Marieskind and Barbara Ehrenreich believe that the women's health movement enjoys coherence, self-consciousness, and public recognition by 1973. The evidence they point to: the existence of twelve hundred groups which identify as part of the women's health movement, the existence of women's health groups and projects outside the United States, the history of a half dozen national conferences on women's health, two national publications devoted to intramovement debate and communication, a distinctive body of literature identified with the movement, and "a growing public acknowledgment of the movement's existence . . . [in] medical journals . . . [and] radio and TV talk shows" (1975, 38).

Another indicator, harder to measure but clearly visible in the records of women's health organizations, was the sense that the movement had forever altered those who participated in it, rewritten their consciousnesses. "We need to be the Ralph Naders now," Belita Cowan said. "We are ready. We've got to be there." Members of the Boston Women's Health Book Collective and the Los Angeles Feminist Women's Health Center were ready, too. They had invented the movement by coming together to change the way health care was imagined and delivered, and they had all recognized the same, simple intoxicating fact: Power creates momentum. Belita Cowan provides a coda for that discovery. "We would all—the whole movement—descend on Washington and we would be a key player and we would influence national health policy . . . You know, it's like, 'they ain't seen nothin' yet'" (Cowan 1991).

On May 20, 1973, when more than one hundred women celebrated the bittersweet end of Jane with a gathering in one of their homes, Nick, the practitioner who had trained some Janes to perform abortions, was struck by the contrast between the revolutionary actions these women had collectively enacted over four years and their appearance as "ordinary women in sundresses and shorts, eating and talking" (Kaplan 1995, 280). Indeed, a group of ordinary women in Chicago had accumulated more power in the past four years than most of them could ever have thought possible. Ordinary women just like them were enacting their ideas in other towns and cities throughout the United States. Yet I argue that it is problematic to depict the growing movement self-consciousness and group activity simply as a process of aggregation. It's certainly true that the movement coalesced as local groups created ever denser linkages and projected themselves through extralocal social practices; but those local groups were energized from their beginnings by a sense that something larger—a movement—was under way, and that sense of a movement, I would argue, came directly from the consolidation and exercise of power. Members of women's health organizations believed that they were responding to, as well as nourishing, an inexorable force. Perhaps Carol Downer expressed that view best, and spoke for many, when she said, "I wasn't leading a movement. I was getting drug by it" (1990).

Chapter 3

On Their Own

Women of Color and the Women's Health Movement

In the early 1970s, Byllye Avery, an African American woman working in the Children's Mental Health Unit at Shand's Teaching Hospital in Gainesville, Florida, was known in her community as someone who had the phone number of a doctor in New York City who performed safe, illegal abortions. She realized this abortion referral was of little use to many women, especially those who had low incomes, because they could never afford the cost of the abortion and travel north to New York. When abortion was legalized, Avery and several friends founded the women-controlled Gainesville Women's Health Clinic (GWHC). Four years later Avery helped to found an alternative birthing center, Birth Place. In the interval she was invited to serve on the board of directors of the relatively new National Women's Health Network (NWHN).

Byllye Avery's life experiences were different from those of many of the women she had worked with at the GWHC, Birth Place, or the NWHN. She was acutely aware of how little information existed about Black women's health and of how the movement she was part of defined issues, strategies, and services with little attention or awareness to the specific needs and perspectives of women of color. As a board member of the NWHN she envisioned a grassroots approach to bring Black women together to define their own health needs and develop their own strategies for change. In 1982 the NWHN announced the beginning of a two-year project on Black women's health with Avery at the helm.

With the help of others who supported her work, Avery constructed a

41

network of about twenty African American women—health professionals, university professors, and leaders and members of community-based organizations—who agreed to plan the project's culminating conference, which was to be held in June 1983. Avery did research about Black women's health and facilitated the formation of local self-help groups in which women could "work together individually and on a daily basis" (Avery 1990a, 78). These groups differed from most of the self-help groups elsewhere in the movement. Rather than focusing on cervical self-examination or women-controlled health care, self-help groups were a forum in which Black women shared their stories and struggles. By summer 1983, more than a dozen self-help groups associated with the National Black Women's Health Project were up and running across the country, in Florida, Georgia, Alabama, Tennessee, Rhode Island, New Jersey, Pennsylvania, Minnesota, Michigan, and the San Francisco Bay Area. Members of those groups joined other Black women at Spelman College in Atlanta from June 24 to June 26, 1983, for the first national conference on Black women's health. The words of Fannie Lou Hamer, legendary civil rights leader, expressed the conference theme: "We're tired of being sick and tired."

Although planners had anticipated only a few hundred participants, more than fifteen hundred women descended on Spelman College that weekend. "They came with Ph.D.'s, M.D.'s, welfare cards, in Mercedes and on crutches, from seven days old to 80 years old—urban, rural, gay, straight—to find something" (Avery 1990a, 78). And find something they did. They found knowledge and strength from each other and the collective energy to build a new organization—the National Black Women's Health Project, which was formally organized in the summer of 1983 and became an official organization in March 1984. Over the course of the next decade, women of color, seeking both autonomy and inclusion in the women's health movement, founded their own organizations: the National Latina Health Organization in 1986, the Native American Women's Health Education Resource Center in 1988, the National Asian Women's Health Organization in 1993. To understand the perspectives, activities, and political goals of these organizations means we must, to use Elsa Barclay Brown's words, "pivot the center" (1988) away from the predominantly white women's health movement to explore how women of color sought to tailor activism to the needs and resources of their own vibrant and diverse communities. In the process, they reshaped the women's health movement and the politics of women's health.

There is no better way to "pivot the center" than to return to the story of Byllye Avery and the National Black Women's Health Project to examine the foundational stories of these women's health organizations and understand the dramatic impact they have had on women's lives and the changing women's health movement. In the period before *Roe* vs. *Wade*, Avery was one of "a handful of women who could help women seek abortions" (Avery 1991). Help, then, meant being able to give pregnant women the telephone number of a doctor in New York City who performed abortions. But Avery and a number of her friends saw the limitations of this kind of help and began to make other plans.

Soon after abortion was legalized, a clinic opened in Jacksonville, about ninety minutes away from Gainesville. Avery and several friends sometimes drove clients there, but at the same time, they began to make plans closer to home. "We used to gather in the kitchen of a woman, I wish you could interview her . . . she was a psychologist at the unit where I worked. And we used to all gather in Judy's kitchen around her kitchen table and dream about having a women's health center" (Avery 1991).

Enacting that dream in May 1974, they founded the women-controlled Gainesville Women's Health Clinic (GWHC). "We had doctors performing the abortions and we had nurses who worked there. But we did it all in a different kind of way. First of all, we made the place beautiful . . . It was a real break at that time, because, if you remember, in the past, our medical complexes used to be real sterile and ugly. And so we made this one pleasing and beautiful . . . more homey and friendly" (Avery 1991). The clinic didn't just look different. It operated differently, too:

> We were able to develop health services within our center in the way we wanted to be treated. That was always the question we asked. How do you want to be treated when you go to a facility? Do you want to greet a doctor who you have never met . . . when you are lying down helpless? We were trying to get rid of some of the hierarchy that existed . . . We started telling women about what the procedures they were having would be like . . . Give them all the information they needed . . . Spend as much time with the person as was needed. (Avery 1991)

For Avery, the key tenet of the women's health movement was always "choice: that we (women) deserve to be respected for the choices that we make" (Avery 1991). Because the Gainesville Medical Society had recently denied Planned Parenthood's petition to open a local clinic that provided abortions, GWHC founders decided *not* to ask for permission. Members of the Gainesville Medical Society found out about the new clinic the same way the rest of the community did: "We just opened it up and they read about it in the *Gainesville Sun*" (Avery 1991). In response to clients' needs for additional services, the ongoing kitchen table discussions led to a decision to open an alternative birthing center, Birth Place, in November 1978: "About two, two and a half years after we opened [the GWHC] we started being drawn in to the birthing movement because if women had trouble with their home births, or if they had trouble with their babies being seen, they would bring them to our doctors . . . That was enlightening. Because we thought, if we are going to be drawn into it, let's see how we can enter into it in a powerful way and . . . we opened Birth Place" (Avery 1991).

Avery remembers her years of involvement with the GWHC and Birth Place as positive and empowering, but there were also challenges: "I learned a lot. But we had our struggles . . . When you get involved in organizations like this . . . you want to feel like you can create a utopia where there will always be peace and love and harmony. Which is very unrealistic." She left Birth Place in 1980 not because of internal strife, but because the facility needed more midwives. "I wasn't willing to go to nursing school," she explains.

There was another reason, too. "An important thing happened to me. I began looking at myself as a black woman" (Avery 1990a, 77). In her next job, Avery headed a Comprehensive Employment Training (CETA) program at Santa Fe Community College in Gainesville. There, she worked with young women who had dropped out of high school; many were Black, and many were still in their teens. "They were having a lot of health problems that I didn't think we got until we were much older. And I started talking with them closely about their lives and how they made decisions. And found a lot of people make decisions by not making decisions. And then I learned that they do make decisions with the best information that they have" (Avery 1991).

Byllye Avery's consciousness as a woman had been well nourished by her involvement with the GWHC and Birth Place. But, she remembers, "the more I worked with young black women, the more I came into my consciousness as a black woman" (1991). Working with the young Black women through the community college helped Avery see clearly the need for women of color to define their own health needs and a vision of empowerment through health activism. Avery had long known that "people look at health in terms of how they live and what is important to them." Now she understood more about the limits of the movement that had been "started and organized mainly by white women . . . white women had no idea about certain issues affecting Black women" (Avery quoted in Scherzer 1995, 4).

The National Black Women's Health Project

When Avery joined the board of the National Women's Health Network in the mid–1970s, her ideas began to evolve. She knew there was a need for more information about Black women's health; for a grassroots approach to bring Black women together; and for a national network of Black women who could work with one another in their own communities to define and advocate for the kind of health care they needed. When the NWHN announced the formation of a two-year project on Black women's health to be led by Avery in 1982, Avery began the hard work of making the connections—connections among African American women who shared the vision of reaching out to and working in their own communities, and the connection between the evolving politics of women's health and the deeply rooted struggle against racism within communities of color. She began talking with Pam Freedman, another African American NWHN member, and she asked friends in the movement to help identify other Black women to join a committee to plan a conference on Black women's health: "I didn't know enough Black women around the country, but I knew white women, and so whenever they would say to me what can I do to help you, I would say do you know a Black woman [who might want to get involved]" (Avery 1991).

Gradually, a diverse group of about twenty African American women agreed to plan a conference on Black women's health. At the same time Avery and her colleagues researched health issues important to Black women and worked to facilitate the formation of what she called self-help groups. "People needed to be able to work together individually and on a daily basis," she recalls. "This gave us the idea for self help groups" (Avery 1990a, 78). "At first . . . we would get together using the regular health education model. Talk about high blood pressure, talk about weight . . . I found out that what women needed is a sense of building self-esteem, a sense of empowerment . . . So many women felt that they had no control over their lives, that things were just happening to them, and that was quite difficult. So we really worked a lot in the psychological domain" (Avery 1991). By the summer of 1983, more than a dozen self-help groups associated with the National Black Women's Health Project were in operation, mainly in the southern United States (Florida, Georgia, Alabama, and Tennessee), but also in Rhode Island, New Jersey, Pennsylvania, Minnesota, Michigan, and the San Francisco Bay Area.

Byllye Avery was a visionary. But even she had not foreseen just how ripe the time was for Black women's health activism. On June 24, 1983, the first day of the conference that Avery and her planning committee had been planning, about fifteen hundred women descended on Spelman College (a historically Black women's college) in Atlanta. Conference organizers had planned for a few hundred participants. By all accounts, the conference was a life-transforming event for many. One woman who later became involved with the Bay Area Black Women's Health Project worked for weeks to raise money—from family, friends, and others—to attend the conference. "I really didn't talk that much that weekend. My heart was literally in my throat. To arrive on that campus and see Black women of every hue, you know, blue eyes, fair skin, dark skin, no hair, dreadlocks, straight hair and permed." From her point of view, all the workshops were powerful; but one had overwhelming significance because it was her first experience of being in a space that was only for Black women. "I was going to this workshop called 'Black and Female: What Is Reality?' . . . for Black women only. I'd never been anyplace that was for Black women only. I'd never been anyplace that was for women only."

The conference keynote was delivered by June Jackson Christmas, former president of the American Public Health Association and medical professor and director of the Behavioral Science Program at City University of New York. Her presentation was hard hitting, focusing on the triple jeopardy most Black women face as a result of "racism, sexism, and the devalued and impoverished existence which they experience" (NBWHP 1994b). The conference catapulted the Black Women's Health Project into the national spotlight, and the NBWHP was formally organized in summer 1983 to carry on the work already under way.

In March 1984, the NBWHP became an independent organization. Its mission statement, published in its news magazine *Vital Signs,* committed the organization to "defining, promoting, and maintaining the physical, mental and emotional well-being of Black women" with four interrelated goals:

1. To enable Black women to understand the concepts of emotional, mental and physical health and the relationship among the three;
2. To provide Black women with the information, skills, and access to resources needed to live healthfully;
3. To facilitate the empowerment of Black women, both individually and collectively, to exercise control over their lives; and
4. To ensure the survival of future generations of Black people through the promotion of health maintenance and prevention. (NBWHP 1985)

The mission statement also clarified the group's relationship with the National Women's Health Network. "This independence was and is not intended to be seen as a move to terminate alliances with any organizations or individuals who nourished us during our earliest days." Instead, the NBWHP aimed "to develop different types of alliances" that recognized the importance of unity in the struggle to ensure the rights of all women to control their health destiny. "This quest for self-definition does not preclude our collectivity with other organizations," NBWHP founders asserted (NBWHP 1985, 2). Women of color needed their own voices and were determined to connect to the larger women's health movement on their own terms.

Health activists came to the NBWHP along many different paths. Julia Scott, a registered nurse, began her work in women's reproductive rights and health through her relationship with another visionary, Edna Smith, who was also a nurse. Smith saw the potential to use newly available federal family planning monies to support broad preventative education about contraception, sexuality, and general health. She persuaded Scott to take the position of director of training for the Boston Family Planning Project in the 1970s.

> I said, oh God, I don't know anything about family planning. Certainly didn't learn it in nursing school. I said, you know I was raised as a Catholic so all of this is supposed to be a sin of some kind . . . and so I hadn't practiced it in my own life. And she said, "Oh, that's the easy part. I'll give you a book on that." She said "I like the way you interact with people and the way you try to pass on information to people" . . . And so I was very excited [by] her ideas of working with a healthy model. (Scott 1991)

After three years of training paraprofessionals and women from the community (the substance of what she was doing was similar to what was happening in feminist clinics), Scott decided to pursue a long-held dream: to become a nurse practitioner. But she balked when she learned that students would practice pelvic examinations on hospital patients under anesthesia. Scott questioned whether those patients had signed releases giving permission for the students to do pelvic exams; she was told that the general surgical release covered the procedure. "So I said, 'well you know, ethically I cannot do that . . . ' and a couple of other people agreed with me and we said we were not going to do that. And they said, 'Well, the only other option is to go on the wards and ask patients.' I said 'no, there's another option. We can examine each other.' I said I am willing to be a subject and we can tell each other whether it hurts and, you know, whatever." Scott's refusal to perform pelvic exams on anaesthetized women mirrored the concerns of activists in a number of feminist clinics who advocated women-centered pelvic exams and pelvic exam instruction. Scott argues that her stand grew from deep roots in her own experiences; "I'd have to say that growing up as a woman in the United States you kind of get sensitized to a lot of these indignities pretty early on in life" (Scott 1991).

In her next job, at a community-based organization in Newark, New Jersey, Scott helped in the process of applying for a grant from the Ms. Foundation, where she was later hired as field director for reproductive rights. One of her responsibilities was to develop coalitions between white women and women of color around reproductive rights. In that context, she saw firsthand how few white women understood the interconnectedness of reproductive health and rights issues as these play out in the lives of most women of color.

A group of people such as African American women and Hispanic women and Native Americans who have been subjected to sterilization abuse, you know, the guinea pig kind of thing, and with the birth control pill and the excessive use of hysterectomies in our communities. We very seldom have the luxury of coming together and organizing on just one simple piece, that being the right to abortion, but we see that within the broader women's reproductive health agenda. (Scott 1991)

That lack of understanding on the part of white women translated into the movement's failure to squarely address key issues about race and health:

And there's been a real reluctance on the part of the white women's health movement and the reproductive health movement to be as concerned about some of those other things as they are about abortion rights. And indeed, when we lost the right for Medicaid funding for abortion, it was a clear signal for most women of color in this country that the white women's movement is not concerned about issues of women of color. (Scott 1991)

Scott first met Byllye Avery when Avery approached the Ms. Foundation for funding for the NBWHP. Scott loved Avery's ideas; she wrote them up for the Ms. Foundation Board, which agreed to help fund the Atlanta conference, and she attended the event, "not only as a foundation representative, but as an African American woman." "I was just so thrilled at the idea of an organization that was specifically for African American women. Where you can sit up, just let your guard down. Where everybody was just totally accepted. And I guess that's the thing that still overwhelms me about this project even given all the problems we have had, conflicts with training and all this other stuff. I still feel it's the one place where you are really accepted for what you are" (Scott 1991).

Scott is acutely aware of the many differences among African American women—"the color of your skin, the texture of your hair," the kinds of access available to you "because of the way you look or talk," and class issues (Scott 1991). She saw the NBWHP strive to understand, work with, and overcome those differences, and that striving inspired what she calls her "lifelong commitment" to the organization. As a member of NBWHP's board of directors in its early years, Scott took part in discussions about the organization's plans to influence public policy in Washington, D.C. While she worked for the Children's Defense Fund (also in Washington), she helped to raise money for NBWHP from the Ford and Ms. Foundations.

By 1986 more than fifty NBWHP self-help groups were functioning throughout the United States, and local chapters of the organization had formed in a number of cities. In 1988, the NBWHP established the Center for Black Women's Wellness in Atlanta to provide health and other services to Black women in housing projects across the city. A "community-based self-help program," the center has offered wellness education, self-help group development, social service information, vocational and educational training, health screening (including Pap smears, breast self-examination, pregnancy testing), and other primary health care services. Beginning with its active participation in the 1985 "End of the United Nations Decade of Women" forum in Nairobi, the NBWHP developed international programs and linkages, too. In 1989, NBWHP founded SisteReach, an international program "to support the global movement of women of color working for self-empowerment and self-determination." The program provided support and technical assistance as women outside the United States sought to "develop a corps of self-help health facilitators for outreach in their communities" (SisteReach n.d.). By 1993 there were SisteReach programs in Brazil, the Cameroon, the Caribbean, and Nigeria.

As the 1990s dawned, the NBWHP was sponsoring 130 self-help groups in twenty-four cities, and that year, with Julia Scott at the helm, the NBWHP Public Policy/Public Education Office opened in Washington, D.C., to broaden the national reproductive rights agenda and to improve the health status of Black women, their children, and their communities. The organization's accomplishments were stunning. Rapid growth and diverse programming did take their toll on the NBWHP. Like many other women's health movement organizations, its resources were stretched thin and internal conflicts and political differences required attention, resolution, and a growing organizational savvy.

Issues of *Vital Signs* were remarkably open about these problems as part of the organization's commitment to open and honest sharing. In February 1989, the newsletter reported that "these past months have found us struggling with the meaning of words like leadership, transition, commitment, change, confusion, and the feelings they inspire" (Ahron and Ward 1989, 4). The challenges were difficult, ranging from conflict between Byllye Avery and another organizational leader, Lillie Allen (who developed the NBWHP's Black and female programs), to organizational development issues concerning budget, staffing, and administration of the organization's many different programs.

Ultimately Avery announced that she would take on a new organizational role as founding president and step down as executive director. She wanted to relocate to Boston and focus her leadership talents on fundraising, public relations, and outreach. In full view of NBWHP members, organizational leaders admitted both the difficulties they had faced and their optimism about the future. It has been a difficult "transition period . . . for quite some time . . . [The NBWHP] has entered a new period that requires the organization to proceed along its course in a *different* manner. The knowledge that all non-profits (and even many for profits) undergo such changes has helped to increase our optimism regarding our future." At the same time, the organization had to cut its national staff by half "because of a growing annual deficit" (Avery 1990b, 2).

Julia Scott, who had been working to organize a newly funded public policy office in Washington, D.C., now became interim executive director. A national search was initiated for a new director as she shuttled back and forth between Atlanta and Washington, D.C., working to stabilize the organization. Scott was philosophical about the difficulties facing the organization, "What happened in our organization, I think is very typical of non-profits and of women's leadership. We want to be all things for all people . . . In your attempt to do it all you make some . . . mistakes. And all of this was the growth and development of a non-profit" (Scott 1991). The NBWHP had reached its adolescence, she says, and although the move into adulthood was complicated, they "did not push it under the carpet or have these sophisticated ways for buying people out . . . We fought it out in a very public kind of way. Because we felt we had a duty to women, certainly to African American women, to be up front about what our shortcomings were and what we were struggling for" (Scott 1991).

The NBWHP survived that period of transition, and in 1994 marked its tenth anniversary with a conference and homecoming under the theme "We Are the Ones We've Been Waiting For." A proclamation by the governor of Georgia declared July 1, 1994, National Black Women's Health Project Day in that state (NBWHP 1994a, 8). The proclamation's clauses recapitulate the organization's history:

> [D]uring the 1970s, the women's health movement recognized the dramatic need to address the fact that health risks for women have changed within the context of revolutionary changes in life-styles, changes in family and work relationships and changes in the ways women perceive themselves . . . [T]he National Black Women's Health Project was founded because the women's health movement had not addressed the needs of Black women effectively . . . [O]ver the last decade, the National Black Women's Health Project has been a tireless and determined voice on the issue of Black Women's Health, challenging America and championing the cause of affordable, equitable and quality health care for Black women, their families and communities. (NBWHP 1994a, 8)

The following year, the NBWHP board consolidated its operations in one office in Washington, D.C., "where we can join like minded national organizations working on issues important to us and our community" (Budu-Watkins and Avery 1995). Julia Scott replaced Cynthia Newbille, who had served as

NBWHP executive director for four years and wanted to run for public office in Virginia.

A Century of Black Women's Health Activism

The women who spearheaded and sustained the organizational and social movement work that led to the formation and maintenance of the NBWHP came of age during the civil rights and women's movements. But a longer tradition of public health campaigns, stretching back through the twentieth century, informed their activism (Davis 1981, 1989; Giddings 1984; Hine 1985, 1989; Hammonds 1986; Smith 1995; Roberts 1997; Ross 1998). This record of involvement in women's health and reproductive rights has only recently captured the attention of scholars and activists, including Loretta Ross, once program director for the NBWHP. In a seminal article, Ross (1998) tracks the struggle to its beginnings almost one hundred years ago in the efforts of women's clubs affiliated with the National Association of Colored Women (NACW). The NACW supported birth control and the idea of voluntary motherhood and later worked toward the establishment of family planning clinics in Black communities (Ross 1998, 168).

The racist ideology of the mainstream, white-led birth control movement, and especially its connection to the rising eugenics movement, complicated the issue for Black women. Nevertheless, granny midwives, licensed health care providers, and community workers provided birth control information and services (as well as abortions) to women in their communities. Later, leaders such as Shirley Chisholm (the first Black woman elected to Congress), Frances Beale (head of the Black Women's Liberation Committee of SNCC), and writer and activist Toni Cade Bambara advocated for Black women's reproductive rights, while revolutionary Black Power organizations defined birth control and abortion as genocide against the Black community and called on women to be "birth warriors" for the movement.

Ross argues that Black women made significant contributions to the reproductive freedom movement even as they fought against racism within it. Groups such as the National Black Feminist Organization and the Combahee River Collective, founded in the early and mid–1970s, acted as springboards for a Black feminist analysis of race, gender, and class. In the middle and later 1970s, when predominantly white organizations failed to prioritize, and sometimes even to support, the efforts of women of color to address issues such as sterilization abuse and the effective denial of abortion rights to poor women by Congress (through the Hyde Amendment, which prohibits the use of federal funds to defray the cost of the procedure), racism diluted the effectiveness of the reproductive rights/women's health movements. But the activism of women of color for improved health care and reproductive rights continued unabated, becoming more connected to a growing international women's health movement. Ross identifies the conference that closed the UN Decade for Women in Nairobi as "the watershed event of the decade [the 1980s] for African American women" (1998, 189), the capstone of a period that saw the formation not only of the NBWHP, but also of the National Political Congress of Black Women, the National Organization for Women of Color Program, and the Coalition of African American Women for Reproductive Freedom.

While many Black women flocked to health movement organizations explicitly identified as Black women's organizations, Black women also worked in mixed-race and predominantly white women's health movement organizations. Their contributions to these organizations are becoming more visible as scholars move away from simple references to the reality that many health movement organizations were predominantly white and middle class and toward organizational analyses that explore the dynamics of race and class within feminist organizations. For example, Ross expands our understanding of Jane in an interview with Lois Smith (a pseudonym), who explained how it felt to be one of only a few women of color involved in that group:

> When I arrived at the facility [she accompanied another woman], I saw that the clients were predominantly Black, but all the workers were white. Even while I was waiting for my friend, I began counseling the women, telling them they would be all right. When I joined the collective our primary problem was the illegality of what we were doing. This produced extreme secrecy and paranoia, but in a sense, it helped us bond as a group. It wasn't a Black or a white thing, but a women's need. (Quoted in Ross 1998, 179)

Women of color joined Jane one at a time, Smith said, "so we could never develop a critical mass, or even three to four of us, to get together to talk about what we were doing" (179).

In a 1990 survey of women's health organizations, African Americans constituted 15 percent of the total staff of fifty women's health movement organizations (Morgen and Julier 1991, 6). Black women have served as directors of several feminist health clinics (including Brenda Joyner of the Feminist Women's Health Center in Tallahassee, Florida, and Viola Pina of the New Bedford Women's Health Services in Massachusetts); both clinics explicitly declare themselves multiracial organizations in their mission statements,[1] and both sponsored programs and community outreach activities that confronted racism head on.

As discussed at greater length in chapter 9, the relationships between women of color and white women in women's health movement organizations often proved tense, textured by racism and often class differences. Those struggles produced some movement-wide changes—the formation of groups such as NBWHP, for example—greater awareness of racism among white women, and new coalitions between organizations. But progress continues to be slow and uneven. Julia Scott observes that there have been many instances in which mostly white organizations failed to understand the politics of race as it intersected with the politics of women's health.

> You know at some point you've got to have white women understanding the issues so that we're not always the one to bring it [our issue] up. And I believe that until the white women's health movement or the white women's movement period deals with their poor white sisters and really understands what it is like to be poor and without money, I think they'll get it a lot quicker. I think the divisions between the races are such that it is always going to be like an effort to put yourself in somebody's else's place . . . I think if white women look at their poor white sisters and the lives they have to live, they'll get the connections across racial lines. (Scott 1991)

Some of the differences between white women's health movement organizations and organizations such as the NBWHP may be obscured by a shared vocabulary that includes such concepts as self-help and empowerment. However, groups may share vocabularies and aspects of their basic political perspectives but fashion quite different meanings, programs, and organizations from the lexicon they share. A striking example of this is how the concept of self-help is used in different sectors of the women's health movement. In many of the organizations and publications of the white women's health movement, self-help is first and foremost a reference to women taking decisions about their bodies and health into their own hands, and often quite literally. The concept was first used to talk about cervical self-examination and soon afterward, menstrual extraction. The concept and practice of self-help as it has developed within the National Black Women's Health Project has a different referent and meaning, as NBWHP member Sharon Gary-Smith explains. According to Gary-Smith, NBWHP self-help groups were "designed to provide a safe, validating environment for us to learn how to come together to share our stories, to be appreciated for the struggles we have all participated in, to review our circumstances, and to make decisions designed to change our lives and our health circumstances" (Gary-Smith 1989, 6).

The emphasis on talking, sharing, telling stories also encompasses the recognition that Black women always faced "a multiplicity of issues—whether from racism and sexism, classism, or substandard housing, chronic financial limitations and unemployment." Therefore, unlike in the white women's movement, "support groups for Black women would have to require a broader definition of our problems and a specially designed program . . . one that provides a forum to participate in dialogues with sisters and results in taking action to make change in our lives . . . [Self-help is] a chance to make a place for all of us to explore our collective history, to analyze our past and to identify our struggles and triumphs as we move to wellness" (6).

Clearly, both gynecological self-help and self-help as it is interpreted in the National Black Women's Health Project are about women taking control of their individual and collective bodies and, by extension, their lives and gaining and sharing knowledge among women. However, the NBWHP defines self-help more broadly (far beyond reproductive health and the physical body) and within a matrix that sees gender, race, and class as fundamentally interconnected in Black women's lives. Within the white women's health movement, women often shared knowledge about their bodies in a very hands-on way. The vocabulary of self-help is immersed in the physical body and aspects of reproductive health.[2] Within the NBWHP, self-help is first and foremost about women sharing their stories, information, and struggles. In *Body and Soul: The Black Women's Guide to Physical Health and Emotional Well-Being,* a 1994 publication of the National Black Women's Health Project, editor Linda Villarosa defines self-help as part of a "spiritual revolution in America" (1994, 386). Nowhere in the ten-page chapter entitled "The Self Help Revolution" are cervical self-exam, breast self-exam, or menstrual extraction even mentioned.[3] Self-help— women sharing their stories and experiences—is a powerful tool, Villarosa claims, to break "what founder Byllye Avery called" a dangerous "conspiracy of silence" (xiv).

Another difference that distinguishes the ideology of the NBWHP from some of its sister health organizations in the 1980s concerned the critique of professionalism that was so striking in many predominantly white health movement organizations. While health professionals, including physicians, who were sympathetic to the movement were welcome in both the feminist health clinics and the health advocacy organizations that emerged, the politics of the movement included a strong critique of the professional dominance of health care, a critique that was less salient in women of color health organizations.

There are a number of reasons for this difference, not the least of which is the fact that for many women of color access to basic health care had been historically, and for many remained, limited. Instead of demanding that doctors, public health officials, and other health care professionals cede their power to ordinary women, women of color health activists were often fighting to expand professional health services into their communities. Moreover, a long history of health advocacy and activism on the part of some African American health professionals, including women, meant that partnerships between professional and nonprofessional women of color were far more important than the critique of professionalism. Finally, given the depth of racism in the health care system, male and female health professionals of color tended to be honored, rather than decried, and seen as allies in the long effort to extend the benefits of the U.S. health care system to communities whose need for these services had never been sufficiently met (Hine 1985, 1989).

The story of the NBWHP, like other foundational stories of the women's health movement, has strong characters, a fascinating plot, and a meaning that resonates deeply for the women whose lives have been touched by the organization. And it is a story that does not end simply by telling the history of the NBWHP. Rather, the story of the NBWHP is inextricably linked to other tales, other organizations. It is to one such story that I now turn.

Other Stories/Other Voices: Organización Nacional de la Salud de la Mujer Latina/ National Latina Health Organization

For Luz Alvarez Martinez, one of four cofounders of the National Latina Health Organization, the work of the NBWHP provided direct inspiration. Alvarez Martinez first became involved in the women's health movement early in 1980 after a classmate in the prenursing program at the local community college told her about a medic training course offered by the Berkeley Women's Health Collective (BWHC). Alvarez Martinez decided to take the course and to volunteer at BWHC. She found the course "exhilarating." The strong feminist organization offered her more than instruction in health care procedures. "I said, this is perfect . . . I am going to get the education that I need about other women," including lesbians, about whom she felt that she knew nothing (Alvarez Martinez 1991).

Unlike many of the others in the medic course (who were young or students), for Alvarez Martinez life was already full. Wife, mother of four sons, and student, she had to leave BWHC's medic training just before completing the course. But she continued to work with a group of women from the health collective who were planning a satellite clinic to serve women of color in south Berkeley. It was through her work with this group that Alvarez Martinez had first heard Byllye Avery talk about plans for NBWHP's first national conference. From that moment she was determined to attend the conference.

> I thought, oh my God, I have to go. So somehow we scraped together some money. I borrowed money. We did some fund-raising. I had never been across the country before, and here I am with my four children. But I went. And oh God, that is really what changed everything for me. I didn't know it at

the time. It did have a tremendous effect on me, just seeing Black women do what they had done. I had never seen women of color do anything like that. Sure it was happening all the time, but I had never experienced it. (Alvarez Martinez 1991)

Two years later, Alvarez Martinez, served on a panel organized by the Bay Area Black Women's Health Project to discuss health and reproductive issues for women of color. Afterward, "Alicia Bejarano came up to me, very excited about the workshop that had just happened. And in Spanish she was saying that this kind of thing has to happen, she said, for Latinas . . . And it was right there that the light bulb went off. And I remember turning to Paulita [Ortiz] and this woman kept talking and I said, Paulita, this is it . . . and that's where we started talking about it" (Alvarez Martinez 1991). As excited as she was by the idea of working with a group of Latinas to form their own group, these plans had to wait until her return from a trip. She left the next day as part of a NBWHP delegation to Africa, a trip that was valuable for what she learned about the international women's movement.

When Alvarez Martinez returned to California, she, Alicia Bejarano, Paulita Ortiz, and Elizabeth Gastelumendi formed the National Latina Health Organization, which celebrates its founding as March 8, 1986, International Women's Day. Their mission was to raise the consciousness, improve the health, and foster the empowerment of Latinas: "The National Latina Health Organization was formed to raise Latina consciousness about our health and health problems. The NLHO promotes self-help methods and self-empowerment processes as a vehicle for taking greater control of our health practices and lifestyles. We are committed to work toward the goal of bilingual access to quality health care and the self-empowerment of Latinas through educational programs, outreach and research" (NLHO n.d.). Alvarez Martinez remembers the early history of the NLHO as hard, fulfilling work. She credits the NBWHP with being an excellent model for the work they had to do: "We worked hard. It wasn't easy. But for me, the whole thing was about the empowerment of Latinas. And for me, my experiences with the Black Women's Health Project really had a lot of effect and influence on how I saw things, and what I wanted to have in this organization. I felt we could learn so much from their experiences" (Alvarez Martinez 1991).

Latinas faced different issues, though, and their stories emerged from different historical, economic, political, and cultural contexts. And NLHO founders drew strength from these differences—in language, ancestry, immigration status, and sexuality—Alvarez Martinez says.

I am first generation, Paulita is second generation Mexican American. Alicia is from Ecuador and came here as an adult. And Elizabeth is from Peru, also came as an adult here. So we had pretty different backgrounds . . . Paulita grew up as a migrant farm worker with her family. I grew up in San Leandro which is a pretty white area. So we were pretty different. Paulita grew up in the fields, I grew up in this white city and the other two grew up in their own countries. It was very interesting. (Alvarez Martinez 1991)

The organization was committed to inclusiveness across all these differences. For the NLHO, bilingualism was critical, both as political statement about culture and identity and as means of outreach. But despite its embrace of difference, the organization focused on specific socioeconomic and cultural issues:

The history of Latina women is filled with struggle to preserve our families, our communities and our own identity . . . As daughters, we are the unwelcome ones; as wives we lose our identities and become a second class citizen; as members of our society we are trained to take a decorative and servile role. Moreover, as members of a prevalent white society, we are considered incapable of being anything but domestic servants. Even our language has been used to humiliate and oppress us. (NLHO 1988a, 6)

The concepts of consciousness-raising and self-help keyed the program from the very beginning: becoming empowered to take responsibility for one's life and health was a process that could occur collectively with the support and encouragement of other Latinas, as women recognized their own personal feelings in the experiences of others. Alvarez Martinez explains,

It was sharing the experiences with each other. Seeing that you're not the only one that is confronting whatever it is. You're not crazy. You're sharing your stories, sharing your experiences. And seeing how some have been able to do something about their situation. All of it . . . And of course, in all the classes, all the presenters on different topics would have to be Latinas . . . because that's part of the self-empowering process. Having someone just like us up there. (Alvarez Martinez 1991)

Beginning in spring 1988, the NLHO sponsored a series of community health education courses entitled "Latina Health Issues . . . Better Health through Self-Empowerment." The courses, which trained students to coordinate and facilitate other classes, addressed such topics as mental health, patient's rights, birth control, sexuality, *curanderismo* (a form of traditional healing), teen pregnancy, domestic violence, alcohol abuse, and language barriers. The concept of Latinas helping Latinas proved an effective outreach strategy.

Sometimes NLHO classes drew family members, even of different generations. Alvarez Martinez's sisters attended some sessions, and her mother, who was seventy-nine, came to a class on sexuality.

A conference in September 1988 designed to bring together individuals and groups concerned about Latina health care galvanized the young organization, welcoming "All Latinas . . . housewives, lawyers, students, domestics, doctors, women on welfare, professional women, migrant women . . . all of us" (NLHO 1988b, 5). More than 350 women gathered to discuss and strategize issues affecting the health of Latinas. By all accounts, the conference was a huge success, both because it reinforced a strong feeling of solidarity among those who attended and because it exposed fault lines about differences that the organization knew it had to resolve. For example, although support for sexual diversity was a foundational teaching of the NLHO, some Latina lesbians were disappointed that their straight sisters did not support their issues. As Carmen Vasquez reported in the organization's newsletter, the workshop "Unlearning Homophobia" attracted only thirty participants, most of whom were lesbians. This pattern—of lesbians believing they were not fully included or accepted in organizations dominated by straight women—was certainly not unique to the NLHO.

As the organization grew, the cofounders discovered that their vision was shared broadly. "The thing is, once you put an idea out there and it's a good idea, it just takes a life of its own, " said Luz Alvarez Martinez (1991). None of the organizers had any experience in seeding a national organization, but the good idea had its own momentum, and its members had an abiding commitment to make the organization work. Soon NLHO chapters opened in a number of cities. One of its projects, Latinas for Reproductive Choice, fostered open discussion of and advocacy for reproductive rights issues. Its launch date was October 3, 1990, the thirteenth anniversary of the death of Rosie Jimenez, the first woman—a Latina—documented to have died from an illegal abortion after Congressional passage of the Hyde Amendment. At a press conference, NLHO announced its intention to "break the silence on reproductive rights issues within the Latina community. . . We will no longer stand on the sidelines and let others decide our fate" (Latinas for Reproductive Choice 1990–91, 9). In addition to education and mobilization of support for Latina reproductive rights, the organization planned to monitor how decision makers voted on crucial reproductive rights legislation and to increase representation and participation of Latinas in other health organizations and directorates. It also sought to educate and dispel myths about reproductive issues affecting Latinas.

Statistics showed how important such advocacy was. NLHO members pointed to an abortion rate among Latinas of 42.6 per 1,000, compared with

26.6 for non-Latinas. Latinas in the age range of fifteen to forty-four comprised 8.4 percent of the population, but they accounted for 13 percent of abortions (Larson 1991). The myth that they do not have abortions because of their religious beliefs contributed to the misinformation that has historically left Latinas out of the abortion debate. But "access to abortion is only half the issue for Latinas," NLHO's newsletter declared. "Reproductive choice for us is much more than abortion—it is the ability to have healthy babies when, and if, we want. It means the freedom to choose to have one child or 10. Or even none. Reproductive choice means access to culturally relevant, quality health care and information, education about sexuality and contraception for our daughters, and access to alternative forms of birth control, regardless of cost" (Latinas for Reproductive Choice 1990–91, 9).

The freedom to choose "to have one child or 10" was particularly important for Latinas because of the history of widespread sterilization abuse of this community. Sterilization rates as high as 65 percent had been reported among Latinas in some areas of the United States; in New York, the rate of sterilization of Latinas was seven times higher than for white women and almost twice that of Black women (9). In fact, mobilization against sterilization abuse by Latinas, and particularly by Puerto Rican women in New York in the mid–1970s, led to the formation of CESA, the Committee to End Sterilization Abuse, an organization that, at least historically, is a precursor to the NLHO.

Like other women's health movement organizations, the NLHO has always scrambled for funds necessary to build organizational capacity and support programs and activities. Some of its earliest support came from the Noyes Foundation (San Francisco), and the Ms. Foundation (the contact was made through Byllye Avery). Although the organization could not afford full staffing, it was able to use a unique strategy to pay Alvarez Martinez as NLHO's first director. She worked for a large corporation that allowed its executives to contribute their time to community organizations while they remained on the company payroll. Alvarez Martinez, with the support of her supervisor, a woman she calls a "very strong feminist," was paid for nine months to serve as director of the NLHO. It was notable that the company let her do this even though she was a clerical, not a management, employee.

Although the ideology and actions of the National Latina Health Organization are framed within a gendered social analysis and critique, the organization does not label itself feminist. "There's a real strong feeling with the organization not to use the word feminist, because it's a white woman's issue. And some of the things that we've done are not always recognized as feminist," Alvarez Martinez explains. For example, the NLHO opposed a California state ballot measure for a single payer health system because it excluded undocumented immigrants. It also vigorously opposed California's Proposition 187, a ballot initiative that barred undocumented residents from all public services and programs, including health care, education, and social services.

When Prop. 187 passed, the NLHO reassured newsletter readers. The article "Don't Panic" enumerates grassroots and legal challenges to the initiative and promises that the NLHO "will continue to work with other local, state, and national organizations to stop the inhumane, racist action of Governor Wilson, the creators of Proposition 187 and all those that support the initiative" (NLHO 1995, 1). Members of the NLHO maintain strong links with local and national feminist organizations, including feminist health organizations, with other organizations for women of color, and with Latino community-based and professional groups. For Alvarez Martinez the bottom line is that Latinas define their own issues, control their own organizations, and work in coalition from a position of their own making.[4] These values have also informed the work of another important women's health organization, the Native American Women's Health Education Resource Center (NAWHERC). Unlike the NLHO, the ancestry of this organization founded by Native American women was not tied directly to the NBWHP or any other feminist organization. But its roots were deep in other cultural and political soil.

Native American Women's Health Education Resource Center

A long history of abuse and neglect by government agencies, including the Indian Health Service (IHS), informs the struggle for high quality health care that respects individual and cultural values in Native American communities. In 1985 a group of women living on or near the Yankton Sioux Reservation in South Dakota took a bold step when they met to talk about health and other issues of concern. The process began, as it did so often in the women's health movement, with informal discussions at the home of Charon Asetoyer, a Comanche woman who was married to a Dakota Sioux man. They had moved back to her husband's reservation in 1985, two years after his father had passed away. "It is a tradition to hold a memorial on the anniversary of a loved one's death for the following four years," Asetoyer says. "It was to be a temporary stay, until our commitment was over (Asetoyer 1994, 22). Women in the community, curious to meet her, began to drop by: "I took that opportunity to invite others to . . . talk. Before long a group of women were meeting regularly in my home to talk about 'women's things.' We moved the meeting to an empty bedroom in our basement. Our conversations centered around problems that women and children were having in the community and what we might do to address them" (22).

By 1986, the basement bedroom housed the office of the Native American Community Board (NACB), a newly incorporated nonprofit organization whose activities had always been determined "by the women who have come through our doors" (1994, 22). A woman stopped in to ask about Fetal Alcohol Syndrome (FAS); she was worried that drinking during her pregnancy had contributed to difficulties her son, now a teenager, was having in school. NACB launched a task force on FAS, which became the formative project of the new organization. Slowly, and with community participation, the women developed programs to address the myriad health problems they were facing.

Very soon, and with so much activity, the group outgrew its small headquarters. Asetoyer had been impressed by the large old house of the National Black Women's Health Project in Atlanta. "It all seemed so right," she remembers. "Why not for us too?" (Asetoyer 1994, 22). NACB had no money for a house, though, not even enough for the six-thousand-dollar fixer-upper they found and hoped to buy in nearby Lake Andes. Ultimately, they did secure the funds to buy the house; once again, a women's health movement organization was aided during a formative moment by sister health activist organizations. It began with help from Alvarez Martinez and Byllye Avery and continued with additional support from others in the movement.

In 1987 Asetoyer attended a conference sponsored by the National Women's Health Network in Washington, D.C. It was there that she met Luz Alvarez Martinez of the NLHO. Among the many topics they discussed was Asetoyer's hope that they might someday be able to buy the house to contain the burgeoning activities of her organization. Alvarez Martinez suggested that Asetoyer appeal for donations during introductions at a conference luncheon scheduled for the following day.

> At lunch I tried to avoid Luz: it seemed too hard to stand up in a crowded room of women I really did not know and ask for money. But Luz found me. Still, when it was my turn to introduce myself, I started to sit down without making my request for donations. Luz kept encouraging me to go ahead and make my request. Before long, all the women in the room wanted to know what we were arguing about. So I went ahead and asked for their help. Then I saw Byllye Avery of the National Black Women's Health Project, across the room, reach into her pocketbook and pull out her checkbook. Byllye held up the first check and announced to the room, "I donate $100." The pocketbooks opened and the checks piled up. It was like a dream: the house was soon to become a reality. I left the conference with about half the money we needed. (22)

Community members pitched in to clean, paint, and decorate the house, and in February 1988 the NAWHERC opened its doors, the first women's health organization located on a reservation in the United States.

U.S. government policy has historically confiscated tribal land and under-mined traditional Native economic, cultural, and political institutions, creating poverty and social conditions that lead to health problems for Native peoples from birth to old age.[5] For reservation communities, health problems are extreme. Asetoyer calls it "natural that health issues should come up first" for a Native American community organization (22). In a historical sketch of NAWHERC, Asetoyer compiles a daunting catalog of health problems facing the women and families in Native communities: infant mortality rates as high as 23 per 1,000 in some areas; diabetes that affects 70 percent of those over forty; higher than national average rates of many chronic illnesses; high inci-dences of alcoholism and domestic violence; and high rate of involuntary ster-ilization of women (22). Poor funding, bureaucratic neglect, and geographical isolation complicate access to basic health care for Native Americans; and en-vironmental health problems—ranging from poor quality housing, often with lead-based paints, to exposure to toxic waste and to unsafe water supplies and sewage disposal systems—are rampant in some communities.

NAWHERC programs often developed in response to individuals contact-ing the organization with specific questions or concerns. Others grew out of workshops organized to elicit more formal, community-wide activities. A NAWHERC brochure from the early 1990s indicates breadth of programming: community organizing and leadership development; a domestic violence project; AIDS prevention; child development; adult learning; assistance to groups working on toxic waste issues; cancer prevention; fetal alcohol aware-ness and advocacy; a food pantry and nutrition programs; scholarships for Na-tive American women; an information clearinghouse; and work on reproductive health issues. The Resource Center documents abuses carried out by the In-dian Health Services (IHS), Job Corps, and other agencies on which Native American women depend for services and health care. Under its broader or-ganizational umbrella, the Native American Health Board (NAHB), the Re-source Center publishes the quarterly good-health newsletter "Wicozanni Wowapi," which circulates information about upcoming events and conferences, fundraising projects, and healthful hints.

Beyond the many programs directed at serving women and families on or near the Yankton Sioux reservation, the NAWHERC has played a critical role in mobilizing Native American women around issues of mutual concern, espe-cially reproductive rights. In 1990, the organization hosted a three-day meet-ing, "Empowerment through Dialogue," that attracted thirty Native women from eleven Northern Plains Nations. At the conference, the women estab-lished a reproductive rights coalition whose platform affirmed Native rights to age-, culture-, and gender-appropriate information about sexuality and reproduction; all reproductive alternatives, including the right to choose the size of one's family; affordable and culturally oriented health care and free and/or affordable abortions; programs that address domestic violence, sexual assault, AIDS, nutrition, prenatal chemical dependency, sterilization abuse, and infant mortality; informed consent for all medical procedures; the freedom to parent in a nonsexist, nonracist environment; and the power to determine the members of each nation (NAWHERC 2000).

By 1994 the Reproductive Rights Coalition included more than 150 women from twenty-six tribes (NAWHERC 1994a, 1). The newsletter reports that the third annual meeting of the Native Women's Reproductive Rights Coalition included traditional dancing and storytelling, workshops on AIDS, Depo Provera, sexual abuse, and self-help gynecological exams, and discussions of the criminalization of alcoholism in Native American women and environmental health issues.

Beginning in the early 1990s, NAWHERC began a research and advocacy campaign around the promotion of Norplant, an implant contraceptive, by the Indian Health Service. A report, issued in June 1992, documented serious health risks and "inconsistencies in the delivery of Norplant . . . within the Indian Health Services" (Lewry and Asetoyer 1992, i) and called for more research and close monitoring of the device. The following year NAWHERC released a second report on Depo-Provera and Norplant, reiterating serious concerns about how these contraceptives are distributed by IHS and advocating strict protocols to safeguard Native women clients.

> This report was developed to present the deep concern of the Native American Women's Health Education Resource Center (NAWHERC) staff and other health advocates. After extensive research into the matter, we believe the current system employed to distribute Norplant and Depo-Provera by the Indian Health Services (IHS) may lead the unknowing or the unscrupulous to inflict great damage on Native American and Alaskan women, given the history of the drugs and of the IHS . . . Our report is a constructive effort to ascertain the accountability procedures of the IHS with regard to Norplant and Depo-Provera; it is not intended as a witch-hunt. It was created with the interests of the Native American and Alaskan people at heart . . . When controversial drugs are combined with a precedent for reproductive rights abuse by the administering agency, the concerns of health advocates everywhere become evident and must be explored. (Krust and Asetoyer 1993, 1–2)

The Resource Center serves as policy watchdog and as clearinghouse for educational materials for tribes and agencies throughout the United States and

Canada. Its reach and scope are international. Accredited as a nongovernmental organization in 1994, NAWHERC participated in the 1994 International Conference on Population and Development in Cairo, where it presented "The impact of population, development, environment, health and reproductive rights within indigenous peoples' communities" (NAWHERC 1994b, 5). NAWHERC has played an important role in building a global movement for indigenous reproductive rights and in advocating a vision of health and social justice for Native women and families.

National Asian Women's Health Organization

For Mary Chung, the need for an organization that addressed the health needs of Asian women was both personal and political. A community activist born in Korea, Chung immigrated to the United States in 1980. Marked by the suicide of her older sister, she recognized the urgency of powerful advocacy work for health information, high-quality health services, and changes in health policy as they affect Asian women. The road from vision to organization was swift. In September 1993, in Oakland, California, Chung founded the National Asian Women's Health Organization (NAWHO), a nonprofit, community-based health advocacy organization committed to improving the physical, emotional, mental, and social well-being of women of Asian decent. Acknowledging that the needs and concerns of Asian women are "at the same time specific and diverse, and that they must be addressed within community, cultural, and linguistic contexts," NAWHO conducts research and promotes the development of affordable, accessible, and culturally appropriate reproductive and sexual health services (NAWHO 1993–94, 1).

In its first several years, the new organization pursued five goals: to foster advocacy by and about Asian women's health concerns; to conduct research on Asian women's health; to educate Asian communities about the needs of women and girls; to develop policy analysis and goals to implement change at the community, state, national, and international levels; and to develop self-help processes and activities (NAWHO 1993–94, 3). NAWHO employed six staff members, including Executive Director Mary Chung. Four interns and a host of volunteers also worked on a Southeast Asian Women's Health project in three northern California counties; planned for a NAWHO conference in October 1995; participated in the California Coalition for Reproductive Freedom group and the Women of Color Coalition for Reproductive Health Rights; and helped organize a number of international conferences.

The board of directors brought a wealth of community and professional experience and national diversity to NAWHO. Of the nine members, five were immigrants—from Korea, Kenya, Japan, India, and the Philippines; two traced their ancestries to China; and Byllye Avery, of the NBWHP, served in an honorary capacity. Links to the women's health movement and to other health organizations that advocate for women of color are apparent in the long list of supporters and donors in NAWHO's first report, including the National Black Women's Health Project, the National Latina Health Organization, the National Women's Health Network, nine foundations, and many different groups and individuals.

In 1995, at the Miyako Hotel in the Japantown section of San Francisco, NAWHO hosted a three-day national Asian women's health conference, the first of its kind. More than five hundred people attended the meeting, whose theme was "Coming Together, Moving Strong." The San Francisco Board of Supervisors endorsed the conference by declaring Asian Women's Health days. "There are those who believe that the Asian American community is apolitical, that we do not vote, that we have no interest in organizing around the very issues we will be discussing this weekend," Mary Chung told participants. "But by our very presence here today, we will prove them wrong. It is here that we begin a dialogue among Asian American women, health care providers, advocates and policy-makers, to break down the barriers of stereotypes, of racism, of sexism, and of silence, that stand between Asian American women and healthy, safe lives" (Chung 1996, 11).

In 1995 NAWHO also released its first research-based publication, *Perceptions of Risk: An Assessment of the Factors Influencing Use of Reproductive and Sexual Health Services by Asian American Women.* The report raised concerns about "increasingly hostile developments in immigration, welfare, and health policies [that] threaten to further undermine the extent to which Asian American women and girls feel comfortable and safe in accessing and utilizing health education and services, particularly in the area of reproductive and sexual health" (NAWHO 1995, 4). And it refuted those stereotypes of racism, sexism, and silence against which all the organizations founded by women of color struggled:

> The first [misperception] is that Asian America is a homogenous community; the second is that this "community" is educated, economically successful, and would not benefit from advocacy in the areas of health, education, and socioeconomic empowerment. These stereotypes are reflected in health-related policy and programs, which have limited their effectiveness in assessing and responding to the health care needs of Asian American women and girls. (NAWHO 1995, 4)

Focusing on the higher poverty rate of Asian and Pacific Islander Americans compared to white Americans, the report revealed that more than 20 percent of those populations lack health insurance. One-third of them speak limited English and so confront language barriers as they attempt to access health services. These combined realities mean that many do not get preventive health care, Pap smears, prenatal services, or mammograms. The report also found that a large proportion of refugee women either used no birth control at all or had been surgically sterilized (NAWHO 1995, 5).

NAWHO's core effort is the Asian Women's Reproductive and Sexual Health Empowerment project, which combines research, education, and advocacy. In 1997 the organization released a second survey-based report. It revealed that almost half of Asian American respondents had not accessed any reproductive health service within the past year, and that one-fourth had never seen a reproductive health care provider in their lives (NAWHO 2000). NAWHO also sponsored a National Policy Summit on Depression and Asian American Women.

In June 1996, the NAWHO newsletter reported that cancer, especially breast, cervical, and lung, is the leading cause of death among the three most populous Asian ethnic groups (Chinese, Japanese, and Filipino). The organization's innovative program on breast cancer, launched in 1996, combines training, public policy, education, and coalition building to reduce cancer mortality among Asian American women. NAWHO also sponsors two training programs for health care providers, one in Los Angeles and one in the Bay Area, emphasizing the need to increase screening practices such as breast self-exams, clinical exams, and mammograms.

NAWHO's concern with Asian American health needs extends to men as well. In May 1999 the organization released a study of Asian American men's reproductive health habits. Virtually nonexistent before this study, statistics revealed that, contrary to model minority stereotypes, 87 percent of Asian men are sexually active and yet 89 percent had never seen a health care provider for reproductive services, such as family planning or STD treatment and education (NAWHO 1999). An alarming number think they are not at risk for sexually transmitted disease like HIV/AIDS. This misunderstanding, Mary Chung points out, also puts the health of their Asian American women partners and families at great risk.

In 1996 NAWHO moved its offices from Oakland to San Francisco. Its second conference, held in 1997, on the theme "The Quality of Our Lives: Empowering Asian American Women for the Twenty-first Century," was held in Los Angeles. One hundred scholarships to Asian women and girls increased participation by refugees and immigrants, who along with hundreds of others attended workshops and listened to a wide variety of speakers. The NAWHO

Leadership Network emerged from the conference; it has created cooperative agreements with the Centers for Disease Control and Prevention to coordinate programs on diabetes, immunization, and tobacco control. That year, NAWHO was selected to represent Asian American health concerns at a meeting with President Bill Clinton and Vice President Al Gore.

The organization then moved its yearly conferences to Washington, D.C., seeking to involve leaders of federal agencies and representatives of the Clinton administration in its discussions. In 1998 NAWHO organized a Women of Color Policy Briefing for media representatives, funders, and advocates. Among the other participants were the National Abortion and Reproductive Rights Action League (NARAL), the National Black Women's Health Project, and the National Latina Institute for Reproductive Health. Now, like the other women's health movement organizations that offered it support and encouragement, NAWHO was playing a key role in creating and building on linkages among women's health organizations and between these organizations and the women, the health professionals, and the public policy makers it hoped to influence.

Coalitions and Partnerships

Beginning in 1983 and over the course of a single decade, the face of the women's health movement changed dramatically with the formation of the National Black Women's Health Project, the National Latina Health Organization, the Native American Women's Health Education Resource Center, and the National Asian Women's Health Organization. Now women of color had their own forums from which they could serve women and families in their own racial and ethnic communities;[6] challenge their marginalization in the U.S. women's health and reproductive rights movements; and represent the concerns of U.S. women of color in high-profile international conferences such as the International Conference on Population and Development in 1984 and the United Nations conference in Beijing in 1995. Through linkages and coalitions that addressed racism within the women's and reproductive rights movements and within the larger society, they believed they could multiply the impact of their separate organizational agendas. As early as 1985, under the auspices of the Religious Coalition for Reproductive Rights, the Women of Color Partnership was created as a "vehicle by which African-American, Latin American, Asian-Pacific-American, Native American, and all Women of Color in this country can become actively involved, as decision-makers, in the reproductive choice movement." The partnership focused on six areas: abortion, birth control, teen pregnancy, prenatal care, child care, and medical abuses against women of color (Fried 1990, 293).

In 1992 a coalition "comprised of Indigenous, African, Latin and Asian American women" founded the Women of Color Coalition for Reproductive Health and Rights (WOCCRHR) to "address concerns specific to women of color which were not being addressed by the mainstream U.S. women's health movement" (U.S. Women of Color Delegation to the International Conference on Population and Development 1994, 7). In March of that year, WOCCRHR protested "uneven power relationships between the long-established reproductive rights organizations and the newly established women-of-color reproductive rights organizations" in NOW's planning of a national March for Reproductive Rights (Martinez 1992, 1). In 1994 the WOCCRHR prepared a position statement for the upcoming International Conference on Population and Development. The statement represented the views of leading activists including Byllye Avery, Julia Scott, and Cynthia Newbille of the NBWHP, Charon Asetoyer of the NAWHERC, Luz Martinez Alvarez of the NLHO, Mary Chung of the NAWHO, and fourteen other women of color from a wide variety of progressive organizations.

> We (the Women of Color for Reproductive Health and Rights WOCCRHR, and the U.S. Women of Color Delegation to the ICPD) wanted to bring attention to the similarities between the Southern conditions of women in this Northern country [the United States] and women in the Southern countries, and to urge our government to act decisively in addressing and rectifying unjust policies and power imbalances within our society and worldwide. (U.S. Women of Color Delegation to the International Conference on Population and Development 1994, 4)

As a result of the work of organizations such as those profiled in this chapter, the voices of women of color are significantly more audible as their organizations advocate for a health care system that has been challenged to admit and reform its legacies of exclusion, inequity, and harm. NBWHP, NLHO, NAWHERC, and NAWHO and their sister organizations, through their effective activism, have succeeded in breaking the silence that isolated women of color within the women's health movement. The voices of women of color echo through the movement as they advocate for the needs of women and families in their communities; contest racism, sexism, and class inequities in the health care system; and challenge white women to incorporate their perspectives in organizational and movement activities and publications. The legacy of racism within the reproductive and women's health movements remains, but it is contested and there are alternative voices. Moreover, predominantly white women's health organizations have been challenged to better address the injustices of racism and the needs of women of color. Thirty years after the women's health movement became a significant part of the progressive political landscape, the movement is represented by a diverse group of organizations that work individually and in various partnerships and coalitions to ensure that women have a strong voice in determining their reproductive choices, influencing the health care they receive and articulating health policy concerns that matter to them over their life span.

Chapter 4

Into Our Own Hands

*Feminist Health Clinics as
Feminist Practice*

By the early 1970s feminist activism and a growing movement to legalize abortion had attracted women from all over the country to an emerging
women's health movement. By one estimate, there were at least one thousand
organizations directly involving women in various forms of health activism
(Ruzek 1978). Some women who worked at free clinics (about 150 of them had
opened since the mid–1960s) or in centers associated with the community
health movement advocated new ways of providing services to women (Marieskind and Ehrenreich 1975; Cousineau 1987). Others developed and dissemi-
nated educational materials about women's health. Still others promoted
self-help, patient advocacy, community organizing, or information and counseling services for women in need of reproductive health care and for survi-
vors of rape and domestic violence. Some provided illegal abortions or worked
in networks to refer women to abortion providers. And in some of the hundreds of communities where feminist health activism took root, women-
controlled health centers or clinics were established to provide new kinds of
reproductive health services.

Many women-controlled health clinics were organized either on the eve of
or the immediate aftermath of *Roe* vs. *Wade*, the most important historical
marker in understanding the emergence of the clinic movement.[1] Once abortion was legal, feminist health care activists immediately sought wider access
to respectful and inexpensive abortion services,[2] and in a number of communities they took matters into their own hands by organizing women-controlled
health clinics. The few clinics that predated *Roe* vs. *Wade* were either in states

that had already liberalized their abortion laws or their services did not yet include abortion. The Vermont Women's Health Center, the Berkeley Women's Health Collective, the Haight Ashbury Women's Clinic, the San Francisco Women's Health Center, the Santa Cruz Women's Health Center, Aradia Clinic (Seattle), and the Women's Clinic (Eugene, Oregon), most of them based in the free clinic/community health movement, opened before the 1973 *Roe* vs. *Wade* decision. But after the legalization of abortion, women organized health clinics in all corners of the country. Suddenly, clinics dotted the map: In 1973 Womancare was established in San Diego; the Women's Choice Clinic in Oakland; the New Bedford Women's Health Services in southeastern Massachusetts; the Women's Health Services in Colorado Springs; the Women's Health Clinic in Portland, Oregon; and the Emma Goldman Clinic for Women in Iowa City. The following year saw the founding of the Tallahassee Feminist Women's Health Center and the Gainesville Women's Health Center in Florida, the New Hampshire Women's Health Clinic, and the Elizabeth Blackwell Clinic in Philadelphia, to name just a few. In those heady early years of the movement clinics were operating in many of this country's largest cities, but also in or near university communities and in selected smaller towns. Many of these post–*Roe* vs. *Wade* clinics provided abortions. Those that did not provide abortion services offered pregnancy testing and abortion counseling and referral as a primary activity or in tandem with well-woman gynecological and/or family planning services.

We do not know for sure exactly how many women-controlled health clinics operated in the United States in the 1970s, but several sources suggest that there were about fifty by 1976 (LAFWHC quoted in Farber 1976; Ruzek 1978; Davis 1991). Feminist clinics never accounted for the majority of women's health movement groups. But while they were not the movement's most common organizational form, they were vanguard organizations that were fertile soil for many of the movement's innovations. The creation of feminist clinics, alternative social movement-based health services, was and is an important form of feminist practice. The acts of envisioning, creating, and sustaining alternative health clinics tested the tenets of feminist theory and demanded new forms of practice. While all women's health movement groups self-consciously aimed to create organizations that practiced what they preached about women's empowerment, the clinic sector of the movement was most intentional about actually embodying in organizational practices the political values that were at the core of the movement.

What made these clinics feminist? First, the concept of control by women. The feminist critique of health care charged that men, particularly male professionals, dominated health service provision and medical research and monopolized knowledge of (thus exerting control over) women's bodies and reproductive decisions. Women-controlled health clinics set out to reassert women's power to make their own choices. In (most) feminist clinics in the early 1970s, women-controlled health care meant that women owned, operated, and made the decisions in clinics they founded. It also meant that many of these women were not medical professionals.

Self-help was the cornerstone of the feminist clinic. At the most basic level, it offered women information about their bodies. But that was only the beginning. Over and over again, the foundational stories of the women's health movement rehearse the same message: in the validation of their own experiences through the experiences of others, women found a transforming power, the chance to become women whom they "loved becoming." Training in breast self-examination, knowledge of the risks of different birth control methods, even such radical acts as cervical self-examination, only represented means toward the end of empowerment. The principle of women-controlled health care extended to practices such as a strong preference for female providers and extensive use of nonphysician or nonprofessional health providers, from lay health workers to nurses or nurse practitioners, occupations more commonly filled by women.

An essential element of the critique of male-dominated health care was the belief that the system overmedicalized the routine passages of women's reproductive lives: birth control, abortion, pregnancy and childbirth, menstruation, and menopause. For most of human history, women had managed these events with the help of lay health providers—shamans, midwives, herbalists—who were almost always other women (Gordon 1976; Ehrenreich and English 1978; Marieskind 1980; Lorber 1984; Petchesky 1984). Feminist clinics sought to restore that partnership between consumers and providers of health care. For many in the clinic sector of the movement, the critique of male- and physician-controlled health care was part of a more general critique of hierarchy within the system: the subordination of women as patients (from the Latin, to suffer) and the subordination of women-dominated health care occupations (lower status and lower paid) to those usually reserved for men. This critique of hierarchy, coupled with the ideology of participatory democracy so characteristic of the social movements of the 1960s (Breines 1989), informs a cluster of organizational features common to grassroots alternative organizations. Community control was one of them. The value placed on egalitarian relationships between health care consumers and providers, and among those who staffed the clinics, was another. Many feminist health groups were originally organized as collectives; consensus decision making was their ideal.

Feminists criticized the organization of capitalist health care that put the profits of doctors, hospitals, pharmaceutical and insurance companies, and others above people's need for health services. The feminist response was to provide free, low-cost, or sliding scale-based services (fees based on a client's ability to pay) whenever possible. But the value attached to providing low-cost care collided with another cherished value—paying women decent wages. Clinics varied in how they resolved the conflict between the need to generate revenues to stay afloat and/or to pay decent salaries. Some organizations, notably those affiliated with the Federation of Feminist Women's Health Centers, were committed to establishing viable financial bases that would allow women-owned and controlled businesses (clinics) to survive: "We're too poor to offer 'free' services to anyone," Carol Downer told me in her interview. Generally, the FFWHC set moderate fees for most services, although some of the federation's clinics provided education and counseling at no cost. However, this policy generated internal criticism within the movement, with some arguing that the Federation of Feminist Women's Health Centers were not doing enough to ensure that all women could afford the services.

Another fundamental difference between feminist and mainstream health clinics came down to the feminist definition of health care as a highly politicized issue. The male- and physician-controlled health system that over-medicalized women's lives was organized to guarantee the profits of a few rather than the health of the many, they charged. That same system was highly complicit in exerting subtle and not-so-subtle forms of control over women through definitions of women's proper roles and the use of scientific and medical rationalizations for women's subordinate role in society.

The publications of the women's health movement analyzed sexism, and in some cases also racism and class, as structures implicated not only in the ways health care services were delivered, but in access to high-quality health care of different populations, based on their control of resources and their ability to influence medical decision making and research. Publications of women of color health movement organizations were far more likely to define the politics of women's health in terms of gender *and* race, ethnicity and class. Feminist health clinics often incorporated this analysis of the system into their community health and education programs, their staff training, and their mission statements and goals. Moreover, many clinics included political advocacy (around reproductive rights, health care access, women's health issues) and community organizing among their goals. Education, service provision, advocacy, and political involvement often went hand in hand as activities that would lead to the ultimate goal: women's empowerment.

Feminist clinics provided services in ways designed to empower and educate women. For example, the traditional practice of draping a woman during a pelvic exam was abandoned in favor of women being able to see the exam in process. Without draping it was also possible to routinely incorporate showing a patient her cervix during a pelvic exam (the provider uses a flashlight and mirror to enable the client to see what, traditionally, only the doctor sees). Common or routine gynecological conditions such as vaginitis were often treated with home remedies such as yogurt and vinegar and water or betadine douches (easily available over the counter and at little expense) before expensive pharmaceutical remedies were prescribed.[3] Preventive health care was the priority, unlike the curative-focused care that was standard in most physician offices. Concern about how little was known about estrogenic drugs led feminist clinics to prescribe lower dose oral contraceptives than was common in many doctors' offices or traditional family planning clinics, and to encourage the use of barrier methods of birth control (such as the diaphragm, cervical cap, or condom) over oral contraceptives or intrauterine devices (IUDs).

Another important difference between the women-controlled and mainstream women's health services had to do with the way birth control and abortion services were organized. The idea that women should make informed choices about both what form of birth control to use and whether or not to carry a pregnancy to term (or have an abortion or put the baby up for adoption) was at the core of business as usual in feminist clinics. Contesting the physician-knows-best attitude and affirming women's right to choose meant that women were given extensive information about family planning options, including abortion, and that information was presented in a self-consciously nonjudgmental or nondirective manner. Provider-patient relationships were redefined to encompass greater mutuality and respect. This could mean that a doctor would be introduced by her/his first name if clinic practice was to address the patient by her first name. Or it could mean that the doctor's role was to present information so the patient could play a key role in making decisions about her health care. Rather than simply doing procedures—a Pap smear, a bimanual pelvic exam, an abortion, for example—the health provider routinely explained what she/he was doing and why. Feminist practices transformed abortion services, from the most basic fact that abortion became a simple outpatient service to a series of carefully considered service features, including the use of patient advocates to provide information and support during what was sometimes a difficult emotional experience.[4]

The earliest women-controlled clinics re-envisioned women as empowered consumers and providers of health care. As social movement organizations, they committed themselves to women's self-determination and to the creation of viable alternatives to profit-driven male- and professional-dominated health institutions. Clinic politics did, of course, vary in different communities. They were shaped by the political histories and experiences of founding members; ideological struggles over the organization's structure; racial, ethnic, and class composition; and the political culture of the community, including the presence or absence of other feminist, civil rights, gay/lesbian, or left political organizations. Pressure was unrelenting as they responded to internal political divisions, struggles over issues having to do with homophobia and racism, and external assaults by local medical communities and the growing antiabortion movement.

That the Vermont Women's Health Center was one of the first sites in the country of lay-controlled artificial insemination services, for example, bespeaks a higher degree of political commitment to issues of lesbian health care than may have been present in some other clinics. The Somerville Women's Health Project and New Bedford Women's Health Services oriented and organized many of their services and policies to meet the needs of working-class women who represented a higher proportion of their clients than in clinics located in university communities. Clinics in racially and ethnically diverse communities faced more pressure to articulate and then put into practice a politics that addressed issues of racism within the clinic and in their communities. But because the clinic sector of the women's health movement was relatively interconnected; because the movement was embroiled in political debates and divisions, for example, over feminism, racism, and homophobia; and because similar external pressures often affected local clinics, important facets of what happened within individual clinics were frequently echoed in sister clinics, creating a sense of shared struggle and history.

The organizational histories of the clinics track the dynamics of change as it created and continually revised the lived experience of being in a social movement. These were hybrid organizations (Ferree and Martin 1995), not just in the familiar sense of incorporating both alternative and mainstream principles, but also in the sense that they are simultaneously sites of political involvement (politics) and workplaces (work). Beginning in the 1960s, the United States witnessed unprecedented growth in grassroots alternative organizations that were also workplaces, from food, bicycle, car repair, and other business collectives to free and feminist health clinics (Kanter 1972; Rothschild-Whitt 1976; Ryan 1992). Typically, such organizations aimed to achieve common goals (social change, the provision of goods and services) in ways that valued community, empowered individuals and groups, and explicitly recognized the personal needs and objectives of collective members.

Concern with process and the desire to build workplaces that reflected (and didn't just aim toward) the empowerment of staff define the work cultures of these organizations. Instead of basing personnel decisions (hiring, remuneration, advancement, and job separation) solely or even primarily on criteria such as specialized training or certification, previous experience, seniority, or merit as evaluated by a superior, collectivist workplaces often supplement these criteria with others that are personal or political (friendship, a person's need for a job, the importance of diversity). Rather than insisting that workers leave their personal needs and political commitments at home, collectivist, and especially feminist, workplaces tend to encourage workers to express those concerns in their organizational lives. Thus, a major defining characteristic of feminist clinics was their commitment to also being feminist workplaces.

Feminist health clinics challenged the impersonality and instrumentality of the bureaucratic norms and procedures so pervasive in traditional workplaces. Their fundamental philosophical premise, that the personal is political, invited sexuality, interpersonal relations, feelings, political concerns, and the family—private issues, according to mainstream organizations—into the public realm of the workplace. Their ideology acknowledged that personal identity is infused by power relations: The individual, they believed, is situated within a matrix of social relations, based on gender, race, ethnicity, and class, that shape and constrain individual experience. They tried to incorporate these understandings in their organizational practices.

Women who work in feminist health clinics rarely think of themselves as just doing a job. For most, the workplace was also a site of political and emotional engagement. Many women interviewed for this book have said they sought work at the clinics because it offered them the opportunity to pursue both personal and political goals: "making social change," "confronting patriarchy," "empowering women." They expected these organizations to offer them respect for their work, opportunities for growth, and excitement—"the thrill of being part of something new," as one clinic veteran said.

Common values and cooperative work toward new organizational forms forged intense bonds among staff and fierce commitment to the enterprise (Morgen and Julier 1991). Many women's clinics used consciousness-raising tactics in their staff training or in staff meetings, further intensifying those bonds. Plainly, such organizational practices explicitly invite self-disclosure and public discussion of feelings. Even when consciousness raising wasn't on the agenda, workplace meetings tolerated, and in some cases encouraged, a discourse that incorporated the personal and the political into the work culture. Coworkers often greeted each other with hugs and kisses. Meetings might be interrupted to attend to the personal feelings or problems of a staff member. Unlike the bureaucratic model that confined personal problems to workers' homes and home lives, here women shared their personal concerns openly; and this sharing was explicitly valued as usefully challenging the boundaries between the dichotomies (personal and political, private and public) feminists defined as part of the structure of gender oppression.

A decision-making model that favored face-to-face staff meetings, often lasting several hours, ratcheted up the emotional tenor of meetings. "Everything that we believe in I think everyone believes passionately," one clinic worker said, "and so we have this collection of passionately believing women . . . You've got seventeen or eighteen wildly opinionated, judgmental, passionately believing people and you know as soon as we start getting down into discussion there's going to be tears and fuss and bother and it's going to be hard." Conflict bred intimacy, too.

Staff members weren't just close to each other. They also identified very closely with and spoke of *loving* their workplaces, investing their "hearts and souls" there. Research on commitment in communal organizations (Kanter 1972) and participatory democracy groups (Mansbridge 1973, 1980; Rothschild-Whitt 1979, 1986) has demonstrated both the cost and rewards of such involvement, which can be emotionally draining, meaningful, and personally fulfilling all at the same time. Serious conflicts over personnel issues, particularly over hiring and firing and over race and class differences, confronted clinic staff with some of the most wrenching memories of their lives in the movement.

The challenge in these workplaces was to reconceive personnel as persons. With livelihoods, identities, and everyday social relationships on the line, it becomes almost impossible, even in bureaucratic organizations, to circumvent the real, personal outcomes of personnel decisions. Nevertheless, since Max Weber, mainstream organizational theory has articulated and reaffirmed the importance of subordinating the personal dimension of personnel issues. Robert Merton's formulation is typical: "Relations among members of a bureaucracy are impersonal and rule governed in order to maintain the organization and to prevent the *disintegration* of the bureaucratic structure which would occur should these be supplanted by personalized relations" (1968). The transformation of persons into mere employees or personnel may be seen as the central achievement of bureaucracies, the linchpin for the subordination of the individual to organizational needs.

In women's clinics, distinctions between organization and staff, and between organizational and personal needs, blur. First, as participatory democracies, the clinics are driven by the ideas, actions, sentiments, and values of current staff, who tend to feel highly invested and to sense congruence between themselves and their organization because they have participated in shaping its rules, goals, and practices. Second, many feminist organizations have explicitly sought to organize work in ways that maximize the autonomy, skill development, and satisfaction of individual workers. Finally, because hybrid feminist workplaces tolerate and indeed create organizational forums for emotional discourse, the distinction between the private expressive and public instrumental selves also fades (Glennon 1979, 18). In the absence of "feeling rules" that enforce boundaries between personal feelings and work decorum, feminist workplaces articulate an ideology that idealizes the integration of personal, political, and organizational needs (Hochschild 1979, 1983).

But enacting that ideology was difficult. In women-run clinics that rented space, hired staff members, met local occupancy and licensure requirements, and provided vitally important health services, the time and energy that enacting these organizational ideals required often seemed to drain resources that were already scarce given the compelling needs of clients and the need to provide services that would generate the revenues the clinic needed to pay salaries and survive. The creation of counterbureaucratic social relations in organizational structures based on the principles of participatory democracy becomes even more challenging as those organizations cross the boundaries of race, ethnicity, and class. Although conventional workplaces may have diverse staffs, the realities of gender, class, and race-based occupational segregation mean that dominant power relations are often reproduced in work organizations. In feminist health clinics, diversity plays out in the context of contesting (ideologically if not in actual practice) dominant power relations, as women from different races, classes, and ethnic groups struggle to become organizational equals.

Moreover, because feminist clinics provide alternative health care, often including abortions, they often operate within a hostile external environment. Antichoice political groups, government agencies ranging from departments of public health to zoning boards, and, in some cases, physicians, hospital administrators, and mainstream medical organizations have worked to shut down or significantly restrict the activities of women-run alternative clinics (Morgen 1986; Simonds 1996; Hyde 1992). A hostile outside environment increases the stress level within the feminist workplace, where staff members routinely face financial (including payroll) uncertainties, brave antichoice demonstrators, and battle regulatory groups. Although these pressures sometimes lead to internal division and disagreement, particularly when the problems are protracted, the condition of being embattled by the system that clinics are trying to change can also inspire cohesion and fierce commitment. Problems caused by internal conflicts are often quite different. These demons operate within the workplace, through competing values, actions, ideals, and assumptions of women who otherwise feel close to each other and who share an ideological commitment to the enterprise.

In the founding and operating histories of the feminist health clinics, women sought to expand the repertoire of organizational categories and choices. They tried to make decisions based on complex personal, organizational, and political considerations; and they took into account whole sets of nonbureaucratic criteria as they tried to create empowering, holistic, and humane social relations. These alternatives to bureaucratic organizational practice may make decisions messier, harder to carry out, and more time consuming, but the rewards—greater member identity with the organization, active engagement in its tasks, feelings of empowerment and the excitement of working everyday to implement ideals and values—seemed to bolster the spirit of innovation necessary in groups that work against the grain of conventional organizational practice.

All the women-run health clinics that opened in the early 1970s—whether they flourished, persevered against odds, or eventually closed—enacted, to some degree, these tropes and patterns of collective structure. The feminist workplace is an important part of the glue that holds the clinic sector of the movement together. Everything else about the clinics depends on the particular women who founded them and on the specific circumstances of their sites. But the hybrid clinic workplace, with its collectivist ideals and the extraordinary interpersonal demands that embodied those ideals, existed at some super-local level, as an outline or scaffold for the performance of tasks and the expression—both by providers and consumers of health care services—of feelings. And its stories, multiple, fluid, situated narratives, always flowed toward change.

In the remainder of this chapter I narrate the stories of four community-based feminist clinics and of clinics associated with the Federation of Feminist Women's Health Centers. These clinics illustrated some of the organizational diversity represented in the clinic sector of the women's health movement. In part 2, I focus on the dynamics of political and organizational change in feminist clinics during the 1970s and 1980s.[5]

Berkeley Women's Health Collective, Berkeley, California

In September 1970, a group of about thirty women medics (lay health workers) at the Berkeley Free Clinic, spurred by "feelings that women's health needs were not being met in either the community or at the Free Clinic," mounted a vigorous campaign within the Free Clinic to offer their version of feminist health care to women one afternoon and evening each week (Berkeley Women's Health Collective [BWHC] 1971).[6] By February 1971, they had succeeded. "Women's Clinic is on Wednesdays from 1 p.m.–11 p.m. at the Berkeley Free Clinic, 2339 Durant (at Dana)," posters announced to the community. Below these words was a screened print of eleven women with arms linked. Two appear to be women of color.

The medics, who ranged in age from nineteen to thirty, matched the print. Mostly white and middle class, they worked hard to prepare themselves to provide high quality, egalitarian health care by women, for women. They studied, along with materials produced by the Boston Women's Health Book Collective, *The Birth Control Handbook* (Cherniak and Feingold 1974), a widely distributed publication of a radical health education group in Montreal. At the core of their politics was the belief that health care was a universal right. Their collective focus was demystification—demedicalization—of services and promotion of preventive medicine. As one active member explained in 1973, "we want not only to reclaim our bodies emotionally from 'experts,' but also to learn technically how to care for ourselves. We want to be treated individually with respect; to be told exactly what our illnesses are, what the treatment is, what medicine we are being given, and what it is doing to us. We want to be related to as whole persons, psychologically as well as physically" (Barfoot 1973, 91). Recruiting both professional and nonprofessional friends to share what they knew about diagnosis and treatment of routine gynecological problems, the medics enlisted two young men as clinic physicians (they were unable to find a woman doctor), hammered out an organizational structure (all decisions were made in meetings of all members of the collective), and opened for business.

About forty volunteers ran the BWHC in its earliest months. They served as receptionists, answered phones, screened appointments, helped clients with their medical herstories, provided counseling, worked as lab techs or in the pharmacy. Four doctors and one nurse staffed clinic shifts. Services included birth control, pregnancy, and nutrition counseling; pelvic examinations; and rap or consciousness-raising groups. At first, only doctors did pelvic exams. With experience and training, however, health workers began to assist at the procedures, and eventually some nonprofessional staff performed pelvic exams by themselves. The women also incorporated cervical self-examination into their work.

From the beginning, the philosophy of the clinic was that health care should be provided on a "free or at least a pay-as-you-can basis" (91). There were no set fees for services; clients were asked for donations of what they could afford. Most services were provided by laywomen trained in one of four function areas (information and referral; pregnancy counselor; well women gynecology/medic; mental health and well baby pediatrics). Function groups held orientation and intensive training sessions for volunteer health providers, who worked six to fifteen hours a week. A small group of women received (very low) wages to work in and, sometimes, to coordinate different function areas. Paid staff were also expected to volunteer beyond their thirty-two hours/week of compensated time.

Early on, some BWHC founders wanted to separate their services from the Berkeley Free Clinic, which was by now a venerable institution within the community health movement. The collective debated the issue vigorously (Cody 1990). Although members recognized the value of alternative clinics as vehicles for "radical social change," they decided against establishing an independent organization because they believed that it would limit their capacity to change the larger health care system: "Alternative institutions alone cannot force existing institutions to change and become responsive to the health needs of the community," the women explained. "We have access to very limited resources and a small amount of community influence. If we use these resources to maintain a women's health center at this time (an alternative which can meet only a small part of existing needs), we will be left with no energy or opportunity to challenge and affect the decisions of existing institutions" (BWHC 1971, 1). Their discussions recapitulated one of the perennial paradoxes of the women's health movement: Was the provision of health services an end in itself, or did women-run clinic care only help empower a few clients, leaving most women to be ignored, abused, or humiliated by the mainstream medical hierarchy? This allocation-of-resources question surfaces again and again. The danger of cooptation, of becoming part of the system they were challenging, was always obvious to many in the clinic movement.

In May 1972 the BWHC received six thousand dollars from the Berkeley City Council to help pay for the weekly women's clinic at the free clinic and to enable the group to rent a storefront that became the site for meetings, abortion counseling, health care counseling and referrals, and training and outreach activities at much extended hours. The clinic grew steadily, and as services expanded, new volunteers joined the collective. With growth and diversification, BWHC members faced organizational challenges that forced them to revise work assignments and to change the protocols for participatory decision making. By late 1973, the women decided to end the huge (and long) all-collective meetings that included all paid and volunteer staff and constituted the clinic's policy-making body. In place of this unwieldy instrument, they created several function groups and a steering committee with at least one representative from each function group, as well as "anyone else who wants to come," an open invitation that guaranteed organizational transparency.

In the fall of 1974, after considerable lobbying, the clinic won a large grant from the Alameda County revenue sharing program. Now the women reversed their earlier decision to remain affiliated with the Berkeley Free Clinic and began the search for a location for their own health center. By early the following year, they had bought and moved into a new building. The number of paid staff rose to seventeen. The organization was still evolving an organizational structure that honored collective process as it tried to balance efficient provision of services with efforts to change the larger health care system. Members decided to limit paid jobs to one year in most instances, so that more women could secure employment at the clinic (at the subsistence-level salary of about three hundred dollars a month).[7] Political disagreements fed anger and frustration within the collective. Clearly, growth had costs.

For many, however, the costs were tolerable. As one woman reported: "The energy [from 1973 to 1976] was wonderful. Really being part of the health collective was having the best of all worlds in many ways. You had, you know, this incredible group of women to be friends with. You could do political work and serve women at the same time. And it was . . . for many of us, the central part of our lives . . . I was really happy there, even though there was so much strife." Like other hybrid feminist clinics, BWHC mixed political and personal passions with work and, at least for some of the people some of the time, represented the best of all possible worlds. BWHC also tried one structural iteration after another as it worked to create an organizational schema that could accommodate almost one hundred people in collective decision making and still meet the pressing need for clinical services and educational outreach. One site of contention, commonplace in the clinic sector, emerged between paid staff and volunteers as it became apparent that the social distribution of knowledge privileged those who were compensated for their work. They put in longer hours and naturally learned more about clinic operations.

With the Bay Area Medical Committee for Human Rights, BWHC members persuaded the local hospital to stop requiring payment up front for emergency room services. This collaboration led to a long-term project—the development of *A People's Guide to Hospitals: Berkeley/Oakland,* a publication that described patients' rights, hospitals' policies, and strategies for securing free or affordable care. Over the years, political projects varied, but they were always central to BWHC's mission. And there were always debates about how to allocate time and resources to direct services and to organizing and advocacy work to change the larger health care system. Like many other feminist groups in the mid to late 1970s, BWHC members struggled with issues around sexuality, ranging from tensions between straight women and lesbians to political debates about separatism. But these debates did not tear the collective apart as conflicts over race would several years later.

By late 1976, the BWHC presented this statistical profile: Staff saw two thousand mostly low-income women and children each year in the gynecology and pediatrics clinics; responded to thirteen thousand requests for information, referrals, or counseling; contacted at least four thousand people in outreach efforts; and trained 150 volunteer health workers (Oppenheimer 1976). Its annual budget, mostly derived from county revenue sharing funds, amounted to $80,000. But despite its achievements, BWHC was not meeting the goals the collective had set for participation by and services to women of color. Staff members and clients were still predominantly white. This was a serious internal criticism, and in August 1976, BWHC held a meeting to discuss it. Because clinic policy had been to recruit paid workers from the ranks of volunteers, and because almost all volunteers were white, BWHC concluded that its hiring practices effectively marginalized "black and third world women": "The meeting was difficult for many people and a lot of anger and defensiveness was expressed. We had to continually remind ourselves that racism is not easy to confront and that we are all victims of an unnatural process that conditions us to oppose and oppress each other" (BWHC 1976). As a result of this meeting, BWHC decided to open up hiring to women outside the collective. It also recommended that clinic function groups undertake political study on understanding racism.

It wasn't easy, though, to provide health care and to achieve political purity at the same time. The first African American woman hired under the August guidelines quit within a few months, citing inadequate training and inability to focus on the political work and services that were her priority. In February 1977, BWHC shut down for two weeks so that members could resolve the many difficulties that beset them on a day-to-day basis. By the end of the shutdown, a new organizational structure was in place, with a smaller and more stable decision-making body and multiple mechanisms through which collective members could challenge decisions they found problematic.

That spring, BWHC received its first large grant from a private foundation, which the collective used for building payments, a new roof, and salary increases. Members decided to extend job lengths from one to three years in order to "increase efficiency within the staff and to make a more meaningful commitment to affirmative action." And in May 1977, the collective pledged to "attempt to establish and maintain a minimum of 50% third world women and 50% lesbians on the paid staff" (BWHC 1977). Although BWHC hired more women of color and increased the number of paid positions, members soon faced yet another financial crisis. Each emergency brought new and different policies for decision making, division of labor, and hiring (for racial diversity). By the end of 1978, the collective had twelve paid positions, six held by women of color and six by white women. Three members of the paid staff were lesbians. But struggles over sexuality, race, and class persisted, and many believed that the pursuit of racial balance was changing the BWHC in fundamental ways. "People were hired because they were CETA-qualified, because they meet the diversity requirements," said a woman who volunteered at the clinic from 1973 to 1975 and worked as a paid staff member from 1975 to 1977. "But they didn't have the history, they didn't have the commitment, and they didn't really understand what had been valuable about the health collective that had been created."

Ten years after its founding, the Berkeley Women's Health Collective looked dramatically different than it did in its earlier years. It had developed a more secure and diversified financial base and it supported a staff that provided a wide range of health care services. But turnover among volunteers and paid workers alike continued to be high, and problems seemed intractable: "Each new population of BWHC members is confronted with the same issues with which the BWHC (and most other alternative organizations) have struggled from the beginning. The most frequent of these issues are: collectivity, accountability, racism, classism, the split between paid and unpaid workers, volunteerism, goals and priorities, political education, and our relations with the community" (BWHC 1977). Such internal divisions over race and class played out in the context of radical change in the larger political landscape.

During the 1980s, the BWHC confronted a series of financial crises related to the rise of the New Right and to conservative economic policies ushered in by the election of Ronald Reagan at the beginning of the decade. Newsletters from the period bristle with information about the politics behind clinic funding problems, which resulted from cuts in local, state, and national monies for health care, particularly in community-based health centers. The passage of Proposition 13 in California (the father of the state-level property tax cut movement) slashed state funding for health care services and for the Medi-Cal (Medicaid) program. In July 1982 the BWHC newsletter identified "Reaganomics" as a major source of projected funding problems, especially cuts and changes in family planning and community health programs.

Despite the effects of budget cuts, the collective was able to realize a goal that gained urgency as the struggles around race and racism escalated in the late 1970s. In August 1982, BWHC opened the South Berkeley Women's Clinic, located at the South Berkeley Community Clinic, which was designed to meet the needs of women of color. The new clinic would be open one afternoon a week. Its mission: "To provide culturally relevant, low cost and/or free, holistic and traditional health care to Black and Third World women; to encourage women to become educated health care consumers . . . ; to provide on-going educational forums which address the social, emotional and physical needs of women; to help combat the high rate of infant mortality in Alameda County" (BWHC 1982, 1).

During these difficult years, the BWHC stopped functioning as a collective (though it retained its original name) and, like many other feminist clinics, adopted an organizational structure that included a director and modified in significant ways the consensus-seeking decision-making policies that conformed so perfectly with the theory of the women's health movement but that had hampered practice. It wasn't just the intrinsic difficulties of collectivism that forced these changes. Across the United States, women's clinics were struggling against powerful forces promoting cooptation. The most obvious and powerful way in which state agencies exercised influence on the BWHC and on other women's clinics was through selective funding of activities. Because of the radical asymmetry between its resources and power and the resources and power of small grassroots organizations, the state could use economic leverage to shape clinic activities and structures, for example, by directing funds to the provision of (certain) services and refusing to support community education, community organizing, health advocacy, or other projects that involved social activism. Yet despite continuing financial problems and ongoing internal organizational struggles, the clinic is still operating from the same building and offering many of the same services, although it is now called the Berkeley Women's Health Center.

Concord Feminist Health Center, Concord, New Hampshire

In October 1974, New Hampshire's first women-controlled clinic, then called New Hampshire Women's Health Services (NHWHS), was founded to "translate feminist principles into services for women" (Concord Feminist Health Center [CFHC] 1989).[8] The clinic opened after a year of discussions by women who wanted to provide an alternative to the hospital-based abortions that were the only option for most women seeking pregnancy termination in the state. The group worked closely with a local (male) doctor who helped develop medical protocols, trained the staff, and served as the clinic's medical director until his death in 1987.

Although provision of abortion services was the clinic's primary goal, the clinic added women-controlled gynecological care by health workers and a nurse practitioner (from family planning to well-women services) in 1975. Unlike many other feminist clinics that were struggling to create and sustain nonhierarchical or collectivist organizational structures, the NHWHS was run as a "traditionally structured women's health organization" (Malasky 1979, 1) with an external board of directors and hierarchical relations between lay and professional health workers. This structure changed in 1977 when, after travel to and increased contact with other feminist health groups, including the Federation of Feminist Women's Health Centers and Women's Community Health in nearby Boston, staff of the clinic began to understand the "contrast between women who were seeking to radically change the way health care is delivered in this country and others who seek to provide much needed services without really challenging the system in which they provide those services" (1). Building on months of intensive discussion, and without internal conflict, NHWHS devised a structure of governance that was worker controlled and incorporated a council of five directors who made policy decisions, regular collective meetings, and a variety of committees. The external board of directors dissolved itself after staff agreed on the new organizational structure.

Now the clinic closed every Thursday for a full workday of meetings and administrative tasks. Agendas covered topics such as funding, interpersonal conflicts, planning and evaluation of services, and political education. Sometimes the staff met as a whole; sometimes the women gathered in "management function groups" to discuss financial, medical, or personnel issues. "By sharing the work load and the decision making, a lot of skill sharing goes on and a lot of personal growth as well," a staff member wrote in the clinic's fifth anniversary publication. "We can think of no good reason to restrict involvement because of a person's title or staff position. Instead of limiting control, our goal is to empower ourselves—all of us—to take control and to participate in all facets of decision making. And closing our doors on Thursdays allows us to do just that" (Downey 1979, 2).

In 1978 NHWHS began to publish *WomenWise,* a twelve-page quarterly to keep readers informed about the clinic's programs, services, and political perspectives, and about issues in the larger women's health movement. That year, the organization also began to sponsor small self-help groups—ten such groups, of four women each, formed between 1978 and 1980 (Bruce 1981, 360). The clinic added the word *feminist* to its name to become the New Hampshire Feminist Health Center (NHFHC). "We have always had a feminist philosophy of empowering women," they explained in *WomenWise,* "but as we evolved, the philosophy became clearer. We had lengthy discussions about the possible alienating effects of the word 'feminist' but decided that we were secure enough . . . to come out as who we are and always have been" (Malasky 1979, 2).

In 1980 NHFHC opened a branch in Portsmouth. The creation of the Concord Center had been relatively uncontested. In Portsmouth six years later, things were different. During the early 1980s the New Right, and the antiabortion movement in particular, was emboldened by the election and then presidency of Ronald Reagan. "Members of a hostile medical community and Seacoast-area anti-abortionists" resisted the organization of a local clinic (Butler 1984, 2). Changes in federal health regulations meant that staff had to seek approval from a regional health policy body that provided a forum for those hostile doctors and antichoice forces. One week after staff members began to see clients, the angry father of a teenager who was seeking an abortion invaded the workplace, threatened staff members, threw the furniture around, and began a campaign of harassment against the center. Despite such opposition, the Portsmouth clinic survived. Originally, the two branches operated as a single corporation with one board of directors. In 1985 they separated officially but remained connected through the New Hampshire Federation of Feminist Health Centers. After the split, the founding clinic changed its name again. From now on, it would be called the Concord Feminist Health Center (CFHC).

Both clinics endured harassment by foes of abortion, a new political reality that confronted most women's health centers as the antichoice movement gained resources and political support during the Reagan years. "As we look back over our last ten years," center staff remembered in their anniversary review, "we have many feelings. There is the sadness of our sister clinics who did not survive the intensified pressures that have threatened abortion providers and women-run clinics in particular . . . We . . . renew our commitment to reproductive freedom for all women and to end oppression of women everywhere" (3).

Among its many accomplishments, the Concord Feminist Health Center helped bring the cervical cap into the arsenal of barrier methods of birth control available in the United States. Staff members were introduced to the cap by a nurse practitioner who had obtained a supply of the devices and fitted herself and some of her friends. Although the cervical cap had been widely used in this country in the 1930s, it had dropped out of sight since the 1950s, except for experimental purposes (Bruce 1981, 359). The feminist health groups that lobbied the FDA to approve the reintroduction of the cervical cap did so with the goal of making safe, effective barrier methods of birth control more widely available. Following pressure by these groups, the FDA initiated a four-year research period during which distribution of the cap was restricted to health providers approved for participation in the study. The Concord Feminist Health Center was one of the first sites in the country to receive approval to supply the cervical cap, and it began to do so in 1981 (NHFHC 1982, 1).

Debates and divisions over structures of decision making continued to plague the staff, and in 1983 the center experienced an "organizational earthquake" (Nye et al. 1994, 1) when the staff directors fired six staff members "summarily . . . without due process" (Spangler 1992, 9). One of the women who was fired explained:

> The way the health center was structured when I first got involved was, you know, very traditional, with directors, very hierarchical. Although it was engaged in some processes of change it was very slow. And as a fill-in [someone who worked clinic shifts but was not regarded as a full staff member] I

got hired in the bottom of the structure and then, true to my nature, I immediately started challenging it. For example, fill-ins were not allowed to go to staff meetings. And I started to go . . . and that eventually escalated to the point that I got fired . . . along with five other women. And then there was this massive convulsion that happened in the health center.

Over the next several weeks, the fired workers sought legal advice and mobilized their support among the remaining staff members, and after a marathon (fourteen-hour) binding arbitration session between staff and staff directors, the fired workers were reinstated and the directors announced their collective resignation (Spangler 1992, 9). In a reversal of the process of job stratification that gripped most feminist clinics during the 1980s, the result of the attempted firing was a flattening of CFHC's organizational structure, the disbanding of the directors' council, and the initiation of "a fully non-hierarchical, collective structure of management" (Nye et al. 1994, 1). In 1987, the collective implemented an affirmative action policy to encourage diversity—by hiring more women of color, lesbians, and women over forty—in a staff that, for most of the center's history, had been predominantly white, young, and straight.

By the late 1980s, the Concord Feminist Health Center was still offering physician-provided abortions and using advanced registered nurse practitioners and physician assistants to perform a variety of other gynecological services. Lay health workers still did much of the service provision and other work of the clinic, which continues to rely almost exclusively on fees for services. Fees were carefully calculated: low enough to be classified as affordable, high enough to ensure comfortable salaries for staff members. In 1990 the staff was organized into five teams—abortion services, gynecology services, administration, education and outreach, and overview; members of these teams worked together closely and made key decisions together. After three years, committee members rotated to different teams. Given that staff turnover was relatively low in the late 1980s and early 1990s, job rotation facilitated learning about CFHC's many functions and the development of new skills. But one woman I interviewed believed that the organization lost the benefit of accumulated expertise and individual talents by requiring job rotation.

In 1989 the Concord Feminist Health Center drafted new goals:

to survive as a women-controlled health center; to value ourselves as able, intelligent women and to encourage personal/political/emotional/educational/professional growth among ourselves; to provide a supportive, respectful environment for staff and community; to recognize the importance of continuing to work on issues of oppression and incorporate this into the work we do at the health center; to provide health care for women of all ages, races, classes, and sexual preferences; to be active politically, challenging the laws and attitudes that are oppressive to women. (CFHC 1989)

As the 1990s dawned, women who had been with the center for several years were proud and protective of the "cooperative nature of the organization right now." However, another staff member noted that clinic services involved less consciousness raising, self-help, outreach, and community organizing than in past years, and observed that CFHC was less outward looking, less identified with the larger movement than in the past.

I think in some ways the whole feminist health movement has been somewhat co-opted by the medical establishment and family planning and Planned Parenthood. So I think each separate organization is really pushing not only to stay alive but to grow. So everyone is really focused on what they themselves are doing . . . Health care has changed a lot. Things we were screaming for years ago doctors now do in their offices, so we are not so radical anymore. So sometimes people [clients] don't see the difference and sometimes we don't see the difference.

Another staff member suggested that the pressure to operate a sustainable business had affected the clinic, as the need to pay salaries and provide benefits that honored the devotion and seniority of the health workers became more and more obvious. A third argued that the organization was changing "because the rest of the world is changing." She believed that the rightward movement of the country and the organizational fallout from the huge battle between the directors and the rest of the staff early in the 1980s had fostered a different orientation at CFWC. "In terms of political services we have done some closing in. But we do a lot of processing, we seem to have internalized the revolution . . . I think in a sense the health center is holding some sort of star, because the fire that was outside went out . . . Hopefully someday we'll have some kind of better environment where we can translate that outward again without draining ourselves, when we can do that and feed ourselves like we did at the beginning of the women's health movement."

In the fall of 1994 the Concord Feminist Health Center celebrated its twentieth anniversary. An article about the anniversary in *WomenWise* summarizes key aspects of the organization's history:

Through the decades, staff members have striven to articulate these [feminist] values in everything from the Health Center's embrace of the word *feminist* in its name, to the way it provides healthcare services; from its pioneering collective structure and decision-making style, to its hiring practices and political advocacy . . . Much effort is invested in fostering a comfortably homey and non-threatening atmosphere, in offering clients lots of information upon which to base their own health care decisions ... The Health Center has consistently acted out of its commitment to being an *accessible* service provider ... never turning a woman away, a policy which has cost the Center approximately half a million dollars over twenty years ... Along with an unwavering commitment to affirmative action in hiring, there is a commitment to create and sustain a workplace where diverse individuals are able to be themselves. (Nye et al. 1994, 1, 10)

Twenty years after its founding, the Concord Feminist Health Center was still located in the same renovated house. Its staff of fourteen served more than 3,500 women a year on an annual budget of about $750,000. In addition to abortion and gynecology services, CFHC offered free contraceptive counseling, held workshops on different forms of oppression, sponsored a monthly lesbian health clinic, published *WomenWise,* and participated in the reproductive rights advocacy movement. In their clinic brochure, the women acknowledged the many wise women who had been healers in the past and projected themselves as "a continuation of this spirit of sharing information and experiences so that all women may become like the 'wise women' of their heritage—sensitive, caring, powerful and wise" (CFHC n.d.).

The Emma Goldman Clinic for Women, Iowa City, Iowa

The Emma Goldman Clinic, founded in September 1973, had its roots in an abortion referral collective that had operated within the University of Iowa Women's Center from 1971 until abortion services became available in Iowa City following the *Roe* vs. *Wade* decision.[9] In addition to doing and teaching cervical self-examination and referring women to states in which abortion was legal and to illegal abortion providers, collective members, like the Janes, themselves performed some early pregnancy terminations. The university town was home to a vigorous grassroots feminist community. Self-help groups had sprung up there after visits from Carol Downer and other representatives of the Los Angeles Feminist Women's Health Center in 1971 and 1972 (Iowa City had been the site of the First National Conference of the Gynecological Self Help Clinics of America in October 1972). One of Emma Goldman's founding members also helped to plan a second such conference late in 1974 in Ames, Iowa, home of Iowa State University.

Plans for the Emma Goldman clinic began the day the Supreme Court legalized abortion. One of the founders recalls, "We heard about it [the Supreme Court decision] mid-morning in classes or wherever we were and we all rushed back to the Women's Center to be together" (Emma Goldman Clinic 1993, 1).

Thus began months of many long meetings and even more self-education about women's health care needs as the women envisioned, discussed the politics of, and took the practical steps necessary to open a clinic to do abortions and well-women gynecological care. One of the founders offered five thousand dollars from an insurance policy she cashed in when her husband died. The money was used to buy a house that ultimately became the first feminist health center in the Midwest and the first outpatient abortion clinic in Iowa (Emma Goldman Clinic 1993, 1).

In part because the collective did a lot of groundwork to build cooperative relationships with municipal agencies and the local medical establishment, Emma Goldman encountered less opposition than many other clinics. "The city was pretty cooperative," one clinic founder remembers. "We went and talked to neighbors and we did well on that. [Two of our members] went and talked to the head of the university hospital gynecology department and they were supportive and there was a woman gynecologist, who may have been in her fifties at the time, who was kind of supportive. We had a real open, let's-work-with-anyone-we-can-attitude." It is not that there were *no* problems. When they approached the bank for a loan the loan officer denied it immediately. Another founding collective member recalled, "We never saw our attackers. They would come in the form of health inspectors and electrical inspectors, people under the guise of doing their jobs who did an exceptionally thorough job" (Erickson, 1996). But, ultimately, their pragmatic approach and perseverance paid off. Less than nine months after the legalization of abortion, they opened their doors and began providing services.

Connections between the clinic and the mainstream medical community were ongoing, another founder explains.

> Some of the doctors came over and trained us to do pelvic exams and fit diaphragms, and we trained doctors in town who were willing to learn from us how to fit diaphragms . . . There was very little hostility. There was curiosity. They were interested in us. They invited us to come to talk to the medical students about self-help and our clinic. We went [there] several times. Emma Goldman Clinic was responsible for creating many changes over at the university hospital which they embraced . . . simply because we existed and we articulated ideas about what women wanted in their medical exams. Like when they put in birthing rooms and when they initiated a patient advocacy system over there. They started hiring women to teach doctors how to give pelvic exams from the patient's point of view, how to present themselves and how to touch women and how to do the exams without hurt or embarrassment.

But relatively smooth relationships with area doctors and neighbors of the clinic did not mean that the group experienced no conflict. "Our worst fighting was among ourselves," one clinic worker reports. Eleven of the twelve women who founded Emma Goldman were white; one was Cuban American. They were all young, in their twenties. At least half came from working-class families. Most had grown up in Iowa and were then, or had been, students at the university. Many had participated in antiwar activities and in feminist consciousness-raising groups. Their early debates repeated discussions under way among other feminist health activists across the country. "Should we get our politics together before we open the clinic or open the clinic and work out the politics as we go?" they asked. Some members of the group felt that if they tried to iron out all their disagreements in advance, the clinic would be doomed. Others feared that on-site abortions would "bog them down in services" and compromise the self-help and education emphases they envisioned for the clinic. Once they had decided that the clinic would provide abortions, another contentious issue arose: Should they hire a male doctor to perform abortions? (Because they could not find a female physician, they did hire a male.)

Like other feminist health groups, collective members argued about class and sexuality, money, and power. Even the clinic's name occasioned debate—between those who wanted to honor Emma Goldman and those who worried that Goldman's name would signal a particular (socialist) political stance. In fact, so few people in the community knew who Emma Goldman was that callers often asked to speak with her when they telephoned. The decision to use the name Emma Goldman was a "conscious political decision," one that resonated to group members who foresaw that for the clinic to succeed they would have to be much like Goldman: "political, ornery, stubborn" (Erickson 1996).

The founding mothers of the Emma Goldman clinic were intent on establishing a "women-owned collectively, operated" organization (Emma Goldman Clinic 1993, 1). They opted for the egalitarian principles of consensus decision making and equal pay for all, and their commitment to these ideals was strengthened just before they opened the clinic when four representatives visited the Los Angeles Feminist Women's Health Center (LAFWC) for training. Two of the women found conditions in LAFWC's hierarchically structured workplace so oppressive that they refused to participate in the training program. Of course, their position elicited strong criticism from Carol Downer and FWHC staff. This negative encounter "really set a tone, and when we got back to Iowa we were at odds with the FWHC for years."

During the mid to late 1970s, Emma Goldman's staff fluctuated from twelve to twenty-five workers, including both full- and part-time employees, all of whom earned the same hourly rate and participated in collective decision making.

The clinic provided well-women gynecology and contraceptive services; first trimester outpatient abortions; training in self cervical and self breast examination; psychotherapy; massage; lesbian health services; prenatal and natural birthing classes; and counseling; and it operated a speaker's bureau for outreach and community education, including self-help demonstrations. "We felt like pioneers," one woman remembers, "and [believed] we were building a whole movement that was going to change women's lives."

Some lay health workers were trained to fit diaphragms and to do well-women screening. And they were trained to consult the doctor if anything seemed out of the ordinary. "We were a little worried that we might get busted for practicing medicine without a license," one woman recalls, "but it never happened. We never diagnosed anything, that was key."

Like most feminist health collectives that experienced the constant challenges of consensus decision making in their efforts to become a fully egalitarian structure, Emma Goldman morphed through a series of organizational changes as it faced increasing financial troubles and powerful assaults from antichoice forces in the late 1970s and 1980s. As one woman involved during that period remembers, "We were always restructuring. There were always problems. It was like a Medusa . . . It was gut-wrenching" (Erickson 1996). Collectivism worked less well as new staff members replaced clinic founders who moved on to other jobs and as the size of the staff grew.

In 1985, Emma Goldman relocated uptown to offices that had formerly housed a pediatrics clinic (Erickson 1996). That same year brought the clinic's biggest crisis to date, the loss of the malpractice insurance they had carried through the National Abortion Federation. They needed to find another carrier, something that was difficult because they were not operating under the license of a physician. For several months there appeared to be no solution. One member, recalling the meeting at which they faced the stark reality of probable closure, remembers the meeting lasting for hours until it was almost dark outside. But "no one turned the lights on"; there appeared to be no way for the "clinic as we knew it to continue" (Erickson 1996).

They did survive, but survival meant significant changes. They negotiated with a male physician who agreed to become their medical director, which meant that residents and other doctors performing services would be insured under his license. The malpractice insurance crisis "and rapidly rising health costs [forced the clinic to decrease] its staff size, and non-management positions were developed in addition to a ten-woman collective management team" (Emma Goldman Clinic 1993, 9). The changes did not mean they lost their commitment to being an alternative workplace. But the realities of survival forced changes in organizational structure. By the mid 1990s, one of the then codirectors of the clinic, acknowledging that some of the changes were compromises, nevertheless believed the clinic retained its commitment to a feminist agenda, "When I see us in the nineties and the compromises we've made and the survival we've enjoyed. It's payback time. We have a successful business . . . We have positioned ourselves by whatever compromises to be an institution . . . that we can use to promote the ideals of feminism that we still hold" (Erickson 1996).

Like the Concord Feminist Health Center, Emma Goldman was an early advocate of the cervical cap. The collective published *The Cervical Cap Handbook* in 1980 and won FDA approval as a research and training site. Emma Goldman continually added new services. In 1983, staff inaugurated an artificial insemination clinic and incorporated PMS counseling into their offerings, and four years later they initiated HIV counseling and anonymous testing.

During the 1980s the clinic adopted employment practices that encouraged diversity and broadened the clinic's mission, which now encompassed "participating in the struggle to end all forms of oppression including: ableism, ageism, classism, heterosexism, racism, and sexism; oppression based on religion, ethnic or national origin or body size" (Emma Goldman Clinic 1993, 3). That was a tall order, but by the fall of 1993, Emma Goldman had gone a long way toward fulfilling it. The clinic now employed thirty-three paid full- or part-time staff members, four associate directors, and a medical director, and it still had many volunteers. Both African American and Latina women worked at the clinic, among them Francine Thompson, the first woman of color to serve as a co-director at Emma Goldman. "Although much has changed over these past years," an article in Emma's periodical noted on the occasion of the clinic's twentieth anniversary, "the underlying philosophy held by the founders remains unchanged: the belief that women must have the option to be active participants in their health care; that they have the right to accessible information and choices. We continue to have hours of arduous meetings, and to struggle with balancing feminist ethics with fiscally sound business practices" (Emma Goldman Clinic 1993, 9).

In 1990 the organization's annual budget grew to $500,000, and a staff of twenty-five served five thousand clients a year, with four women codirectors in the areas of operations, health services, personnel, and community education and relations. Gayle Sand, community education and relations director, had helped found the clinic and worked there from 1973 to 1978. In 1985 she returned to Emma Goldman because she "missed the melding of the personal and the political in a women-powered setting" (11). Sand kept that job until 1996, when "increased regulation and competition meant the Clinic would have to function more efficiently . . . [leading to] reorganization from co-directorships to an Executive Director and an external Board of Directors" (1). Beyond clinic services, Emma Goldman staff did lobbying, community organizing around health issues, and clinic defense in response to antiabortion harassment. A 1996 fund-raising letter made it clear that the clinic continued to suffer the effects of antiabortion activity, the consequences of which included cancellation of its worker compensation coverage because of "escalating violence at clinics nationally." But the organization hewed to its founders' commitment to the "ideals of participatory health care, informed medical consumerism, patients' rights, women-oriented health care delivery and the larger ideals of the feminist philosophy: political, economic, and social equality and the right to choose our vocations and lifestyles. We believe that controlling our bodies and health is a first step in controlling the quality of our lives" (2).

Women's Community Health Center, Cambridge, Massachusetts

Women's Community Health Center (WCHC) in Cambridge, Massachusetts, was conceived in August 1973, when Jennifer Burgess and Cookie Avrin met at a self-help presentation in Worcester, a community about an hour west of Boston.[10] Carol Downer was there, on a tour demonstrating self-help. When a small group of women indicated they wanted to organize their own self-help group, Downer suggested that they hold a citywide conference to mobilize support for a local feminist health clinic. Burgess and Avrin planned the November conference, at which about 150 women agreed to establish a "women-owned and women-controlled health center."

By January 1974 clinic organizers were getting together twice a week, once to do self-help and health education, and once to take care of "business and the nitty gritties." Membership in the core group was fluid, but the project persisted, funded, in part, by a fifty-dollar-a-week gift from the Los Angeles Feminist Women's Health Center (WCHC 1975, 4). That spring the group filed for incorporation. They were spending most of their time raising money, negotiating details of clinic services and structure, and searching for health care professionals who would work with them. Proceeds from benefits by Boston-area feminist poets and singers and the sale of the speculums, and a five-thousand-dollar grant from the Boston Women's Health Book Collective (authors of *Our Bodies, Ourselves*) enabled WCHC organizers to rent space, install phones, and begin paying one of their members a salary of twenty-five dollars a week. WCHC enjoyed a rich political environment. The Boston-Cambridge area was home to vibrant feminist, left, and civil rights organizations and to other feminist health groups, the Somerville Women's Health Project as well as the Boston Women's Health Book Collective.

Less than a year after Burgess and Avrin began their discussions, Women's Community Health Center was providing gynecological services. By this time, the women had closed the collective to new members "to try and catch up with ourselves" (5). In the fall of 1974 WCHC organizers traveled to women's health conferences in Montreal and in Ames, Iowa, and despite fiscal constraints that were already very obvious, they returned home filled with energy and looking forward to "the time when all women will control our bodies and our lives" (2). Self-help was the cornerstone of their philosophy: "every woman learning and sharing her knowledge, as well as demystifying the medical profession and her own body" (2). The clinic sponsored self-help presentations and beginning and advanced self-help groups; offered pregnancy screening and counseling; provided telephone referrals and outreach and community education; and performed gynecological exams and abortions.

During its second year, eighteen active members, some of whom had children, ran the collective. It was their habit to organize services around all the needs of staff and clients, so WCHC rotated responsibility for childcare in the clinic along with other administrative, clerical, and client-centered tasks. Collective members attended women's health conferences (one of WCHC's most successful outreach events was a yearly women's health weekend) and documented their many close connections with the movement, including their new commitment to serve as the Northeastern Coordinator for WATCH (Women Allied to Combat Harassment), an organization founded to monitor and combat the harassment of feminist clinics.

In 1975, through a member of the Boston Women's Health Book Collective, local women medical students approached the clinic, "asking that WCHC help improve the teaching of gynecology, and especially of the pelvic examination. The collective initiated the innovative "Pelvic Teaching Program," in which, at first, WCHC staff members served as "paid pelvic models" who helped medical students learn how to conduct exams respectfully. But WCHC workers objected to the program design. "Although we gave active feedback as the exam was being performed, the physicians were the major instructors . . . We had very little control over the teaching session . . . We did not agree to their approach to health care as looking for disease. We felt exploited" (WCHC 1976a, 19). The collective redesigned the program the next year, expanding it from one to four sessions, drafted formal contracts with the medical students that made collective members their sole instructors, and offered the new format to medical schools at a higher fee. None expressed interest. WCHC concluded that the increased political content—in which staff members firmly believed—was too threatening. Clinic staff also believed that the first version of the program contributed to the "support of a health care system that needs *radical* change. We have discontinued [it] . . . and we *strongly* discourage other groups of women from participating in similar programs (20).

Costs at WCHC were defrayed by client fees and donations, an arrangement that rendered the organization's financial picture uncertain. In 1975 the collective began the process of securing a clinic license, which was required by the state of Massachusetts if the clinic was to be eligible to bill insurance companies and Medicaid for health care services. Licensure, they believed, would also support fundraising efforts and encourage referrals from other community agencies. The process was long and arduous, and indeed it drained the clinic of financial resources and staff members of energy. But they were open about their financial problems and shared their analysis of the licensing situation with members and supporters in their annual reports and special fundraising letters.

The collective was determined to survive in a way that "does not oppress the women who work here." But ten full-time staff members earned only $85 for a work week that averaged forty-five to sixty hours, an effective hourly wage of about $1.50. And despite these "below subsistence wages," the clinic failed to make full payroll six times that year (WCHC 1976b, 6). Collective members blamed the shortfalls on a decrease in clients and in self-help presentations during the summer months, and on the limitations imposed by their unlicensed status: They could not advertise their services until the clinic license had been granted.

There were other reasons for their problems, too. WCHC refused to use volunteers on whom most feminist clinics depended. Political principles rationalized that decision; they defined volunteerism as a tradition that demeaned and devalued women's labor. And political reasons also explained why they refused to seek support from foundations or other sources because "we have seen community health services depend upon limited foundation and government monies followed by a subsequent severe . . . shock to those facilities when the funds dried up. We will never put ourselves in a similar position of dependence upon those institutions" (7). This fierce political independence had consequences: Its refusal to risk cooptation by seeking outside support guaranteed that financial worries would haunt Women's Community Health over the entire period of its existence.

In its third year, Women's Community Health Center (now a collective of thirteen members) found it "impossible for all women to have an active ongoing role in all areas of the Center's work" (WCHC 1977a, 3). After several different attempts to balance efficiency with their commitment to self-help and "nonalienating" work structures, members finally agreed that a steering committee should coordinate the clinic's work and develop clear political and program priorities. As they abandoned their consensus-based decision-making model, they nevertheless expressed their determination to maximize "input and control from the entire group" (4).

With another bold stroke, the clinic adopted a needs-based salary policy, in effect a sliding scale for wages. In theory, the change made sense. In practice, workers still earned subsistence-level (at best) wages. Citing larger political-economic realities, the collective admitted that it hadn't been able to deliver on its promise to make WCHC a "good place for all kinds of women to work" (14). "The current medical system makes it difficult for any independent, innovative health center to survive financially, especially in the face of expensive requirements for becoming licensed and restrictions on advertising," collective members argued. "Economic conditions work against the survival of small, antiprofit businesses. Business profits and tax money are not used to provide human services such as community controlled health care and day care. While society exploits us daily as workers and consumers, we are struggling not to continue these patterns in the ways we work together" (14).

In spring 1978, after WCHC had moved to a new location to meet licensure requirements, the state of Massachusetts finally granted the collective its long-sought-after clinic license. Nevertheless, as antiabortion forces within state agencies mandated compliance with ever more restrictive and costly regulations, WCHC could only tell stories of limited triumph in its fifty-two-page Fifth Anniversary Annual Report (1979). Red tape and continuing fiscal constraints worsened after 1980, and in July 1981 WCHC announced to its extended family that the center would file for bankruptcy. Collective members blamed the closing on the "continuous financial struggles of the Health Center" and noted that its immediate cause was "an unusual and severe drop in . . . women coming for services" that spring, which depleted the center's small savings completely" (Ponge and Stein 1981, 1). The clinic's valedictory letter details a series of problems, including high staff turnover and an inability to pay enough staff to keep the center afloat (WCHC had twenty employees in late 1979; by January 1981 that number had dropped to five). Collective members placed responsibility squarely at the feet of the right: "The effects of Reagan, the conservative climate and the current economy are hitting small businesses hard . . . In large part, we see the Health Center as a victim of the New Right and depression economics, and are enraged that so many years of good, hard, productive work still leave us with no other option" (2).

Although the collective's financial problems were by no means unique, its radical stance against private or state funding certainly played a role in the clinic closure. The lengthy battle for a clinic license, coupled with the legislative successes of the New Right in Massachusetts, demonstrate that WCHC operated in a most inhospitable local environment. Moreover, the collective held fast to its allegiance to feminist organizational ideals. "There were probably a half dozen political points that were integral to the health center's identity," a long-time member reflected many years later. "One was that it was women owned and controlled, that it was controlled by workers . . . Not having dependence on outside money was a political stance." WCHC rejected the idea of working with volunteers because collective members were determined to act out their principles. "We always saw ourselves as an institution of social change. That was a real critical part of our identity right from the beginning."

External assaults and internal divisions kept collective members on an emotional roller coaster in the clinic's final months. But the five women interviewed all believed that WCHC had enriched their lives and the life of the community. "We were one of a whole series of voices that were saying to women—you can do this for yourself and you really can have some control," one member recalls. "And however that has trickled into later definitions of feminism, we were part of that stream and we were pushing hard. I think we pushed definitions of what a workplace should be, and did a lot of things that most workplaces don't do that were positive for the women who worked there." Feminist workplaces tried to reconceive organizational decision making as a process that acknowledged antibureaucratic values and empowered human relations. Their collectivist ideals demanded extraordinary personal investment, and many women in many clinics eventually found themselves exhausted by the politics of feelings (as well as by the politics of politics). But years later, most honor and value even "what was trying and difficult and intense and debilitating . . . We were very much part of a historical era . . . Because I was in the middle of it. I am like the stone that dropped in the water and I don't know where the ripples went."

Feminist Women's Health Centers: The Federation of Feminist Women's Health Centers

All the women-owned, women-controlled affiliates of the Federation of Feminist Women's Health Centers (FFWHC) provided abortions and gynecological services under the banner of self-help.[11] Although other loose confederations of feminist clinics (for example, Rising Sun in the northeastern United States) arose during the 1970s, no other movement organization created a national entity with constituent units, and until the National Black Women's Health Project instituted self-help affiliates and formal chapter/national memberships in the 1980s, the FFWHC was the only multiple-site group in the larger women's health movement.

Carol Downer, Lorraine Rothman, Frances Hornstein, and the other women who founded the FFWHC set out to create an organization and feminist clinics that espoused a unified ideology and identifiable politics, in effect to build a movement-within-the-movement. "Unlike most Free Clinics," Frances Hornstein, a member of the Los Angeles Feminist Women's Health Center (the first of these clinics) board of directors, explained in 1974, "our goal is *not* to provide an alternative health delivery system . . . We do not want to coexist with the medical establishment, we want to take it over" (1974a, 75–76). Their radical agenda was tested by local medical societies and state regulatory agencies across the country as, differentiated both by their formal affiliation and by aspects of their philosophy and practice, FWHCs opened in other California cities and elsewhere.

In the early 1970s, new clinics radiated out from Los Angeles elsewhere in California and then across state lines. First, Lorraine Rothman and others started the Orange County FWHC. Then "women who had worked at the L.A. FWHC moved to Oakland to help start the Oakland FWHC. That summer Los Angeles had a summer institute; they invited women from all over the country to come and train at the Health Center . . . to learn self-help, health worker skills, and how to start a Feminist Women's Health Center . . . and out of that, the Tallahassee FWHC started in 1974" (Hasper 1981, 267–268). Chico was next in line. One evening a week, the Free Clinic in that northern California town operated a clinic for women, referring those who wanted abortions to the Oakland FWHC. "Oakland had so many referrals from Chico it suggested a clinic start here," Hasper says. "They did a self-help group for us and showed us menstrual extraction and we got very excited" (268). Excitement always led to action in the FFWHC, and the Chico clinic opened in February 1975. Atlanta (1977); Concord, California; and San Diego quickly followed suit. In 1979, Southeast Women's Health Clinic in Portland, Oregon, affiliated with the FFWHC and began to provide abortions.

By 1981, according to Hasper, affiliation with the federation meant that women seeking care at any FWHC would get standardized health care with built-in accountability by clinics to the larger umbrella organization. "The Federation is founded on the principle that we agree on our political strategy, our goals, and our internal workings. We are accountable to each other . . . We standardized our clinics. Now you can go into any of the FWHCs . . . and get the same health care" (268). But there was conflict within the federation as well as critique of the federation from other clinics. In 1976 the Tallahassee and Detroit FWHCs signed and published in a feminist newspaper a resolution that declared that the Oakland FWHC was "not a FWHC" because of politics that made them unacceptable to the larger group. Several years later the Tallahassee FWHC left the federation after a bitter dispute with Downer over their own political alliances and decisions.

Within the highly structured environments of the federation-affiliated clinics, self-help evolved to mean much more than just looking at one's own cervix. It meant diagnosing and treating with home remedies such common conditions as vaginitis monillia, or yeast. And it included menstrual extraction, by far the most controversial of the federation's activities, one that allowed women to terminate pregnancies without resorting either to doctors or to illegal abortionists. But despite its relative ease—Lolly and Jeanne Hirsch, in *The Monthly Extract,* asserted that, for normal, healthy women, menstrual extraction is "simplicity beyond imagination"—the FFWHC advised caution.

> The Advanced Self-Help Clinics have also found that there is no way for a woman, by herself, to know *her* exact uterine position as well as other disqualifying conditions. Sisterhood is Safety, Safety is Sisterhood. In addition, continued research with Del-Em indicates that group experiences, knowledge, cooperation and sisterly concern improves the kit's efficiency. It would be irresponsible, here, to give step by step written directions in menstrual extraction . . . if this movement is to succeed it will [do so] only through SISTERHOOD. Groups of sisters learning from sisters and helping other sisters to fully realize their control over their own bodies is a very meaningful and workable concept. (FFWHC 1981c, 6)

The Federation developed a prototypic health service model that was institutionalized beginning in 1973, with the development of FWHCs' well-women services and the inauguration of the participatory clinic, "an educational process which enables women to arrive at their own conclusions" about their health (FFWHC 1981a, 87). The participatory clinic brought trained lay health workers together with four or five women who shared similar health concerns to create a "peer-oriented non-professional context" in which the women learned to do vaginal and cervical self-exam, breast self-exam, and other self-help procedures (1981a, 87).

Carol Downer wanted to spread the word of self-help beyond the United States. She and her colleagues traveled to Canada, Mexico, England, France, Germany, Italy, Northern Ireland, Belgium, Denmark, and New Zealand to demonstrate self-help (Ruzek 1978, 54). But it was the enactment of their revolutionary politics at home through such instruments as the participatory clinic that, throughout the 1970s and into the 1980s, drew fire from California's Board of Medical Examiners and Departments of Health Services and Employment Development. Downer's writings teem with references to revolution, taking power, challenging the enemies of women, creating solutions to women's oppression. To register disapproval of the clinic's self-help emphasis as well as its use of lay health workers, for example, the Los Angeles Regional Family

Planning Council (a private organization of physicians, hospitals, and Planned Parenthood representatives) withheld family planning monies from the LAFWHC for years, even after all the other California FWHCs were receiving such funds. Both the Tallahassee FWHC and the Chico FWHC had to resort to filing antitrust suits against local obstetrician-gynecologists for their attempts to block clinic operations. Their shared experience of such attacks led the federation, in conjunction with some other feminist health groups, to found WATCH in 1976. FWHCs used the model of the participatory clinic for years, only changing the protocol when their continued receipt of state family planning monies and Medicaid reimbursement for services was jeopardized by medical community opposition to the extent to which lay women were providing health services.

But strenuous opposition to the FWHCs also came from within the movement. Typically, that opposition focused on how FWHCs structured the workplace and on Downer's ideas about leadership and her own leadership style. At a time when most other feminist health clinics were adopting collective organizational structures, the FWHCs' hybrid bureaucracies seemed retrograde to many activists. Directors, regular staff, and contract workers received different base wages and enjoyed different degrees of involvement in information sharing and decision making. To those who might object to such hierarchy, Hornstein responds that although FWHCs' designated leaders to make policy decisions and to represent the organization, the leadership group was open to "any woman who came into the group" (Hornstein 1974b, 32). Workers had to earn access to the leadership group, however, by accruing points based "on the amount of time [women] spend at the center, on their initiative, and on how quickly they learn skills" (33).

Policies related to revenue generation also differentiated the FWHCs from other feminist clinics. FWHCs did not strive to provide abortion services at the lowest rates possible, but set fees at moderate levels that would generate sufficient operating income to serve as the basis of the clinic's budget. Frances Hornstein acknowledges that FWHC protocols for funding and organizational structure are unpopular with independent clinic operators, but she insists:

> The women's movement has weakened itself by refusing to recognize leaders among our own people. We have adopted pseudo-equalitarian principles which have prevented many women from exercising their talents, abilities, and skills to their fullest capabilities. We must be aware of these differences and use them. This does not mean that we value each other any less as people. It does mean that we recognize and value leadership. It means that we value women who have more experience than others, that we utilize and

appreciate women who have skills and talents. As Carol Downer put it, "Leaders are people who help groups achieve their goals." (31–32)

But criticism of the federation was intense within the movement. In June 1974 a group of eleven women who had worked at the Orange County FWHC and had either quit or been fired aired their criticisms in a feminist newspaper, *off our backs*, decrying their "common experiences of exploitation and oppression from a supposed 'feminist' organization, the FWHC" (Leste et al. 1974, 2). The women detailed working conditions they found intolerable: very long hours of work for very low pay, which might be suspended when revenues fell short; exclusion from decision making on the grounds that they had not shown sufficient commitment to feminism (as demonstrated by even longer hours in the workplace); nonexistent grievance procedures; distrust of staff by leadership; leadership's belief that workers' complaints demonstrated the absence of feminist consciousness or inadequate commitment to the FWHC.

Later that year, in response to these public charges, Downer explains FFWHC policies in *The Monthly Extract*. What makes the FWHCs feminist, she argues, is

> *Not* total collectivity, *Not* the absence of hierarchy, *Not* the meeting of each woman's needs at any given moment, *Not* the absence of sexism, racism, homosexism or ageism. RATHER the Feminist Women's Health Center is feminist because 1) The FWHC is women-controlled, 2) the FWHC is working towards achieving feminist goals (i.e., gaining power for women on this earth) through not only hard work and sisterly concern, but through daily confrontation with the male power structure. ADDITIONALLY, the FWHC: 1) provides good health care for women *right now*, 2) provides job opportunities for women to work in an all-women organization that is working for feminist goals. (Downer 1974, 10–11)

Antagonism between FWHCs and other clinics exploded onto center stage at the November 1974 conference of women-controlled health projects in Ames, Iowa (where organizers hoped to establish a FWHC). Conceived as an open forum for clinics' philosophies, policies, practices, and long-range goals, the conference attracted women from all over the country. Although Downer herself did not attend, her daughter, Laura Brown, director of the Oakland FWHC, and other FWHC staff members represented the organization. On its last day, a delegation of women from some independent clinics issued a statement protesting the FWHCs' failure to engage in respectful, open dialogue about differences within the movement, a failure that created "resentment, frustration and anger at this conference." The statement also thanked the Feminist

Women's Health Centers for "bringing us self-help"; for "some of the most original and exciting research going on in the field of women's health"; for "investment of energy, time, and money in giving so many of us a good start in understanding our bodies, ourselves and our power and in helping us set up our own health projects, clinics and centers"; for "helping us to recognize the immediate and long-term necessity of developing a comprehensive global communications network"; and for "seizing our power back from the patriarchal system which uses and abuses women throughout the world" (First Annual Women-Controlled Health Projects Conference 1974, 1). Despite such soothing sentiments, many who worked in independent clinics, particularly those in California, remained so hostile to the FFWHC that they refused to refer clients to them for abortions.

Carol Downer agreed that significant political disagreements produced the antagonism between the FWHCs and many of the independent clinics. But her analysis is premised on a different set of political values.

> There was a quite a marked philosophical difference between clinics that decided to become FWHCs and those I would roughly clump as community based health centers . . . And there were hard feelings. Community based health centers accused us, me in particular, of being imperialistic. We thought they were short-sighted and wanting to have a post-revolutionary job in a pre-revolutionary world . . . Most of the criticisms I've heard revolve around hierarchy . . . I might say it was the difference between being organized and disorganized . . . It's hard for me to understand why anyone who goes into a political arena doesn't want to be as organized as they can possibly be . . . if you are really serious about what you are doing. Because otherwise you are at the mercy of these larger forces which are organized. (Downer 1990)

Carol Downer refused to pretend that the revolution in women's health care had already happened. With her radical politics and her radical colleagues and a series of FFWHC health manuals [*How to Stay Out of the Gynecologist's Office* (1981); *A New View of a Woman's Body* (1981); *A Woman's Book of Choices* (1992)] she hoped to make the revolution and rewrite all the protocols of health care for women. The Federation of Feminist Women's Health Centers clearly saw itself as the leading information clearinghouse of the women's health movement (The Boston Women's Health Book Collective surely would have contested this perception). FFWHCs produced—and distributed widely across the country—written materials and films, videotapes, and slide shows about self-help. They offered training sessions for women who wanted to work at feminist health facilities. And they traveled to communities where women were organizing health projects to offer onsite advice and consultation.

The FFWHC continued to grow through the 1980s, when opposition from the state and organized medicine paled in comparison with increasingly violent attacks by an emboldened antiabortion movement. Throughout the decade, staff of the various FWHCs rallied to help clinics most under fire (and the fire was literal) as affiliates suffered dramatic revenue losses and incurred huge additional costs for security, insurance, and facility repairs after vandalism, fire bombings, and arson. Although such attacks succeeded in closing some clinics, most FWHCs survived, joining other feminist health care and abortion providers in a hearty defense of women's reproductive choice. In the early 1990s, Carol Downer stepped down as executive officer of the Federation, and in 1993, FFWHC moved its national offices to Eugene, Oregon. But it soon became too costly to staff the federation office, and although the FWHCs stay affiliated with each other and in touch, national networking and political work have been much reduced.

Some Concluding Remarks

In its formative years, participants in the clinic sector of the women's health movement experienced themselves as pioneers, revolutionaries whose organizations could model a new, empowering alternative health care, a platform from which to promote change in women and the society at large. They didn't just think, believe in, and formulate their ideology. They felt it, too, powerfully, and their passionate political commitment to movement goals moved mountains. The metaphor used by one of the founders of the Emma Goldman Clinic for Women is that of giving birth, an act done in the context of familial relations: "It is like giving birth to a child and you have to come together as a family to do that" (Erickson 1996).

After the act of creation, as this chapter has described, the course of organizational life brought highs and lows, lots of routine, and many accomplishments. But the constant was change itself. How could it not be? It came with this radical territory, surfacing as a continuous need to define and redefine the collective enterprise, the alternative service, the organizational mission and priorities. Besieged from within by the continuous need for change, these politicized workplaces were besieged from without by other political actors—the mainstream medical establishment, the state, and the New Right—that wanted to protect the status quo. Part 2 explores the ways in which women's health clinics resisted and accommodated the various pressures from these powerful political actors.

Part II

The Politics of Change in Women's Health Movement Organizations

Chapter 5

Against the Odds

Patterns of Organizational Change in Feminist Clinics in the 1970s and 1980s

---

Marked by the sense that the movement was always moving, clinic work unfolded against a background of shifting, competing, often clamoring priorities. The profiles in chapter 4 outline how organizational change arced through the women's clinics. Things were never quiet, life was never dull, stasis couldn't take hold in those workplaces. Women did develop new work structures and invent their own work protocols, but in order to survive they also had to make payroll and pay rent, utilities, medical supply companies, and more. Radical though their vision usually was, on a day-to-day basis they were like many other health facilities or small businesses—they had to staff the clinic, provide quality health care, attract clients, interact with the public and other health providers, maintain extensive records, and cope with both the routine and nonroutine pressures of staying afloat.

Political ideals sometimes came up against the compelling needs of clients for services. Feminist values collided with those of regulators and health providers they had to work with. Debt and/or the desire to address their clients' many needs directed them to seek financial support from individuals, organizations in the community and foundations or to compete for grants and contracts from local, state, or federal sources. The dedication to survive against the odds forced them to weigh pragmatic against idealistic considerations. And in the thick of all these realities collectivities of women, most without either professional or business training, managed to build and sustain over years, in some cases over several decades, viable alternative health clinics and vibrant community organizations. As feminist scholars of organizations Myra Marx

Ferree and Patricia Yancey Martin conclude, feminist organizations were "doing the work of the movement" (1995, 3). Feminist health clinics were and are part of a larger breed of feminist organizations that intentionally combined the work of advocacy and/or service provision and/or political mobilization and/or public education with the development of organizational forms that differed from, were alternatives to, most workplaces and many other social movement or community-based organizations in their institutional environments. The achievements of these organizations are nothing short of extraordinary, but the struggles they faced, both from internal conflicts and external pressures, were intense and complex.

In the following four chapters I examine the struggles of these organizations to survive against the odds. Here I explore overarching patterns of organizational change throughout the 1970s and 1980s. From the earliest studies of the women's health movement to the present (Ruzek 1978; Simmons, Kay, and Regan 1984; Thomas 1999), researchers have created typologies to differentiate among health movement organizations and to compare them with their mainstream counterparts. Ruzek's pioneering study of the women's health movement divides the spectrum of clinic workplaces into traditional feminist and radical feminist settings in an attempt to define distinguishing differences between groups of clinics. The first group follows a mutual participation model, in which paraprofessionals deliver most services, patients are encouraged to learn about their bodies, and doctors retain significant control. The radical feminist setting designates self-help as its cornerstone, encourages patients to accept major responsibility for their health care, and uses the doctor as technician *"only after lay persons have decided what needs to be done"* (Ruzek 1978, 109). Ruzek would agree with Ruth Simmons, Bonnie Kay, and Carol Regan (1984), Jan Thomas (1999), Simonds (1996), and other scholars (Schecter 1981; Matthews 1994; Ferree and Martin 1995; Reinelt 1995), as well as with movement veterans, on this stark truth: Feminist health centers had trouble sustaining their collectivist organizational practices. Subject to regulation by the state, buffeted by the entrenched power of organized medicine and the insurance and pharmaceutical industries, and exposed to the full wrath of the anti-abortion armies, the health and reproductive rights sectors of the women's movement, and especially the clinics, encountered unrelenting opposition. But as they hybridized themselves again and again to meet pressing needs and long-term goals, they consciously sought to preserve their founding ideals.

When I began my research on and participation in the women's health movement in the mid 1970s, it was fully alive: encountering opposition but blossoming. Organizations that Ferree and Martin (1995) call the "harvest of the new women's movement" were in their formative years. Their architects had high hopes. They would empower women. They would prove that bureaucracy, hierarchy, and domination could be erased or minimized in settings where women were in control. They would create what Breines (1989) has called prefigurative social movement organizations that embodied feminism's revolutionized egalitarian social relations. (In Carol Downer's rather dismissive formulation, they were designing postrevolutionary jobs in a prerevolutionary world.)

Many of the women who helped found the clinics had cut their political teeth in the Civil Rights movement and/or the New Left, where ideas such as participatory democracy, the "beloved community," and small-group consciousness raising had been central to organizing efforts (Evans 1979; Breines 1989). Many also brought from these earlier experiences—collectively and individually— memories of sectarianism, endless conflict, frequent power plays, and the dizzying cycle of group schisms and dissolution. They did not want to reenact those patterns, and many believed that women's difference (from men) would save them from such strife. But conventional wisdom, lots of social theory, and some early cautionary notes from feminist scholars suggested that the paths of these alternative organizations would be paved with difficulties. Feminist political scientist Jo Freeman, for example, cautioned women who were striving to build collectives against confusing the absence of formal hierarchy or traditional organizational structures of leadership with true equality. Her research had shown how undemocratic processes percolated in many a structureless small group (Freeman 1972). Others outlined the dangers of co-optation as clinics struggled for legitimacy with or came to depend upon doctors, private funding sources, or state agencies, patriarchal forces all (Ahrens 1980).

Such problems have been well documented in the literature on social movements and social movement organizations. Weberian theory, long dominant, argued that social movement organizations ultimately succumb to political-economic pressures exerted by the larger society. After a charismatic formative phase, they either collapse or conform. Weber's analysis (1947, 1978) captured the imagination of the small group of scholars who had trained their eyes on the dynamics of change in collectivist organizations in the 1960s and 1970s (Bush 1978; Hearn 1978; Rothschild-Whitt 1979; Newman 1980). Although Max Weber certainly wasn't a staple in the reading diet of most feminist activists, it didn't take much day-to-day experience in the movement for them to learn how difficult it was to live out their values in alternative organizational forms. Feminists cared deeply that their organizations practiced what they preached. When organizational problems arose around power, social distribution of information, or division of labor, they focused their discussions on the degree to which their new feminist structures matched and honored their egalitarian ideals. By the late 1970s and early 1980s, scholars, too, were turning their attention to the difficulties feminist organizations confronted as they tried to preserve their collectivist, women-empowering ideology (Mansbridge 1973, 1982; Rothschild-Whitt 1979; Ahrens 1980; Morgen 1982) in complex workplaces that provided sophisticated services.

My own experience as a researcher in a feminist health clinic (between 1977 and 1980) stimulated my curiosity to find out how other clinics were weathering the pressures of staying alive and staying true to their ideals. As difficult as the formative years of the 1970s were, the challenges of the 1980s were far tougher. Recession, Reaganomics, an increasingly emboldened New Right, and complex internal political struggles within feminism tested the wills and resources of these small, mostly community-based social movement organizations. Other abortion providers also faced tough times (Joffe 1986).[1] As the 1990s dawned, I undertook a second stage of research on the movement, moving far beyond the several feminist clinics I knew well from my work in the late 1970s.

In 1990 I initiated a study to systematically investigate organizational change in the movement by doing a survey of extant women's health movement organizations throughout the United States. This study was carried out with the able assistance of Alice Julier, a graduate student at the University of Massachusetts. We gathered names of women's health movement organizations from the mailings lists of the Boston Women's Health Book Collective and the National Women's Health Network, from the appendix of Ruzek's 1978 book on the women's health movement appendices, and from other movement publications. We identified 144 possible respondents. Fifty of them replied to our rather lengthy mail survey about how their organizations and work had changed since their founding.[2] (See appendix 1 for a list of clinics.) At the same time, I continued to interview (and did so for eight more years) forty-five women whose combined health movement experiences included ten advocacy organizations and eleven health clinics.[3]

How closely were these organizations able to enact their founding values and practices over time, and what were some of the focal points of patterned change? In 1990 three-quarters of organizations that responded to our survey defined themselves as women-controlled, and they all provided women-centered services or activities. Two-thirds espoused an explicitly feminist ideology. The organizations remained predominantly white organizations, except for the staff of the several women of color organizations that responded to the survey. Of the total staff of responding organizations in 1989, 73 percent were European Americans, up from 70 percent a decade earlier. The percentage of African

American staff members saw a tiny increase, from 14 percent in 1979 to 15 percent in 1989; however, the numbers of Latinas, Native Americans, and Asian Americans remained very small and had declined slightly since 1979. These statistics likely reflect less a decreased commitment to diversity and more an attenuation of the resources that help organizations diversify, such as the Department of Labor (Comprehensive Employment Training Act [CETA]) funds available in the late 1970s.

On the whole, respondents' staff members were older in 1989 than in 1979. Teenagers have never been well represented within the women's health movement, and their numbers declined from 6 to 1 percent of staff from 1979 to 1989. In 1979 the largest single cohort of employees was women in their twenties; in 1989 the largest cohort comprised women in their thirties—of course, in many cases, these were the same employees, now grown older. In 1979, 25 percent of staff were in their forties or older, but by 1989 more than 40 percent fell into that category.

The absolute numbers of clients served by respondents' organizations grew significantly between 1979 and 1989 with the mean number of clients served per organization almost doubling (from 3,638 to 7,052). In addition to the growth in numbers of women served, survey results suggest that the client profile changed between 1979 and 1989. Half or more of the reporting organizations said they served more women of color, poor women, working-class women, and teenagers in 1989 than in 1979. There was some growth in the numbers of Medicaid recipients and older women served during that period as well.

Budgets grew dramatically between 1979 and 1989, but, of course, so did costs and client loads. For 1979 almost 40 percent of respondents reported annual budgets of less than $100,000; by 1989 only about one-quarter recorded budgets of less than $100,000. For 1979 almost one-half reported budgets totaling between $100,000 and $500,000; and 14 percent had budgets exceeding $500,000. By 1989, 35 percent reported budgets of $100,000 to $500,000; and 38 percent said their budgets topped $500,000.

But the absolute size of the budgets masks serious financial difficulties that struck responding organizations in the 1980s. Health care costs had skyrocketed, especially for insurance premiums (both malpractice and facilities coverage), medical supplies, and physician services. Assaults by the antiabortion movement were very costly. At the same time, government funds for women's health services decreased, and foundations shifted their priorities, often away from women's reproductive needs. Client fees continued to constitute the largest single source of revenue for most clinics, with other important revenues generated by health insurance and Medicaid, private donations, and local, state, or federal grants.

In 1990, fully 26 percent of our sample reported serious budget cuts between 1979 and 1989. Eleven percent found ways to make up for these cuts "without undermining our goals or decreasing our activities." But 15 percent of respondents reported budget cuts that meant "significant changes in our goals and services." Forty percent managed to increase their funding during the 1980s. At one time or another, two-thirds of responding organizations were forced to reduce advocacy or outreach activities (these activities are hardest to fund because they rarely generate revenue). Almost as many had laid off staff; 43 percent had cut services; 38 percent had reduced staff benefits; and 35 percent had cut salaries. Of course, financial difficulties also forced some clinics to close during the 1980s.

Interesting patterns emerged from respondents' answers to questions about their perceptions of change in organizational structure, politics, activities, and priorities between 1979 and 1989 and confirmed the impressions I had gathered from interviews, fieldwork, and organizational documents: Job specialization, hierarchy, and time spent on clerical and administrative work increased for a large majority of respondents. By 1990, 71 percent of the organizations linked salaries to job titles and responsibilities; one-half compensated employees based on their seniority; almost three-quarters had directors; and 69 percent had boards of directors. In 22 percent of the organizations, management teams performed the functions of boards of directors. Only one-quarter of respondents reported that they rotated jobs periodically. Outreach activities had increased and resulted in significant growth in services to women of color (41 percent of respondents reported such increases) and to low-income women (55 percent reported increases). Community involvement and community organizing had increased in almost one-half of reporting organizations. Nearly 50 percent registered increases in advocacy activities and involvement in more legal battles.

Thirteen percent of respondents reported stronger identification with the women's health movement in 1989 than in 1979; twice as many groups, one-quarter of the sample, reported a weaker identification with the larger movement. Most respondents described their sense of affiliation with the women's health movement as unchanged. Both self-help and consciousness-raising activities seemed to be on the decline. Forty-two percent of organizations reported that they did less self-help in 1989 than in 1979; 16 percent registered an increase in such activities. More than one-half of respondents reported a reduction in consciousness-raising activities (which they nevertheless regarded as important). Although about one-half reported no change in their contacts with other feminist health groups nationally or in their communities, almost one-quarter described reduced contact with other feminist health groups. Almost one-half of respondents reported less contested decision making at staff meetings, in part because such meetings were shorter than in the movement's earlier days.

External pressures and the relative availability of resources—from mainstream medicine, the state, and other social movements—powerfully influenced what happened to feminist organizations between 1979 and 1989. We asked respondents what kinds of pressures organizations or agencies outside the women's health movement exerted on them, and whether those pressures undermined or reinforced their goals and ideology. By far the most negative external influence was perceived to come from the political mobilization of the New Right, and particularly of the antiabortion movement. Almost 40 percent of the sample reported considerable pressure on their organizations from these forces. Twenty-seven organizations described direct contact with Operation Rescue, and many others reported considerable pressure from this activist antiabortion group. Only a small percentage of respondents said their goals or ideology had been undermined by such pressure; indeed, the vast majority reported that opposition from the antiabortion movement actually increased their determination.

As health care organizations, a large proportion of respondents were exposed to influence or pressure from the state either through application for or receipt of state grants or contracts or through regulation of their facilities by the state. One-quarter reported considerable pressure from state agencies; 51 percent reported some pressure. Twenty percent reported considerable pressure from federal agencies; 32 percent report some pressure. One-fifth of responding organizations claimed that pressure from state agencies undermined their goals or activities; 14 percent reported that pressure from federal agencies undermined their agendas. But the majority of respondents reported that pressure from state and federal agencies either had little impact on or reinforced their goals and activities.

Fifteen percent of feminist health organizations reported considerable pressure, and 61 percent reported some pressure from "the health care establishment." Almost one-fifth described such pressure as sufficiently powerful to undermine their goals or ideology. That figure is very close to the percentage of respondents who reported significant impact from the assaults of the New Right and the antiabortion movement. On the other hand, a little more than one-half of respondents reported that other feminist groups had either a considerable (11 percent) or some (42 percent) reinforcing influence. And community organizations also had a positive effect on respondents. Three-quarters of the sample reported either considerable (7 percent) or some (64 percent) influence from local groups, with most (62 percent) reporting that such contact reinforced their agendas.

To the extent that our survey demonstrates change in what had been nonbureaucratic features of feminist health centers, particularly between 1979 and 1989, it supports the basic pattern of organizational change predicted by Weber's paradigm of routinization, a process of institutionalization and conservatization fostered, according to his theory, by "the technical superiority of the bureaucratic mode of organizations" and the "objective necessity of adaptation to . . . everyday economic conditions" (Weber 1978). Robert Michels had argued the same position in his seminal study of the German Social Democratic Party (1959). Michels goes farther than Weber, insisting that the process of routinization is inevitable. His "iron law of oligarchy" defines bureaucratization and the displacement of radical by more conservative goals as necessary, indeed unavoidable consequences of the primacy social movement organizations place on survival in what is usually a hostile political-economic environment.

However, the picture and explanation for this pattern of change are more complex than Weberian theory suggests. Scholars of organizations, especially feminist organizational theorists (including my own work), offer alternative organizations more sophisticated ways of understanding and charting their development over time. It is important to note that most scholars paid little theoretical attention to feminist or collectivist organizations until well into the 1980s. Jane Mansbridge was one of a few exceptions. As early as 1973, she was studying participatory groups, and she pursued that interest into the 1980s (Mansbridge 1973, 1979, 1980, 1982). As she acknowledges the practical, moral, and psychological advantages of participatory democratic organizations, Mansbridge also identifies recurring problems: the inordinately long time required for decision making; the emotional intensity of interaction among members; and the persistence of certain inequalities of influence despite democratic ideals and structures (1973). Like Freeman's (1972), Mansbridge's initial contribution was to point to the gap between egalitarian ideals and actual practice in alternative organizations.

The active revision of the Weber-Michels thesis began in earnest when scholars such as Zald and Ash (1966) and Rothschild-Whitt (1976) questioned the inevitability of routinization and goal displacement. They argued that the nature and direction of changes in social movement organizations are conditional, and that radicalization of goals or intensification in democratic procedures can also occur. Rothschild-Whitt notes that small group size, consensus about goals, relatively egalitarian social division of knowledge, nonhostile environment, and membership that is noncompetitive and accommodating can actually facilitate participatory democracy, thus heightening the alternativity of social movement organizations over time (Rothschild-Whitt 1976, 1979).

My own work was strongly influenced by those who questioned the dominant and unilinear model of organizational change. And I had another bone to pick with Weber, Michels, and their adherents, whose analyses of how larger political-economic forces shaped the nature and direction of change in feminist and collectivist organizations I found vague and imprecise. In particular, I explored how the capitalist state—directly through funding and regulation and indirectly through legitimation and support of conservative backlash in the New Right and antiabortion movements and hegemonic ideologies—powerfully affected oppositional organizations whose goals, internal structure, and/or activities were directed at social change (Morgen 1982, 1986). Other scholars have also examined the dynamics of cooptation, focusing on the effects of state funding and other forms of engagement with the state (Matthews 1994; Reinelt 1995) and/or on the New Right (Petchesky 1990; Hyde 1991, 1992, 1995; Simonds 1995, 1996).

In addition to examining the emergence of hierarchy, increased bureaucracy, and goal displacement in feminist organizations, some scholars have elaborated the notion that bureaucracy, as a particular form of hierarchy, is inconsistent with feminist ideals. Perhaps the most well-known version of this argument is Kathy Ferguson's work (1984) that counterposes bureaucratic norms and practices with feminist ideas and strategies, particularly equality, sisterhood, and community, to construct a binary opposition between feminist and bureaucratic organizations. Ferguson argues that all manifestations of hierarchy were anathema to a radical or transformative feminism.

Although many others have since challenged Ferguson (Gelb and Palley 1987; Buechler 1990; Eisenstein 1995), work such as hers reinforced either the bureaucracy or feminism framework that already pervaded the consciousness of many activists and the theories of scholars. Reinelt observes that feminists, both scholars and activists, often measured organizations against a set of opposing characteristics: feminist/patriarchal; collective/hierarchy; democratic participation/bureaucracy; empowerment/power; grassroots/professional; confrontation/co-optation; political/institutional; outside/inside; people/state (1995, 91). She argues that such binarisms make it impossible to envision organizations that include both collective and hierarchical processes, participatory and bureaucratic elements, outside and inside political strategies, grassroots mobilization, and organizing within institutions. Furthermore, Reinelt points out, such a framework assumes that collectivist, participatory organizations are by definition open, democratic, and responsive; and that hierarchies and bureaucracies are always oppressive (1995, 92–93).

As both the clinic profiles and responses to our survey indicate, most of the organizations of the women's health movement developed decision-making structures and other organizational features that combined bureaucratic and counterbureaucratic, hierarchical and egalitarian characteristics. Ferree and Martin make this important overarching argument: "Feminist organizations are an amalgam, a blend of institutionalized and social movement practices . . . A movement organization is . . . by definition, in tension. It is always a compromise between the ideals by which it judges itself and the realities of its daily practices" (1995, 78). In short, such organizations are hybrids.

In the early 1980s, Simmons, Kay, and Regan surveyed many of the then-existing women's health movement groups, choosing from a larger sample twenty-eight organizations that were women controlled, provided women's health services, had local rather than national constituencies, and "espoused an alternative view of health or adopted a nonhierarchical form of organization" (1984, 621). Because they chose from the larger sample those organizations that self-described themselves as collectivist groups and because their study was done before the worst damage of the 1980s political and economic climate had taken its toll, they were able to study a core group of clinics that remained relatively close to the organizational ideals of the early women's health movement. Ranking those organizations from least to most collective, they found that collectivist internal organization was associated with greater task sharing and rotation, with a stronger sense of community, with a higher regard for shared values in recruitment, with lower salary differentials, and with smaller size. But even in the early 1980s a pattern of change was apparent. Hierarchy is more apparent, and respondents indicated that consensus-seeking modes of decision making had been too time consuming, especially once financial pressures forced the clinics to become more efficient in order to survive (630). Indeed, their study provides evidence that financial constraints and the pressures of trying to survive in a hostile larger political and economic environment had been a primary determinant of organizational change for the groups they studied.

Almost a decade later, shortly after the survey I conducted, sociologist Jan Thomas assembled survey, interview, and site-visit data to examine change in fourteen feminist health centers. Thomas found three organizational ideal types among the clinics that she labels feminist bureaucracy, participatory bureaucracy, and collectivist democracy. She argues that feminist ideology was most visible within collectivist democracies (there were three in her sample), where the empowerment of clients remained a core goal, there was little division of labor and critical decisions were made by the group as a whole (Thomas 1999, 107). Her conclusions mirrored those of the Simmons, Kay, and Regan study and our survey—the "hostile climate of the 1980s forced feminist women's health centers to reassess their core beliefs and make difficult decisions regarding ideology and survival" (117).

Each of these studies found that while some features critical to the identity of these groups as oppositional social movement organizations or alternative health clinics had eroded or were muted a decade or more after their founding, other alternative features remained intact. Notably, Thomas's study as well as my own found that feminist ideals remained most alive and well in relation to how services were delivered. Change did not usually mean an abandonment of feminist ideals and principles. Through constant reassessment, and because they were brave enough to make the difficult choices that confronted them, women who worked in feminist health centers altered practices, but not necessarily in ways that they found inconsistent with their political principles; and not necessarily in ways that compromised the vibrancy of their organizations.

Rather, they acted and reacted to constraints and opportunities and guided the hybridization of the clinics. These women were agents of their own and their organizational histories, living out Marx's now famous dictum: they made history, not always under the conditions of their own choosing, but with their sights set on a feminist praxis guided by deeply felt, passionately articulated ideals and values. What is important here is that processes such as routinization, bureaucratization, goal displacement did not simply occur to organizations. Rather, thinking, feeling political actors exerted agency over their lives and the political institutions they built and sustained (see also Acker 1995).

Chapter 6

The Changer and the Changed

The Women's Health Movement, Doctors, and Organized Medicine

In 1971 Belita Cowan drafted a book proposal—"Death of the MDeity"—and sent it to a publisher in New York. There was no market for the book, the publisher told her. But Cowan and other feminist health activists were creating another kind of text, a story in words and actions that spelled change in medicine, particularly in how physicians viewed and treated women. Her working title condensed key themes in the evolving feminist critique of doctors, and especially of obstetrician/gynecologists, as patriarchal, godlike figures who deprived women of the right to be active agents in their own lives and exposed them to harmful effects of routinely used pharmaceuticals (DES, for example), medical procedures (hysterectomies or sterilization performed without informed consent), and clinical research. Movement activists were intent on demystifying health information, demedicalizing key aspects of women's reproductive processes, and deprofessionalizing routine health services. In each of these efforts, feminists took aim at doctors, the guardians of medicine as an institution of social control.

The burgeoning literature of the movement encodes this searing indictment: Doctors enforce the subordination and neglect the basic needs of women, the poor, and people of color. The first edition of *Our Bodies, Ourselves* starts a conversation that continues even today. American medicine, members of the Boston Women's Health Book Collective say, does not "take responsibility for the health of the people" (1971, 123): "Doctors' attitudes toward patients are terribly condescending, especially toward women . . . Doctors withhold information . . . A standard complaint . . . is that they are tired of neurotic women with nothing wrong with them who come in because they are lonely or dissatisfied with life . . . On the other hand, unnecessary and cruel surgery is often performed . . . The medical system is not responsible to the community. It is controlled by the doctors" (BWHBC 1971, 125). Source by source, the same allegations surface: physicians are too wealthy and powerful; the American Medical Association's (AMA) stranglehold on health policy and delivery systems costs too much; mainstream medicine often strips patients of their dignity, their right to information, and their freedom to choose appropriate treatment.

The feminist challenge found its roots in earlier health-focused oppositional struggle that also contested physician control of health care or the care those physicians provided (or did not provide) to those in need: the nineteenth-century popular health movement; the struggle by midwives and by women who sought entrance to medical school early in the twentieth century for the right to provide health care; the crusades of the Black women's club movement for public health services in their communities; and the New Left, Civil Rights, consumer, and community health movements of the 1960s. From different vantage points, each of these antecedents to feminist health activism began the process of politicizing health care and working for change.

Medicine Takes It On the Chin

Women have always been healers. They were the unlicensed doctors and anatomists of western history. They were abortionists, nurses, and counselors. They were pharmacists, cultivating healing herbs, and exchanging the secrets of their uses. They were midwives, traveling from home to home and village to village. For centuries, women were doctors without degrees, barred from books and lectures, learning from each other, and passing on experience from neighbor to neighbor and mother to daughter. They were also called "wise women" by the people, witches or charlatans by the authorities. (Ehrenreich and English 1973a, 1)

Women's health care, Barbara Ehrenreich and Deirdre English assert in *Witches, Midwives, and Nurses,* is "part of our heritage as women, our history, our birthright" (1). In their short, influential book, Ehrenreich and English articulated an impassioned message. Women are not trespassers on a terrain that rightfully belongs to health professionals; instead, we aim to reclaim control of our own (individual) bodies and of an occupation (healer) that we've always, until the last century, called our own. In *Witches, Midwives, and Nurses* and its companion publication, *Complaints and Disorders: The Sexual Politics of Sickness* (1973b), Ehrenreich and English track the suppression of women healers by a sexist medical establishment that defined upper- and middle-class women as sick—they needed intensive oversight by doctors—and working class women as sickening—they threatened public health and there was no profit to be made from their care. In the past thirty years, feminists have built a body of scholarship that confirms, specifies, and elaborates such insights (for example, Leavitt and Numbers 1978; Ehrenreich and English 1978; Reverby and Rosner 1979; Starr 1982; Fee 1983; Corea 1977; Morantz-Sanchez 1985; Apple 1990; Doyal 1995). This scholarship demonstrates the processes through which medical knowledge was used to justify women's secondary place in society; exploit women as consumers of medical care; rationalize racist health practices and a health system that provided class-stratified services; and exclude women from positions of importance within the hierarchy of medical occupations.

The campaign to deprive women of power as providers of health care began in 1859, when the ten-year-old American Medical Association fired the first volley in its attack on abortion. Many scholars now see this campaign as part of a broader plan by physicians to gain control of health care and eliminate competitors, including midwives and other lay health practitioners (Starr 1982; Petchesky 1984). Fifty years later, the Flexner Report, commissioned by the Carnegie Foundation (1910), helped doctors win the struggle to monopolize and professionalize American medicine, reserving its practice for an elite of wealthy (and later middle-class) European American men. For most of the twentieth century, white male professional dominance over an increasingly sophisticated medical care system was entrenched. Technological and pharmaceutical innovation, especially in the period after World War II (Starr 1982), had accelerated to warp speed in the early 1960s (the first successful heart transplant took place in 1964), when the Sabin oral polio vaccine, Librium, Valium, and the birth control pill changed the way contagious disease, mental illness, and women's reproductive health were conceived and treated. But striking medical advances didn't expand access to services for low-income Americans, and in fact, costs skyrocketed with the development and acquisition of new technologies.

Health care became a major political issue in the 1960s, galvanizing social reformers and radicals within and between various radical movements. The Medical Committee for Human Rights (MCHR), for example, allied itself with the Civil Rights movement and the New Left (Kotelchuck 1976), challenged segregation in medical facilities and local medical societies, sent health care workers to the Mississippi Freedom Summer, positioned itself against the war in Vietnam, and supplied dedicated professional staff for emerging alternative health care facilities. The Black Power movement, especially the Black Panther Party, also established health clinics, among other community-based services, in some African American communities (Jones 1998). These actions were part of a prolonged struggle for improved health care access at lower cost; they also challenged basic assumptions of medical practice in the United States, charging that it was not concerned enough with preventive and primary care. The most radical of these groups embedded their analyses of the political economy of health care in a larger critique of imperialism, capitalism, racism, and then, as feminist analysis developed, sexism.

In 1965 Congress responded to the upswing in radical political activism, especially the Civil Rights movement, with legislation that would dramatically affect health care delivery in the United States: authorizations for Medicaid and Medicare and funding for community mental health centers, community vaccination assistance programs, and medical training (McBride and McBride 1994). Over the next several years, that legislation underwrote the establishment of a nationwide network of neighborhood and community-based clinics that offered affordable care to the medically disenfranchised. Now, the poor were to receive medical services, and they were to enjoy a degree of control over its organization and protocols: Federal mandates for Office of Economic Opportunity–funded clinics required that 51 percent of their board members be consumers of the health care they provided. The War on Poverty had begun, and "maximum feasible participation" of the community was one of its mantras. But not all of the new health care facilities were government-initiated or even, in their early days, government funded. The Haight-Ashbury Free Clinic, a grassroots answer to the needs of the youth counterculture, opened in San Francisco in 1967, and by 1972, there would be hundreds of such clinics in cities and towns across the country (Taylor 1979).

Feminist health activists stormed onto this shifting ground with their powerful analysis of the ways the (capitalist) health care system made women suffer. The first edition of *Our Bodies, Ourselves* catalogs its sins: "The prohibitive cost of medical care, the racist and inferior treatment of poor people and black people, the profit and prestige-making institutions of the 'health industry' (hospitals, medical schools, drug companies, etc.), the total neglect of the public or preventive protection, or the fee-for-service, pay-as-you-die economic base upon which most medical practice is based" (1971, 136). As new editions of *Our Bodies, Ourselves* and other feminist health publications appeared in print, no major component of corporate health care went unexamined: from the lobbies of the health insurance, health research, hospital, and pharmaceutical industries to the practices of medical schools, the family planning establishment, physicians, medical supply companies, and commercial medical insurers. This critique of health care rested on a critique of capitalism and of white, upper middle-class male physician control of health care.

This latter charge accurately described reality in the late 1960s as the women's health movement was first organizing. In 1969 women represented

9.4 percent of applicants to medical school, and in 1970 there were only about twenty-five thousand women physicians in the United States (Bickel and Kopriva 1993, 141). In the mid–1970s Dreifus could report that 94 percent of board-certified gynecologists were male (1977). This pattern was deeply rooted. Elizabeth Blackwell, the first woman doctor in the United States, had received her medical degree in 1848, but in the first half of the twentieth century, "more than 50 percent of the medical schools in America still did not accept women and many others had strict quotas limiting female enrollment" (Bickel and Kopriva 1993, 141). As Morantz-Sanchez (1985), Lorber (1984), and others have shown, organized medicine, a mostly white profession, resisted opening opportunities for women to become physicians. First-wave feminists protested that exclusion, and although the second-wave feminists who launched the women's health movement believed that women should have equal access to medical training and medical practice, particularly in obstetrics and gynecology, their politics expressed ambivalence even about women doctors. Always, the movement's ideological focus was the empowerment of women as patients, consumers, active agents in their own health care.

The protocols of obstetrics and gynecology diminished (or infantilized) women in so many ways. Draping during the traditional pelvic exam, activists argued, symbolized the veil of secrecy doctors imposed on women's bodies. But as the movement's foundational stories prove again and again, women meant to tear away that veil. Carol Downer, with other women of the FFWHC explored the female body, made maps of its secret places (as did the BWHBC in *Our Bodies, Ourselves*). Members of Jane learned how to perform abortions. Advocacy groups undertook independent research. Limited information wasn't good enough any longer. They sought answers to their questions and greater control of their medical treatment. In all these ways, they encroached on a well-guarded and profitable terrain, and that encroachment provoked response.

Physicians and Organized Medicine Respond

As feminist analyses of health care proliferated in books and in scholarly and popular articles, as the movement began to score policy victories, as self-help groups and women-controlled clinics opened for business, physicians, especially obstetrician-gynecologists, took notice. In 1974 Barbara Kaiser and her coauthor, Irwin Kaiser, M.D., presented a paper, "The Challenge of the Women's Movement to American Gynecology," at the ninety-seventh meeting of the American Gynecological Association in Hot Springs, Virginia. That such a paper was presented in this venue testifies to the growing influence of the women's health movement. The Kaisers, whose paper was later published in the *American Journal of Obstetrics and Gynecology,* are sympathetic to the feminist critique of medicine.

> The challenge to the masculine stronghold by the women's movement has pushed to the forefront the fact that the medical problems of women are a special case of the social and political problems of women. Failure of many gynecologists and obstetricians to grasp this fundamental truth is one of the factors that have caused the growing rift between women and their doctors and the resentment that so many women feel toward that branch of the medical profession that is supposed to specialize in their particular problems and illnesses. (Kaiser and Kaiser 1974, 652)

The Kaisers understand the central political aim of the women's health movement to be the "redistribution of power" between doctors and patients, and they argue for women's right "to define their femininity in their own terms" (most feminist health activists would not have chosen these words) "and to assume some control and decision functions with respect to the social and personality effects of gynecologic care" (653). They conclude their paper by reiterating that feminist activists want to be "treated like full human beings" and not to have to submit to "demeaning and insulting role stereotypes" (659). Nevertheless, they raise concerns about whether self-help, especially menstrual extraction, might be dangerous and warn of the possibility that "women's groups are simply pooling their ignorance" (660). They urge their colleagues to practice with "more lengthy explanation of medical information, avoidance of an expectation of unquestioned trust, emergence from behind the drapes to teach and demonstrate self-examination to patients, sharing of records and laboratory reports, acceptance of loved ones in labor and delivery rooms, and genuine candor about malignant disease," all leading to what they believe would be a "vast improvement in medical care" (661).

Six physicians, one a woman, responded in print. Dr. Donald Swartz questioned the "broad applicability of generalizations [about doctors]" as well as some of the tactics of the movement, but he urged his colleagues to look beyond such rhetoric to grasp the importance of the health activists' concerns (661). Dr. James Merrill argued that gynecologists must respond to the challenge of the movement because it reflects profound changes in the role of women in the larger society. Dr. Robert Kintch compared aspects of gynecological self-help to the practice of breast self-examination. If doctors teach women how to do procedures such as self–Pap exams, he said, and if women retain their "initial enthusiasm, this movement could possibly be supported."

Another relatively supportive comment came from Dr. Clay Burchell, who reasoned that whether or not the feminist critique of gynecologists was entirely just, the "relationship [between woman and doctor] is changing and needs to be reconciled" (664).

But Dr. Denis Cavanagh dismissed the feminist argument as a product of the "lunatic fringe" of the women's movement and exhorted his fellows not to "forsake the women who are the epitome of stability in our society in order to seek the approbation of the militant feminists who seem to be obsessed with a fantasy that somehow all will be Utopian when the top dog is female" (664, 665). And Dr. Georgeanna Jones suggested that good doctors were already doing much of what feminists want. She urged her colleagues to "ignore the insinuation that gynecologists are prejudiced against women. We are not really talking about men vs. women, but good doctors" (665). Women deserve more information, she observed, but they should never be allowed to take over treatment decisions from their physicians.

The Kaisers's paper and the responses it generated open a window through which we can look at the impact of the women's health movement on organized medicine in the mid–1970s. First, the feminist challenge was compelling enough to necessitate a response from the profession. Second, at least some doctors could agree that women deserved more information about and involvement in their own health care. Third, as Cavanagh's letter demonstrates, some doctors dismissed the movement's charges outright. Fourth, even relatively supportive doctors intended to retain their control of gynecology and obstetrics.

The debate over the merits of the feminist challenge continued at the ninety-eighth annual meeting of the American College of Obstetricians and Gynecologists in 1975, where Virginia Johnson, codirector of the Reproductive Biology Research Foundation in St. Louis, Missouri, applauded feminism for fostering greater "self-confidence, self-definition, and commitment to oneself as an individual," qualities that make women more effective consumers of health care (Pollner 1975, 13). In the debate format of this session, another woman, Dr. Evelyn Gendel, wielded the con gavel—she was assigned to represent the position that feminism had had a negative effect on the practice of gynecology. But her satiric comments left little doubt that she supported key aspects of the feminist critique. Dr. James Merrill went farther than he had the year before and gave the movement credit for "altering hospital policies concerning sterilization and maternity care" and demonstrating that "minor surgical procedures [including abortion] can be done on an ambulatory basis rather than on an expensive inpatient basis" (1975, 34).

Beyond discussions at professional conferences and debates in the pages of journals and newsletters, skirmishes between the medical establishment and feminist clinics and advocacy organizations were often heated. When feminists were seen to seize their privileges, doctors frequently fought back.

Close Encounters of Another Kind

Activists (and most other women) knew little about the usurpation of women's health care by organized medicine in the mid-nineteenth and early twentieth centuries, but they quickly learned how state law and professional control of health care blocked women's reproductive choice in the present. Although some doctors strongly advocated abortion rights, and others even performed abortions or helped patients get safe(r) abortions before *Roe* vs. *Wade,* organized medicine operated as a conservative, self-interested political force, and it was slow to jump on the bandwagon for liberalization (Petchesky 1990, 79). When the AMA decided in 1970 to support repeal of abortion laws, it did so within a framework that sought to guarantee physician control of the decision and the procedure, and it succeeded (124). *Roe* vs. *Wade* makes no mention of abortion on demand. Rather, it acknowledges a woman's right to privacy in the medical choices she makes in consultation with her doctor, who retains power.

As women organized health clinics before and after *Roe* vs. *Wade,* they had to face the hard facts of operational life: licensing laws, reimbursement policies of insurance companies and public agencies, and a host of other regulatory practices guaranteed physicians and other professionals control of health policy, family planning methods, and medical practice. So despite their ideological commitment to overturning professional (and male) control of health care, feminist clinics had to work closely with doctors, often under the license of a physician—and the physician was typically a white male— if they sought to provide abortions, family planning, or many other gynecological services legally and in a way that could be reimbursed by private and public third-party payers.

Interviews with activists across the country suggest that the doctors who worked with or as part of the women's health movement were a more diverse group than one might expect. Many were relatively newly trained; some had established practices in their own communities. Among the specializations of those about whom I gathered information were obstetrics and gynecology, family practice, psychiatry, internal medicine, and in at least one case, pathology. Some served as medical directors of clinics and participated in all phases of decision making and administration. Others performed abortions or provided gynecology services for a few hours a month.

Relationships between physicians and lay staff of feminist clinics varied, depending on the values and beliefs of the physician about the role of nonprofessionals in health care delivery, self-help, and other issues, and the attitudes of clinic staff about how they wanted doctors to function within their organizations. Physicians always had power associated with their licenses, but it would be a gross distortion to suggest that they dictated policy in the clinics. Far from it. At New Bedford Women's Health Services, for example, as well as at other clinics, doctors had to agree with the clinic's philosophy of health care and with examination protocols that included a health worker who served as client advocate, recorded the "herstory," inserted the speculum, and performed the Pap smear and gonorrhea culture. Clinic policy placed clients on the lowest-dose oral contraceptive possible, emphasized barrier methods of birth control, and demanded that physicians work to encourage their use.

Later in the 1970s, affirmative action and changing career goals would bring more women into medical school, but early in the decade most feminist clinics were unable to find women doctors to staff their shifts. So women's health activists found male doctors willing to work in their clinics. Staff of the Vermont Women's Health Center and the New Hampshire Feminist Health Center cooperated with local physicians, Emma Goldman's founding mothers forged close relationships with many physicians who practiced obstetrics and gynecology at University Hospital, and other clinics enjoyed similar comity with area doctors. In some locations, though, organized medicine went on the offensive against feminist clinics, and by the late 1970s and early 1980s, the virulent antiabortion movement had made it harder than ever to recruit and keep doctors. In New Bedford, Massachusetts; Tallahassee, Florida, and Chico, California, local medical communities harassed doctors who worked with feminist clinics—by impugning their competence or threatening their staff privileges at local hospitals.

A case in point: In 1975 the Feminist Women's Health Center in Tallahassee lost three doctors in four months to a campaign of harassment by local physicians. After a newspaper article praised the low-cost, high-quality care the FWHC offered, obstetricians and gynecologists at the community hospital passed a resolution barring doctors with staff privileges at the hospital from performing abortions at the clinic (Carroll 1980, x). Several months later, the FWHC filed a lawsuit claiming restraint of trade against the Florida Board of Medical Examiners and five Tallahassee obstetrician-gynecologists. The suit was settled in the clinic's favor in 1980.

The Chico (California) Feminist Women's Health Center had a similar experience. Threatened with loss of privileges at their community hospital if they agreed to work at the FWHC, Chico's doctors turned their backs on the clinic, which then had to import physicians from as far off as San Francisco and to rely for emergency backup on a doctor who lived twenty-six miles away. That FWHC's insurance company, Norcal, then canceled the clinic's malpractice coverage because local physicians labeled it high risk—it used out-of-town doctors, didn't it?—was ironic but not funny. In 1980 the Chico FWHC filed a $12 million federal antitrust suit against nine Chico obstetrician-gynecologists, claiming that they had conspired to dissuade physicians from working with the clinic, denied its patients medical backup for abortion complications, instigated unfounded investigations by the state, and encouraged Norcal to cancel the clinic's malpractice insurance. Three years later, the suit settled out of court: The Chico FWHC won the promise of medical backup and enough money (the amount was undisclosed) to open a clinic in nearby Redding.

Five years after the settlement, the former director of the Butte-Glenn Medical Society and director of emergency services for the local hospital described the relationship between the Chico medical community and the feminist clinic as "civil"; he added, "It wouldn't be fair to say that the center is considered by doctors to be in the mainstream of medical care. But we work with them and have no problems. In general a lot of physicians ethically do not believe in doing abortions. There is no question that they were threatening to doctors when they opened and that physicians were taken aback by their presence" (Abramson 1988, 8).

That feminist clinics were often threatening and that physicians were at least taken aback by their emergence should not be surprising. The clinics boldly trumpeted the features that distinguished them from mainstream health care providers: the use of nonprofessional caregivers; self-help; emphasis on alternative (nonprescription) remedies when possible; demystification of health information and providers; and clinic administration and control by nonprofessional women. Trailblazers for abortion services in underserved communities, they suffered from the stigmatization that associated abortion providers with immorality and danger. And they bore the brunt of attacks by the growing antiabortion movement.

The organized medical community and its individual practitioners commanded an arsenal of weapons that could be used against the feminist clinics. Physicians are always well represented in health regulatory agencies and oversight committees. In 1972 the Board of Medical Examiners was directly involved in a six-month surveillance of the Los Angeles Feminist Women's Health Center (LAFWHC). In 1976, the same agency, recycled as the Board of Medical Quality Assurance, pursued another investigation of LAFWHC, "finally summarized by a state official as a 'fishing expedition'" (Schnitger 1981, 3). The Los Angeles Regional Family Planning Council, a private organization of physicians, hospitals, and Planned Parenthood affiliates that controlled the disbursement of federal family planning moneys in the city, was able to withhold crucial funding from the LAFWHC for several years—because council members disapproved of participatory clinics that emphasized self-help and peer and paraprofessional counseling.

As a general rule, the more an alternative organization seeks to change, constitutes a viable source of competition for, or embodies a meaningful challenge to mainstream organizations, the more likely it is that the larger context in which it operates will be hostile or undermining. The groups that constituted the organizational infrastructure of the women's health movement frequently competed with doctors for patients, and at the same time, they functioned in an environment highly regulated by the state, professional organizations (especially the American Medical Association), and other private interests, including the insurance industry. Medical licensure laws constituted the most powerful form of regulation of clinic practices, and it was these laws that Carol Downer and Colleen Wilson were accused of violating in 1972 when they were charged with (and Downer was later acquitted of) practicing medicine without a license.

In March 1974, after a yearlong undercover investigation, three lay midwives associated with the Birth Center in Santa Cruz, California, were also charged with practicing medicine without a license. The lay midwifery movement was a close ally of the self-help movement (Edwards 1984; Sullivan 1988), and many in the larger women's health movement took up the midwives' cause, providing political and financial support. After lengthy delays, the case finally came to trial in 1976. The three midwives were acquitted when the court ruled that because pregnancy was not a disease, assisting at childbirth could not be construed as practicing medicine without a license (Ruzek 1978, 60). Soon afterward, the California Supreme Court reconsidered the charges and ruled that lay midwives who assist in labor and childbirth were covered by the state's Medical Practice Act.

Such legal actions had a chilling effect on some feminist clinics. Nevertheless, the principal disincentive for the use of nonprofessional practitioners was not fear of arrest, but the business practices that determined the reimbursement policies of private and public health insurance plans. Most of these plans would cover services only if they were physician provided. It goes without saying that physicians—many of whom were determined to reinforce physician control of health care—have had a tremendous impact on the development of third-party payer policies. As clinics saw how difficult it was to generate sufficient revenues to stay open, they chose to adapt to the requirements of insurance companies in order to ensure health services for their clients.

Health Activists Confront Mainstream Medicine

As doctors and their professional and regulatory organizations worked to constrain the development of feminist clinics, some activists initiated frontal attacks on their territories. The Federation of Feminist Women's Health Centers argued that it was not enough to model alternatives to mainstream medicine. They wanted to replace it, and they were ready to commit trespass (literally) to make their point. Inspections of hospitals, they argued, provided "an important tool for consumers to use to bring about changes in routine practices which are dangerous and/or unnecessary" (Chico FWHC 1981, 14). In March 1977, thirty activists who had gathered in Tallahassee for the first national conference of WATCH entered Tallahassee Memorial Hospital accompanied by a reporter and photographer from a local television station, and inspected the obstetrical unit (Ruzek 1978, 167). When hospital staff asked Carol Downer and her companions to leave the nursery, they did so immediately. But not before they found evidence of what they considered unsafe childbirth practices, including routine use of an internal fetal monitor during labor and delivery, routine separation of babies from mothers after birth, and routine use of Phisohex, a chemical believed to cause brain damage when used at high concentration, and particularly with infants (Chico FWHC 1981, 14).

Within forty-eight hours, the film of the inspection had been confiscated by Florida's attorney general and four WATCH members, including Carol Downer, had been arrested, charged with trespass, and released after posting bond ($1,000). Before their trial in May, the WATCH members won backing from feminist and civil libertarian groups (NOW passed a resolution of support for their action at its annual convention). Local news coverage, however, was extremely negative (FAAR 1977), and the women were convicted of criminal trespass, fined $500 to $1,000, and sentenced to thirty to sixty days in jail. WATCH published an "afterthought" acknowledging that the inspection would have been better received if it had been undertaken in concert with more members of the local community (FAAR 1977). But the organization continued to argue for the value of hospital inspections and later circulated a short guide that recommends what to look for and what to do if objectionable practices are found. WATCH used the guerilla inspection of Tallahassee Memorial Hospital's labor and delivery ward to attract the national media spotlight to the organization and its critique of hospital birthing practices. Activists knew that doctors wouldn't change their routine practices without organized, persistent pressure, and some of them were willing to invite criticism and break the law to keep the pressure up.

Another, ostensibly more cooperative, encounter between feminist clinics and organized medicine was the pelvic examination teaching program, which brought activists into medical schools to serve as models. The goal of pelvic teaching programs—denunciation of the traditional pelvic exam was ubiquitous in the movement—was to "provide a counterbalance to previously held and institutionalized attitudes towards women as passive recipients of medical care" (Women's Community Health 1976a, 19). Educated and politically aware, the activists could participate in the process more effectively, could actually teach students how to perform the procedure thoroughly and with respect. And pelvic teaching programs allowed feminists to share with medical students their larger concerns about provider-patient relationships.

Both Women's Community Health in Cambridge and the Emma Goldman Clinic in Iowa City, for example, established such programs. But early optimism about their power to affect medical education soon gave way to political concerns. From the beginning, the WCHC program—developed after members of the Boston Women's Health Book Collective approached the clinic on behalf of women medical students at Harvard who were displeased with how pelvic exams were being taught—was controversial among staff members who believed that it helped doctors to better manage their patients and who argued that they should instead be working to subvert power relations between consumers and health care providers (Bell 1989).

During the program's first incarnation, clinic volunteers (who were paid twenty-five dollars per session) provided feedback during the physician-taught examinations. But they felt like "talking pelvises" whose "bodies were [deemed] valuable, but our information and skills were not" (WCHC 1976a, 19). So they developed a new program protocol that made the model an active instructor about the pelvic exam and well-women gynecology. Women's Community Health distributed the revised protocol widely within the movement, and after more discussion, members of the pelvic teaching program (PTP) developed a third protocol that more emphatically promoted self-help and a radical perspective on health care. They expected it would be less acceptable to medical schools. They were right. No medical school agreed to implement the third protocol, which admitted only women (medical students and other hospital professionals) to the $750 four-session program. Nevertheless, Women's Community Health strongly recommended that other feminist groups model their PTPs after this third protocol.

Pelvic teaching programs represented both an opportunity and a trap for feminist health groups. This was clear to Susan Bell, a PTP participant who, in an article entitled "Political Gynecology: Gynecological Imperialism and the Politics of Self Help," concludes that "by 'improving' the health care system it may be possible to generate more humane care, but at the cost of strengthening an already oppressive system . . . When it confronted basic power relations and current assumptions about the goals of medical education," pelvic teaching programs lost favor with medical school administrators (Bell 1989, 582). Indeed, such programs did transfer important knowledge from feminists to mainstream medicine and helped change gynecological practices; and over the long term, effacement of the differences between alternative and traditional care adversely affected the sustainability of feminist clinics.

Physicians in the Movement

Some of the most significant relationships between feminist health activists and doctors occurred within the movement, inside clinics and advocacy organizations that also served as breeding grounds for future medical and health care professionals and as way stations for students who sought alternatives to what they were learning in medical school. Several physicians played leadership roles within key women's health advocacy organizations, and many others were instrumental in either the founding or staffing of health clinics.[1]

For example, Dr. Mary Howell, who received the National Women's Health Network's first Physician Service Award, was one of fourteen women admitted to Harvard Medical School in 1958. By the end of their first year, seven of them had left the program. Howell was the only member of her class who was married and a mother. In the late 1960s, she was teaching pediatrics at Harvard Medical School and serving as its dean of student affairs. That women's experiences in medical education still so closely resembled her own spurred her to undertake a survey of 146 women students from forty-one different medical schools in the United States (Ruzek 1978, 85). In 1973, under the pseudonym Mary A. Campbell—she feared that Harvard would "not be receptive to the book's message" (Benjamin 1995, 1)—Howell published *Why Would a Girl Go into Medicine? Medical Education in the United States: A Guide for Women,* a scorching analysis of the ways in which medical education perpetuated sexist beliefs about women patients and imposed overt and covert forms of discrimination on female students.

In a speech at a national women's health conference at Harvard in 1975, Howell made a radical proposal, a school for women only "that would roughly parallel present day medical schools by training physician level providers of health care." The idea, she admits, "imperils efforts to [integrate] into the world of men those qualities that have been assigned to us as women, such as collaborative sharing of effort and responsibility, nurturance, care-giving and personal service to others." But if working within male-controlled institutions compels women to "act like men, identify with men, and adopt the characteristics of competitive individualism that have been traditionally ascribed to men," she says, a women-only medical school, which she compares to single-sex undergraduate institutions, might be the only answer (Howell 1975, 50, 53). Such a medical school was not created. But later that year, Mary Howell, Barbara Seaman, Belita Cowan, Alice Wolfson, and Phyllis Chesler founded the National Women's Health Lobby, which soon became the National Women's Health Network (NWHN). By the time the second edition of *Why Would a Girl Go into Medicine?* appeared, Mary Howell had disengaged from medical education and dropped the pseudonym. Harvard's reaction no longer mattered.

Another physician who left a lasting imprint on the women's health movement is Dr. Helen Rodriguez-Trias, a woman of Puerto Rican ancestry who was born in New York City and grew up in Puerto Rico. Rodriguez-Trias enrolled in medical school there at the age of twenty-seven. Like Howell, she was married, and by the time she graduated in 1960, she had three children. Profoundly influenced by the Puerto Rican nationalist movement, Rodriguez-Trias was no newcomer to politics when she became involved in health activism through her work at Lincoln Hospital in the Bronx, where she practiced pediatrics and eventually served as head of the Pediatrics Unit. She knew firsthand the many health issues women—especially women of color—confronted, and she understood that gender was only one dimension of their interactions with health care services, and that it was tied inextricably to the ways race and class shaped a two-tiered system. Rodriguez-Trias entered medicine "for the people"; even in medical school, in the years before organized feminism emerged, she had a budding feminist consciousness, "I thought of myself as relatively conscious about women's issues when I went into medical school, not in the sense of there being a women's movement with a defined set of women's issues, but like I think I had a woman's consciousness and I'd had children and I was very aware of what it meant to be a mother and how doctors relate to you" (Rodriguez-Trias 1997a).

Rodriguez-Trias was instrumental in the creation of an important New York–based reproductive rights organization in the mid–1970s, the Committee to End Sterilization Abuse (CESA). CESA, and its ally the Committee for Abortion Rights and against Sterilization Abuse (CARASA) took more radical positions than mainstream abortion rights groups, focusing on health and reproductive rights issues of poor women, especially poor women of color. CESA led a broad coalition effort against coercive sterilization practices, common for women of color, and helped to develop a reproductive rights, rather than a simple pro-abortion analysis that had a significant impact both in the changing reproductive rights movement and in the women's health movement.[2]

Ultimately the organization unmasked the vivid realities of ways poor women were being sterilized without their consent, finally pressuring the U.S. Department of Health, Education, and Welfare to issue guidelines for sterilization procedures designed to correct some of the abuses by then widespread in the United States. Noncompliance with even these relatively weak guidelines was commonplace, and Rodriguez-Trias and CESA pushed for stronger regulation that resulted in more stringent guidelines in New York City public and then private hospitals. Based on the success in New York, activists in other communities took up the battle against coercive sterilization. Finally, after considerable pressure from CESA and other groups, the Department of Health Education and Welfare strengthened their guidelines (Krase 1996, 1, 4–5).

CESA's strong insistence on defining reproductive rights broadly was an important early influence on the growing awareness of how racism and class shaped differences in women's health needs and issues. Sterilization abuse might be seen as a human rights issue, Rodriguez-Trias explained, but it was more important to identify whom "it was happening to and why, and to examine what this meant in terms of maintaining society as it is" (Shapiro 1985, 144). Rodriguez-Trias and others in CESA, and later in CARASA, also took aim at the population-control establishment. A charter member of the National Women's Health Network, Rodriguez-Trias served on its board of directors in the 1970s, shaping priorities, emphasizing the need to ensure reproductive freedom and safe, affordable contraception for all, and monitoring national health policy to guarantee that the voices of poor women and communities of color were heard.

When Dr. Mary Howell published *Why Would a Girl Go into Medicine?* in 1973, only 978 (less than 6 percent) of the 16,500 fellows of the American College of Obstetrics and Gynecology were women (Seaman 1975, 43). Some women physicians, like Dr. Terry Brock (a pseudonym), defined themselves as feminists and believed in many of the tenets of the women's health movement. Brock had participated in antiwar, civil rights, and early feminist consciousness-raising activities in college and in medical school, and she worked at several feminist and community clinics in California as a way of extending her political commitments into her early professional life. Only about 10 percent of her medical school classmates were women, Brock recalls, and she felt that she was "being tested all the time" there. Working at feminist clinics proved an "antidote to establishment medicine . . . [T]he health collective, where it was all women, . . . was very supportive and nurturing, more than my experience and training had been" (Brock 1991).

In the early 1970s, Brock served as medical director at a feminist clinic and oversaw a gynecology practice staffed by lay medics. "They were very careful and insecure," she remembers, "so that if there was anything other than routine, I think they would come to me." Brock's assessment is that the medics "got pretty good at doing just regular, general gynecology checkups and doing

Pap smears and solving routine gynecology problems." But even for a feminist, it was challenging to practice medicine in feminist clinics.

> There was sometimes a problem in not knowing how much people knew. Even though there was ongoing training ... and a lot of the people were very bright and they were very motivated ... They had a fairly narrow focus ... They didn't have the background in physiology, anatomy, or pharmacology, or any of the other stuff that I had ... And so there were times when we didn't understand each other on that level ... because there was a big discrepancy in our training and background.

In her year at the clinic, Brock learned "certain ways of dealing with patients that were ... valuable in terms of treating them as equals, or ... sharing information with them, the kind of thing that is not particularly the way we are taught in medical school ... I learned a lot more about contraception and minor GYN problems than I learned in medical school." She left the clinic because she wanted to treat a broader range of medical problems and because she was "ready to make some actual money," but she served as a referral and back-up doctor for the clinic for many years afterward, and she forged lasting personal and professional relationships with "half a dozen" other women during this "very important time" in her life. "Medicine has changed in a lot of ways, particularly women's medicine and obstetrical care, and although it's not like it's moved to the ideal, things are different today. What the women's health movement said and did was a real revelation to a lot of people and it isn't anymore. But it's probably easier for a young woman to find a sympathetic, feminist-minded physician ... than it was twenty years ago."

Brock also observes that issues that seemed so important back then had faded for her by the early 1990s.

> In the years I have been in practice we have always kept a mirror near the exam table. And I used to always, you know, ask if women wanted to see their cervix. People used to say sometimes, occasionally ... "oh yeah." They had never heard of it and were fascinated the way everyone used to be. And then some would say no ... Now I would say over the years the "no's" far outweigh the "yes's" so that I don't routinely offer anymore ... If I find something unusual I am liable to say "hey I want you to look at this". ... I think having a curiosity about it, knowledge about one's anatomy is certainly positive ... But I think that now that it's sort of experiencing the harsh realities of trying to run a practice and take care of a lot of people and make a living, it's sort of like you don't have the luxury ... There was something very nice about it and if people want to do it, it's fine.

Another physician who played a key role in one of the early feminist health clinics is Dr. Mary Jane Gray, a founder of the Vermont Women's Health Clinic, one of the first feminist abortion providers in the United States. Gray joined the faculty of the medical school at the University of Vermont after years of practicing medicine in New York. Both in New York and Vermont she had served on hospital committees that heard appeals from women seeking medical abortions in the years before abortion was legal. Gray came to believe that women, not their doctors, should be the final arbiters of the decision to have an abortion. "People expected me to be sympathetic to them because I was a woman more so than in the beginning I was. At Columbia Presbyterian I was caught up in the refer-them-to-committees-and-evaluate-their-reasons process, trying to decide whether they deserved an abortion or not. And the more women I talked to the more it seemed clear that no one could decide except the woman herself" (Gray 1999). Gray found her views and practices diverging from those of many of her colleagues. "I came into the women's health movement from gynecology, and really from my patients, from dealing with their problems and from finding that some of my male colleagues didn't approve of the things I did. For example, when I first came to Vermont my chair and boss was very upset because I prescribed contraceptives to unmarried women. I realized that I had a different perspective on things than many of my male colleagues did" (Gray 1999).

For years, Gray had chaired a group that worked to liberalize abortion legislation in Vermont, and when that legislation was declared invalid, she sought to set up an abortion clinic at the hospital. But because her colleagues had very different positions on abortion, and because the hospital was involved in merger negotiations with a Catholic institution, it became clear that establishment of a free-standing abortion clinic was the only choice. Gray describes the process, telling a story I heard over and over again about movement organizations.

> The original collective was on a totally first name basis and I didn't originally know who many of these people were or what they did. It was so much an equality kind of thing that people tried to conceal their qualifications. But I gradually became aware that we had a bacteriologist and a pharmacologist and some nurses in the group, and all kinds of people who knew what they were doing and were also trying to get along with everyone as equals and do everything collectively. (Gray 1999)

Within ninety days, the clinic staff was providing one hundred abortions and seeing three hundred patients a month. In 1976, Gray and a colleague published a paper in the *American Journal of Obstetrics and Gynecology* describing the clinic's philosophy, its services, and the internal (between feminists and the medical establishment) and external (pickets and a ballot referendum to outlaw the clinic) challenges its organizers and staff faced over several years (Gray and Tyson 1976). They concede that "a deep philosophical division" existed between "those representing establishment values (a majority) . . . and a small but determined and articulate group of young women" who wanted the clinic to advance feminist goals (761). Gray and Tyson report that "physicians working in the center were threatened initially by the lack of a rigid medical hierarchy coupled with the existence of an atmosphere in which their judgment could be freely questioned." But eventually, "recognition of the genuine concern for the patient felt by all persons working in the clinic, respect for the increasing level of medical information held by all staff members, and the fact that the physician maintained the right to make a final decision in medical matters led to acceptance of the working conditions and a sense of sharing" (764).

Gray locates herself on the border between traditional medicine and the women's health movement: "I was as radical as you could be as a doctor and as conservative as you could be in the movement."

> I was always worried they were going to do something screwy that would get them in trouble . . . I had no great objection to women doing pelvics on each other, but I didn't think they were going to be able to tell as much about what they were finding as people who spend their lives doing it. Yet I always had that kind of wary, what are they going to do next approach. My male colleagues thought I was way out on the fringe, though I had solid medical training so they could not fault me on what I did medically. (Gray 1999)

Gray had confronted more than her share of sexism in medicine, a point she reiterated throughout her interview. There was "a lot of truth" in the basic feminist critique of doctors, she argued, and for years she saw herself as a translator between physicians and women's health activists, a role she felt obligated to play (Gray 1999). Always a pragmatist, she believed that she had "a responsibility to try and speak for women in areas where they had no voice. I wasn't as strong at it as I sometimes think I should have been, but I was as strong as I could be. I was practicing full time and I did have four stepchildren I was raising and a husband who was the old-fashioned helpless kind. So I didn't spend a lot of time philosophizing" (Gray 1999). She took her role as translator seriously, and she believes the movement has made a difference:

> Most doctors thought the women's health movement . . . was sort of a nuisance, and then they realized they were really going to have to change things. There was a time when I was off a lot giving talks to medical doctors, sort of

trying to explain what it was that the women wanted because they were having trouble understanding. Women had an interest in knowing what was going on. They resented the paternalistic approach of men. They wanted choices, things explained and I think they wanted control of their sexual lives without the sense they were being judged by their physician. This was one of the things that bothered women a lot, and it was a time when sexual mores were changing and doctors were often on the conservative side of things. But I think they know now that it is not their business to tell women what they ought to be doing. (Gray 1999)

Another feminist physician/activist is Dr. Margaret Gordon (a pseudonym), a psychiatrist who founded a feminist mental health collective with other psychiatrists, social workers, and psychologists, all of them veterans of civil rights or radical left organizations.

We would talk, really talk about both the way we were treated as women and how our patients were treated. And then over time [their discussions took place over three years] we evolved to this idea we wanted to practice together. That we wanted to do things differently than our training, that we wanted to run our practices differently... And then we had a retreat in which there was a kind of put up or shut up meeting. You know, did people really want to cast in their lots together and become financially dependent on each other and income share and all that. A certain number of people left at that point, saying I want a regular paycheck... But you know I mean, if anyone had framed it as going into business for yourself, I mean that's not how we were thinking, but in a certain way it was what we were doing. (Gordon 1991)

The political histories and investments of this group of white, middle-class mental health professionals guided them to seek out and then work with a group of white, working-class women from a neighboring community who wanted to provide primary health care for women and children. In 1973 the merged groups of middle- and working-class women opened a women's health clinic in a predominantly white, working-class area of a large northeastern city. The mental health collective, incorporated as a nonprofit independent of the clinic, occupied the same building, but the money the therapists earned did not go into the larger pot of the clinic. Nevertheless, they participated in the clinic's activities. "It had been a very organic step from the point of view of the mental health collective to say we wanted to work with the health clinic. They're willing to have us come. I mean, for them, it was an offer of six free part time staff people." Gordon worked "as a regular doc for awhile. I mean at that point I wasn't that far from my internship and could still really do physicals and that sort of thing"; she also served as patient advocate and performed the same tasks the lay (and working-class) staff members did.

Gordon worked with the health collective from the beginning, over a five-year period punctuated by frequent conflicts within the clinic. Tensions emerged, particularly between some of the clinic's paid staff (almost all of whom were working-class women from the community) and members of the mental health collective. Five years after the merger, the coalition collapsed. Gordon agreed in principle with the clinic's egalitarian ideology, but her experience in medical school and her professional training gave her a different perspective on leadership, process, and the work environment. "Part of the ideology was that there shouldn't be an enormous division of labor along professional lines," Gordon says, "and that idea appealed to us, but I think having been through an internship and a residency and you move into a situation [the clinic] that was chaotic and you're used to a certain way—making structure and making things, you know you are work oriented. You are not particularly process oriented. I mean I am about as process oriented as they come for docs." Making structure was the rock on which the cross-class alliance failed. But members of the mental health collective stayed together. "We still exist, and we are still an income-sharing group and we are still a licensed clinic and we are still in business. We don't think we are making revolution anymore. But we practice a fairly radical feminist brand of mental health psychotherapy. And we teach it to others."

Gordon's statement reminds us that many health care providers who practice today have been deeply influenced by the women's health movement. It would be wrong to assume that the only feminist health care practiced in the last quarter century unfolded within clinics that self-identified as feminist. In the 1970s and later, movement organizations funneled many workers into medical school and the practice of medicine. Terry Brock recalls that at a health clinic reunion in the early 1980s, she was stunned by how many lay workers, inspired by the rewards of their interactions with patients and frustrated with limitations on nonlicensed practitioners, had become health care professionals themselves. Margaret Gordon also referred to a cohort of young women, often just out of college, who used "two or three years in the health clinic to figure out that they wanted to go on to professional training and went and did that, including———, who went to medical school and became a doc."

In the last quarter century, the landscape and population of medical schools have changed very dramatically. By the early 1990s, women constituted 18 percent of all physicians and 42 percent of all medical students (Bickel and Kopriva 1993, 141). By 2000, 36 percent of practicing gynecologists were women and women held an astonishing 70.3 percent of residencies in obstetrics and gynecology in the United States, compared with less than 50 percent ten years before, creating what Dr. John Musich, chairman of the Council on Resident Education in Obstetrics and Gynecology calls a "huge issue for male medical students" (Lewin 2001, 1). But such gains don't guarantee equality. Studies in the early 1990s showed that more than half of women physicians experienced regular gender discrimination (Ulstad 1993, 75); that women doctors earned from 59 percent to 63 percent of men's annual mean net income (Bickel and Kopriva 1993, 142); and that women are underrepresented on medical school faculties (42) and in powerful leadership positions within medical institutions and medical research (Taylor 1994, 147–148).

Today's women physicians have been primary beneficiaries of feminism and, in particular, of the activism of the women's health movement. Mary Jane Gray believes that one of the movement's most lasting effects is that it led women to choose careers in health care, a change that transcends just "adding [more women] and stir[ring]." "I think it helped to push more women into the specialty, helped push men into changing their approach to women patients, in trying not to be paternalistic towards them, and pushed [medicine] more toward education and explanation and trying to empower women and give them choices" (Gray 1999).

The question of how the influx of women into medicine has affected health care professions is largely beyond the scope of this book. However, it is important at least to note that some women physicians, influenced by second-wave feminism, have established or rejuvenated women's organizations such as the American Medical Women's Association (AMWA). Founded in 1915 as the Medical Women's National Association, and essentially dormant for several decades, the American Medical Women's Association was revitalized in the 1970s by a "core of active feminists who were tired of their marginality within the profession and women physicians' weak group consciousness" (Morantz-Sanchez 1985, 274–275).[3] In 1982, when the AMWA hired a new managing editor for its journal, the decision to hire this individual was couched in terms that strongly suggest the influence of feminism and the women's health movement on this organization. The new editor is described as having a philosophy "in keeping with the more feminist direction of the organization. Since then, strong efforts have been made to investigate and expose the more hidden difficulties women physicians experience balancing home and careers, as well as to provide a balanced *female* professional approach to some of the important health issues for women which have been raised over the last decade by the women's movement" (343).

In 1990, another group of physicians and other health professionals organized the Society for the Advancement of Women's Health Research and two years later launched a new journal about women's health because of their concern "that the health of all American women was at risk due to biases in medical and health research" (*Journal of Women's Health* 1992, xxi).

Although there was surely considerable overlap between the agendas of these professional organizations and the grassroots women's health movement, their philosophies often clashed. Physician Anne Colston Wentz, editor-in-chief of the *Journal of Women's Health,* used her bully pulpit in 1994 to deride the "antidoctor" attitude she had seen at a series of recent women's health conferences. Wentz's editorial is interesting in part because it shows what has not changed in relationships between physicians and health movement advocates. "Certainly, the thinking was different in medicine 25 years ago, when some of us who were training to be gynecologists wondered why anyone would even want to diagnose her own case of *Trichomonas* vaginitis" [a reference to the practice of cervical self-examination] (Wentz 1994, 249). Wentz alluded to the importance feminism attaches to recognition of differences among women, using that principle to point out what she believes to be unfair generalizations by health movement activists, "Can you imagine, then, my surprise, my discomfiture, my alienation, my sadness, and yes, my anger, to find that women seem to think that medicine and we who practice it are homogeneous. We are thought to be all the same, all alike, and not good" (249). Such charges are inaccurate, she contends, as part of a strong argument about the need for activists and doctors to work more closely together, "We need to get this women's health thing together and have people work together for change. It can't be a we-against-you situation when the bottom line is basically the same. We are not going to be able to reframe women's health without physicians, leaders in women's health, men and women all buying into the idea of change and working together to get the job done" (250).

Rosemary Pringle, a feminist scholar who has studied the changing power and authority of women in medicine over the past quarter century, agrees that even today women physicians are "regarded ambivalently by some feminists" (1998, 1). "There is the heroic past, when they [women physicians] played a key part in the history of feminism, scaling the heights of patriarchal power to gain entry to the profession, enduring ridicule and hostility from male doctors and medical students. And then there is the present, when women doctors, in the main, are seen as a conservative group with little sympathy for feminist causes" (1). Nevertheless, Pringle believes that activists recognize that women doctors "have navigated a turbulent field and both transformed and been transformed by it," that they "may be understood as structuring agents in restructuring the field" (217–218).

Pringle's research focuses on the relationship of physicians and the women's health movement in Britain and Australia, where national health services and labor governments often provided funding directly to women's health centers, thus integrating movement principles more fully into the mainstream system of health care delivery. The situation in the United States is, of course, different, but even as interactions between physicians and feminist health activists have grown less adversarial, the fundamental critique of physician dominance remains the movement today.

A basic principle of feminist health activism, especially in the clinic sector of the movement, was to provide well-women care, to carve out a territory that offered routine, preventive reproductive services, birth control and Pap tests and breast examinations, as well as interventions such as abortion. But women's relationships with physicians extend beyond reproductive health care, indeed beyond well-women care. In the late 1980s and 1990s breast cancer activism politicized women's relationships with oncologists, surgeons, and other doctors involved in the treatment of this all-too-common disease. While extensive analysis of breast cancer activism is beyond the scope of this book, it is important to recognize that this new focus of the movement shifted aspects of the movement's rhetoric and goals, as well as relationships with physicians.

Although the first edition of *Our Bodies, Ourselves* made only brief references to breast, cervical, or uterine cancers, BWHBC included several pages on these diseases in the 1973 edition. In 1975, in *Breast Cancer: A Personal History and Investigative Report*, Rose Kushner, a medical journalist, questioned such practices as the infamous "one-step" protocol that forced women to consent to mastectomy before they were even certain that they had cancer.[4] African American theorist and poet Audre Lorde added her powerful voice to Kushner's when she described her journey through an often-oppressive medical system in *The Cancer Journals* (1980), another now-canonical text of the women's health movement. By 1984, *The New Our Bodies, Ourselves* included a chapter called "Some Common and Uncommon Health and Medical Problems," with much expanded information about breast cancer and breast problems (written by the Breast Cancer Study Group); other cancers affecting women; and chronic illnesses such as arthritis, diabetes, heart disease, and stroke. In 1994, in *Patient No More: The Politics of Breast Cancer,* journalist Sharon Batt writes about her experience of breast cancer, her treatment by medical professionals, and the emerging breast cancer movement. Like an earlier generation of women's health movement activists, these writers challenge the protocols for treatment of women with breast cancer as they make clear they will no longer be, to use Batt's turn of the phrase, patient patients.

Ellen Leopold argues in *A Darker Ribbon: Breast Cancer, Women, and Their Doctors in the Twentieth Century* (1999) that breast cancer differs in important ways from most of the other issues that attracted the attention of health activists. This is "largely a contest between women and the medical establishment," she says (200). It excludes questions of reproductive rights and does not excite the political energies of lawyers, religious activists, or the right wing. Relationships between women and their surgeons and oncologists are often quite different than their relationships with obstetricians and gynecologists, "When the battle joined patriarchy with pathology, a different dynamic arose. Where male authority and expertise were believed to be tied up with life-saving skills, the habitual female response of total surrender was much harder to dislodge. If the physician was all that stood between a newly diagnosed woman and death, it would be not just foolish but possibly suicidal to put sexism over survival. Who would risk it, for the sake of principle?" (249). Nevertheless, Leopold says, although the disease remains very much the province of high-tech medicine, the power of "the surgeon as healer-in-charge has been much diluted" (262).

Breast cancer activists set out to gather and disseminate information so that women can exert more control over the many decisions they face once they are diagnosed, and they could build on the strong foundation of empowerment through information that had long been the heart of the women's health movement. As they clamored for more research, access to mammography (including coverage of the procedure by health insurance), less invasive and radical surgical techniques, and information about and access to alternative therapies, breast cancer activists reprised the first phase of the women's health movement. They demanded that their doctors give them opportunities to be active decision makers in their treatment.[5] They also demanded a place at the table where decisions about research funding priorities could be made. Their presence there dramatically increased monies for breast cancer research.

But feminist health activists have been unable to dislodge the dominant paradigm that underlies most medical research, including breast cancer research—a biomedical model that is innocent of the environmental and social causes of illness and of the ways race, gender, and class hierarchies structure access to disease prevention and treatment. It was almost two decades ago that Byllye Avery and other women of color pointed out that although the incidence of breast cancer is actually lower among African American women, they are far more likely to die of the disease than European American women because they are less likely to have early access to state-of-the-art treatment. Many breast cancer activists believe that there are powerful environmental reasons behind the soaring rate of breast cancer;[6] but most medical researchers prefer to pursue genetic causes and other triggers that are less likely to run up against the interests of corporate America. Despite the long road ahead for health movement activism focused on the priorities of research funding and treatment of illnesses such as breast cancer, the extension of feminist concern to these issues has required new strategies and relationships with physicians.

The Changer and the Changed

There is no doubt that the women's health movement led to major changes in how obstetrics and gynecology are practiced in this country. Because of the complex array of different forces that impinge on medical practice today, it would be difficult to prove a strict cause-and-effect relationship between feminist health activism and health care reform. To use the words of feminist songwriter Chris Williamson, the relationship between the changer and the changed is both mutual and fluid.

Consciousness raising set the stage for women's empowerment in health care decision making. But the rising cost of delivery of services counted, too. Between 1960 and 1990, total health care spending rose at an annualized rate of nearly 6 percent after adjustment for changes in the overall price level as measured by the GDP deflator (Organization for Economic Cooperation and Development [OECD] 1992, 9). During the 1960s, with implementation of Medicare and Medicaid, the rate of growth exceeded 6 percent; between 1970 and 1990 health spending grew at an annual rate of 5.5 percent in excess of inflation, twice as fast as the GDP (9). By 1990 the United States was spending $660 billion a year on health care, almost 12 percent of GNP, as compared with the early 1960s, when health care spending amounted to about 6 percent of GNP (Ropes 1991).

Rising costs translate into a relatively simple reality for ordinary people. Those who are privately insured pay higher premiums and out-of-pocket expenses for services and for prescription drugs and dread the loss of such benefits. For those who rely on government-sponsored third-party insurance (Medicaid, Medicare, Champus), the new reality includes changes in eligibility standards, loss or reduction of benefits, and stigmatization. For the growing numbers of uninsured working families, the new reality makes access to health care an almost impossible dream. At any given moment, about 15 percent of those under sixty have no insurance coverage, with children accounting for more than one-quarter of the uninsured (37). Access to health care and health insurance is even more limited for African Americans and other people of color (Byrd and Clayton 2000). These ordinary people are among the clients who use the services of women's health clinics. Many are unable to pay even reduced or sliding-scale fees.

Of course, rising costs disproportionately impact small health organizations and those with marginal financial profiles. As hospitals and physicians struggle to control expenses for personnel, laboratory services, medical supplies, and malpractice insurance (and pass increments on to their clients when they can't), feminist clinics fight to maintain their ideological commitment to affordable service delivery even as they struggle to stay in business.

Beginning in the late 1970s, but especially in the period following Reagan's election to the presidency in 1980, national policies reversed federal engagement in expanding access to health care, just as the government reduced overall social spending and reinforced a competitive market model for the medical system (McBride and McBride 1994). As part of that competitive model, many hospitals and some physician-owned groups began to develop women's health centers to provide comprehensive primary health care for women. Although changing cultural ideas about women and women's greater political and economic power are usually regarded as partial explanations for these new centers—the demand for which was inspired by the women's health movement—the major driving force in their creation was the increasingly competitive market-driven environment of health care (Looker 1993; Weisman et al. 1995). In fact, women's medicine is one of the major "diversification strategies" hospitals have looked to as they sought to compensate for revenues lost by reductions in in-patient days (largely a response to changes in insurance reimbursement policies) and other shortfalls attributable to changes in demand for and use of obstetrical and gynecological care. For example, as the women's health movement redefined the birthing process as a routine, nonmedical event (except in relatively infrequent cases), many new mothers opted to shorten their postdelivery hospital stays. Later in the 1980s, insurance companies saw this phenomenon as an opportunity to cut costs, and began to enforce very short post-partum stays for delivering mothers.

The new, for-profit women's health centers have adapted some of the ideas and practices developed in the feminist, women-controlled clinics of the 1970s. They aim at a demedicalized look for their facilities, and their rhetoric adopts key features of the feminist model. Patty Looker summarizes the philosophy of what are, in fact, a diverse lot of facilities as

> collaborative . . . based on dialogue between provider and client-team . . . oriented . . . education centered, based on the belief that women want, need and deserve the most current information about all aspects of their health over their lifespan . . . wellness and prevention concentrated. . . comprehensive . . . client focused and empowering, established on the premise that the individual woman knows her situation best and has ultimate control over her own health; gender specific . . . caring . . . and pro-woman, showing by

the character of services delivered that the lived experience of women is interesting, valuable, and worthy of respect . . . Part of this philosophy has been expressed in the predominance of women serving women in these centers. (Looker 1993, 98–99)

By the mid–1990s there were about thirty-six hundred women's health centers in the United States, the overwhelming majority of which focus on reproductive health care (Weisman et al. 1995, 106). Although these new centers have effectively used the ideas of the women's health movement in their marketing campaigns, they are in no sense alternative health care providers. Instead, they operate under professional control; their policies are dictated by hospital boards and administrators or by the physicians—some of them women—who are their owners. For the most part, the professional, administrative, and other staff of these facilities are female (Weisman et al. 1995, 107). They emphasize those aspects of the feminist health care model most amenable to mainstream medicine. A recent study reveals that almost all the new centers endorsed the same goal: provision of services in a caring, sensitive manner that empowers women to take control of their own health care and involves shared decision-making between provider and client (113).

But what is incorporated into this reformed medical model and what is left behind? What does it mean to empower women to take control of their health care in this institutional context? Clear political goals inform the service models and the organizational policies of the feminist clinics; for many of the new women's health centers, especially those linked with hospitals, the underlying rationale is to gain a competitive edge by providing services at a profit. Few deny the economic agenda of the centers. Sally Rynne, president of Women's Healthcare Consultants and director of one of the earliest hospital-sponsored women's health centers, has made a career out of using market research and bottom-line arguments to help hospitals develop strategies to recruit patients from among the 11 to 33 percent of women between the ages of twenty-four and fifty-five who are "disassociated and dissatisfied" with their current provider. This target group, Rynne asserts, challenges hospitals to "match philosophies and programs with the dreams and desires of the marketplace" (Rynne 1989, x). Women's health care has always been a profitable endeavor for modern medicine (obstetrics-gynecology is one of the more lucrative specialties), and today is no exception.

How does this basic difference—a social change goal for the feminist clinics and an economic bottom line for many of the new, hospital-linked or doctor-owned women's health centers—affect how they provide services and work to empower women to take control of their health care? As our 1990 survey indicates, most feminist facilities espouse political goals and incorporate social activism into ongoing organizational activities; they see women's health status and health care as deeply affected by unjust power relations and multiple forms of discrimination. Feminist clinics don't just inform clients about the special nutritional needs of pregnancy, for example. They also seek to help consumers understand the effects of cuts in social welfare programs such as WIC, food stamps, and welfare on women's health, and sometimes they help mobilize women to fight against such cuts. The newsletters of the feminist clinics have more political substance and take a more critical view of health and social policies than the informational materials and newsletters of the hospital-linked and physician-owned centers, and they don't shy away from controversial issues such as abortion. Rather, they proclaim women's right to reproductive choice.

Another significant difference between feminist and mainstream health centers is their client base. Most alternative women-controlled facilities have developed mechanisms to ensure that their fees and payment practices don't exclude low-income women. Although the free or very low-cost services of the 1970s have given way to higher, but usually still moderate, fees, feminist clinics assign priority to serving women of color, low-income women, lesbians, and others who encounter discrimination in mainstream medical facilities. In fact, most women-controlled clinics in our survey reported that they had focused outreach on, and increased the proportion of, women of color and low-income women who used their services.

Hospital-affiliated and physician-owned practices target women who are covered by insurance and command resources to pay for enhanced services that may cost more than those offered in traditional health settings (Kay 1989, 19). In addition to providing reimbursable clinical services to such clients, many facilities sponsor workshops or sell books and videos on topics that range from menopause to childbirth to stress reduction. These workshops and sales may generate substantial revenue. But even when they don't make profits outright, they provide a framework for thinking about health care that comes directly from the mainstream medical model, touting the benefits of estrogen replacement therapy, mental health counseling, mammography, and other revenue-promoting services. Whereas once it was enough for women to detect signs of menopause through such symptoms as hot flashes, changes in periods, and similar bodily observations, now physicians are likely to recommend blood tests that measure estrogen levels and signal the progress of menopause. This isn't demedicalization.

Bonnie Kay argues that one of the legacies of the Reagan-Bush era is an intensive commodification of women's health by and in the proliferation of the new women's health centers. Federal cuts in health and social services funding, twinned with the new emphasis on cost containment and efficiency, have replaced health planning (the assessment of community health needs with the development of services to meet those needs) with health marketing. The result? "A shift from equity to efficiency as the criterion for deciding which services are made available and accessible and to whom. Health care is whatever people will pay for—a commodity for sale" (22). The new women's health centers use the language of prevention and primary care, but their practices skew toward high-tech detection and treatment strategies. Worcester and Whatley exemplify this point with their analysis of how osteoporosis and breast cancer screening substitutes a true focus on prevention with early detection strategies, just one of the ways mainstream medicine has diluted and appropriated the feminist critique in women's health centers that are less about empowerment and more about capturing market share (Worcester and Whatley 1988).

That mainstream medicine has recognized and taken advantage of new strategies to market women's health care is well documented; the new women's health centers represent one of those strategies (Worcester and Whatley 1988; Kay 1989; Benderly 1990; Eagan 1994). It is important, however, to recognize that this market niche did not just emerge spontaneously. It was created by the hard work of feminist health activists who heightened women's awareness of the role they could play in their own health care and modeled successful medical services that expanded women's involvement and choice. Nevertheless, three decades after the foundational stories of the woman's health movement first began to write this text, the feminist, women-controlled health clinic constitutes a very small proportion of women's health care centers in the United States.

The proliferation of hospital-linked or physician-owned facilities demonstrates both the dramatic effects of the women's health movement on mainstream medicine and the resilience and power of mainstream medicine to co-opt the ideology and practices of the movement. It's clear that women today receive more information about their bodies and reproductive health care, and that in some settings they are encouraged to participate actively in their own health care by questioning their providers and asserting their own preferences and opinions. But control of women's health care remains the province of physicians and other health professionals who, although they may manage their patient's care somewhat differently than previous generations of physicians did, still manage it nonetheless.

Certainly, things have changed since that watershed year of 1969. Today, women's health constitutes a separate classification in many bookstores. Osteoporosis, breast cancer, self-esteem, cosmetic surgery, eating and sleep disorders, depression, pregnancy and childbirth, aging—we can buy books on a bewildering range of topics related to the workings of our bodies and minds. There are more women physicians at the end of the century, and there is some evidence that they treat their female patients differently than their male colleagues do. We can now buy Gyne-Lotrimin (for yeast infections) over the counter and save the cost of a doctor's visit, but we're still using a product that turns a huge profit for Burroughs Wellcome and relatively few women first try the less expensive treatments such as yogurt or vinegar and water douches. Hospitals now boast birthing rooms that look more like home; they allow family members to be present during labor and delivery; and they permit mothers to keep their babies with them in their rooms. But most women end up attached to a fetal monitor at some point (and often for long periods) during labor; and most births are attended by licensed professionals, usually doctors, not the lay midwives that the feminist birthing movement sought to put in control of this most natural of women's bodily processes.

And what of the women-controlled clinics? How have they fared in this changed environment? They are struggling for survival as they face not only the old forms of regulation and constraint by organized medicine, but now its direct competition. When women who can afford to pay for services (directly or through comprehensive health insurance coverage) are channeled to the more upscale medicalized women's health centers, business lost by community-based women-controlled clinics decreases their ability to subsidize the care that low(er)-income women need but cannot afford.

Competition has been particularly acute in recent years for feminist abortion providers, principally from Planned Parenthood Federation of America, a longtime provider of women's reproductive health care, but surely not a feminist organization (Benderly 1990; Hartmann 1995). Expanded abortion services are desperately needed in the wake of antiabortion activism that drove many clinics out of business, and most counties in the United States do not have any abortion providers at all. But despite this, an organization such as Planned Parenthood has chosen to open abortion clinics in communities already served by small feminist clinics. As Gail Sands of the Emma Goldman Clinic in Iowa City comments, "Instead of going into 'underserved' areas, Planned Parenthood targets markets that have already been set up for them by the blood, sweat and tears of feminist clinics" (Benderly 1990, 13). Staff at Emma Goldman report that Planned Parenthood representatives told them they must affiliate with that organization or compete with the lower fees that a "corporate chain" could offer (13). Emma Goldman refused to sign up.

The Feminist Women's Health Center in Chico faced the same problem. Even though the FWHC was able to meet the community's need for abortion services, Planned Parenthood established another abortion clinic there. FWHC administrator Shauna Heckert echoes Gail Sands: "They want to go where existing providers have already made abortion acceptable" (13). The financial impact on the Chico FWHC was profound, Heckert reports: "They didn't close us down but they did hurt us." And competition for clients is only one ramification of such doubling of services. When Planned Parenthood moved into Chico, the Feminist Women's Health Center also lost a large portion of its federal family planning funds to the new clinic. New Bedford Women's Health Services lost such funds to a nearby community health center the feminist staff had helped start and to which they referred clients for services they did not themselves offer.

Carol Downer warns of what will happen if the feminist clinics shut down because of competition from Planned Parenthood: "What people don't realize is when the feminist clinics are driven out, there is not going to be any later abortion available. If a woman is on drugs or has health problems, often they'll turn her away. The other providers take the cream. So it's going to have a lot of adverse effects. The feminist clinics and the clinics where women have a lot of control . . . [will] deal with the hard cases, battle the anti-abortion forces" (1990).

Although feminist clinics may represent only a tiny minority of women's medical care centers today, these clinics constitute (as they have for more than two decades) an invaluable source of innovation in medical practice. Moreover, as long as these clinics survive, they embody and exemplify a vision of health care that is different from mainstream medicine. Most important, feminist clinics and advocacy organizations articulate an approach to women's health that is fundamentally different from the biomedical model that is the core of mainstream medicine. Some feminist health activists define their model in terms of its politics—that it is about empowering women, changing social relations of power, redistributing health care resources, and changing the complexion of health policy decision making. Others, including prominent feminist health researchers Sheryl Ruzek, Adele Clarke, and Virginia Olesen contrast the biomedical model with what they see as a social model of women's health—that is, a model that recognizes the social features of health and that links health and health care to gender, race, class, and community (1997).

This politics of women's health, envisioned by countless individuals and organizations associated with the movement over the past quarter century, has had a lasting effect on mainstream medicine (Dan 1994; Ruzek, Clarke, and Olesen 1997; Weisman 1998), but it has also been powerfully affected by the changing political landscape, most particularly the ascendance of the New Right in the 1980s and the entrenchment of neoliberalism during the last two decades. The changer has also been the changed; mainstream medicine and feminist health activism have influenced each other. However, changes in the women's health movement have resulted from encounters with other powerful actors besides organized medicine.

Chapter 7

Neither Friend nor Foe

The State, the Movement, and the
Changing Political Landscape

Feminist health activists understood the overwhelming power of the state to control their bodies. The foundational stories of the women's health movement, and efforts to legalize abortion and to defend reproductive rights, emerged from the struggle to reclaim that power for themselves. The *MDeity*, whose death Belita Cowan predicted, was only the most visible representative of patriarchal control, and although many women felt their powerlessness most acutely in the presence of their doctors, state policies routinely guided those often humiliating encounters in medical offices across the country. This chapter focuses on how the state shaped and absorbed feminist health activism and how it deployed counterforce to the grassroots movement.

The state is a complex set of institutions and social practices that affect people differently, depending on their social location and the resources they bring to their multiple interactions with it. For my purposes, the term encompasses all levels of government, the law, the judicial system, and public social welfare and health bureaucracies. It cannot be understood apart from the larger political culture that dictates its policies and motivates its personnel. Pervasive social unrest marked the early days of the women's health movement, and it grew up during a period when the political landscape still echoed with the ideals and demands of powerful movements of disenfranchised groups. The New Right took root during the 1970s and by the end of that decade, it had begun decisively to influence mainstream politics. But even with Richard Nixon at the nation's helm, state policy was mightily etched with such social concerns as poverty and race and gender inequality, and with such political problems as the lingering effects of defeat in Vietnam, the rising power of OPEC, and continuing fallout from Watergate.

Frances Fox Piven has observed that much feminist theory "evinces an almost categorical antipathy" (1985, 265) to the state as it emulates and reinforces capitalist, patriarchal, and racist social relations (McIntosh 1978; Davis 1981; Eisenstein 1984; Petchesky 1984). The irony, Piven argues, is inescapable: "While women intellectuals characterize relationships with the state as 'dependence,' women activists turn increasingly to the state as the arena for political organization and influence" (1985, 265). As theorists and activists pursue their different analyses, they have become more aware of what Mimi Abramovitz, tracking the move in feminist scholarship away from this reductionist antipathy, calls the state's "paradoxical character" (1988, 10). The state functions as an arena of contestation with and a target of resistance by activists and advocates who challenge its action (and inaction), even as it constrains and shapes their oppositional social movements (Morgen 1990).

Many of the founders of the women's health movement came of political age during a time when the United States was decried as an imperialist power in Vietnam and elsewhere around the world, and when European American legislators and jurists were slowly, and many reluctantly, liberalizing civil and reproductive rights. This oppressive state, the "white, ruling class male-dominated bastion of power," was the target of political critique in the 1960s and early 1970s by the New Left and the Civil Rights, women's, and other progressive movements. But the state also promoted the War on Poverty and, increasingly, such civil rights policies as affirmative action. Activists recognized that the role of the state in the promotion of social justice was a response to the growing power of progressive social movements, and some believed that it could be used as a resource in the long, multifaceted battle for the collective empowerment of women, communities of color, and other disenfranchised groups. Even when state resources could be mobilized to further the goals of social movements, however, there was always risk: A direct relationship with the state—as regulator, funder, legal protector—could lead to cooptation of the transformative change orientation and activities that energized social movement organizations.

State policy on family planning and abortion underwent dramatic changes during the 1960s, beginning with the FDA's approval in 1960 of the commercial distribution of oral contraceptives. Before 1960, only seven states (all in the South) included family planning as part of state public health services; by 1965, half the states covered some birth control programs under their public health services (Solinger 1992, 213). In 1965 the Supreme Court invalidated state laws that prohibited the sale of contraceptives to married couples, and the Office of Economic Opportunity began to receive significant funding for family planning services for the poor. (These were the funds Edna Smith, discussed in chapter 3, captured in her efforts to promote the availability of birth control for women). Even as late as the late 1960s, one of the most powerful arguments for federal support of birth control programs was the desire to halt the epidemic of illegal abortions.

Federal funding for family planning expanded during the 1960s in response to pressure from the influential population control establishment; and in response to growing recognition of dramatic changes in women's lives: declining fertility rates, increased age at first marriage expanding participation in the labor force, and new social mores about sexuality (Petchesky 1990). State support of family planning increased in the early 1970s, too, but by then the liberalization of abortion laws was also under way, culminating in *Roe* vs. *Wade* in 1973. Feminist ideas about the state evolved in this context of changing policies in areas of great importance to women. But there was no single feminist position.

One influential sector of the women's movement had itself emerged within the state apparatus: women whose feminism was expressed through and formed by their participation in state commissions on the status of women formed in the early 1960s in the years immediately following President Kennedy's establishment of a national Commission on the Status of Women. Many of these women saw the state as the primary route for social change; they worked to influence legal reform and to promote legislation that would equalize relations between men and women; and they founded groups such as the National Organization of Women, the largest single national feminist advocacy organization, and the symbol of liberal feminism. NOW committed itself to the goals of legalization of abortion and institutionalization of affirmative action plans that opened health care professions to women.

Many of the women who worked in the clinics came from a different, more radical political background; those who had participated in the antiwar and Civil Rights movements, distrusted the state—its police, its courts, its social welfare agencies, its elected officials—and wanted to work toward the transformation of all major social and political institutions. Their attitudes about the state were also shaped by their growing sense that regulatory agencies had done little to protect women from the hazards of oral contraceptives, DES, the Dalkon Shield, and other products and procedures whose harmful effects the movement uncovered. Moreover, as the state's role in sterilization abuse, especially of women of color, become more widely understood, distrust intensified (Davis 1981, 1988; Rodriguez-Trias 1997a).

For the feminist health activists whose primary goal was to change federal,

state, and local health and reproductive rights policies, there was no alternative to active engagement with the state. Groups such as the National Women's
Health Network, the Coalition for the Medical Rights of Women (in the Bay
Area), DES Action (Berkeley), and the policy office of the National Black
Women's Health Project, represented constituents of the women's health movement in that effort. But in the clinic sector of the movement, which aimed to
be women controlled and free from the dictates and influence of health professionals and political power holders, interface with the state was more complicated. The work of the clinics was constrained, supported, and changed by
evolving relationships with different parts of the state apparatus. In most cases,
the force driving those relationships was money. Whenever clinics received
funds from state agencies, whenever they sought medical licensure that allowed
them to bill Medicaid for abortion and family planning services, they exposed
themselves to the oversight, regulation, and power of the state.

The first story in this chapter focuses on the regulatory and legal appara-
tuses of the state; the second story explores how the state funding exerted
co-optive influences on organizations. Although I want to highlight the vast
power of the state, my argument is not that the state coopted the feminist health
clinics. Rather, I show the processes through which clinics encountered, interpreted, accommodated, and resisted pressures.

Red Tape and Bureaucratic Hostility

Within the women's health movement, the history of Women's Community Health Center (WCHC), in Cambridge, Massachusetts, stands as an
antifoundational story, a narrative of uncreation that, while unique, nevertheless resonates in the organizational lives of many clinics. WCHC, activists agree,
was the focus of unrelentingly political attack by antiabortion forces powerful
enough to influence the operations of regulatory agencies in the city of Cambridge and in the Commonwealth of Massachusetts. Unresponsive, hostile, in-
transigent officials and agencies confronted women's health activists across
the country, and at every level of government.

A women-controlled collective that provided well-women gynecology and
abortion services with a strong feminist self-help orientation, WCHC opened
in 1974. The organization made a firm commitment to consensus decision making, and although its structure changed over time, it resisted hierarchy more
strenuously than many of its counterparts in the movement. During its first
year, WCHC had operated under the licenses of its physicians. Early in 1975,
the collective began the process of application for state licensure as an abortion and well-woman health care clinic. The incentive was financial. Collective
members saw licensure as a way to secure funds from a wider variety of

sources, including third-party (insurance) payers; and they believed that licensure would help the clinic attract referrals from other community agencies. In their second annual report, they predicted that the process would be "involved and complex"; they expected it to take about a year (WCHC 1976b, 3).

This history of that process is reconstructed from interviews with clinic staff involved during that period, as well as from such documents as annual reports, press releases, and correspondence with sister organizations. Clinic workers always saw the battle for licensure as a political struggle. "Women's health centers all over the country are working toward ending the medical monopoly of health care and taking back our control over our bodies. Restrictive zoning ordinances, selective enforcement of health department regulations and enactment of legislation requiring woman-owned facilities to comply with economically discriminatory building codes, are all ways that feminist health centers are being harassed" (WCHC 1977b, 1).

The first step for WCHC was to demonstrate need for the clinic's services within the area.[1] Collective members composed and filed a seventy-page application, supported by thirty letters from local agencies and individuals, and in June 1975 the Massachusetts Department of Public Health issued the Certificate of Need. Next, the clinic had to secure approval for its operation from the Cambridge Building Department (CBD). But it was difficult (almost impossible) to get consistent information from city officials about regulations around zoning and building. After a long struggle, they figured out which forms to file and what kinds of supporting documents to present. Shortly after the clinic completed this round of paperwork, CBD reported that it had lost the application. So WCHC sent the materials in again.

Late in June 1975, an electrical inspection uncovered a few minor problems that would be enumerated and explained in a letter from CBD, health collective members were told. The letter arrived a month later and WCHC made the necessary changes. In July 1975 WCHC received a Certificate of Inspection—a clean bill of health—from the Cambridge Fire Department. CBD then reinspected the building and promised a follow up-letter. A month passed. When WCHC representatives inquired about the promised letter, they were told that their documents had been lost, and that they must resubmit their application. But before they could do so, they must once again wait for specific information about building deficiencies and zoning status. It was perfectly clear now: WCHC was a moving target. With every step forward, clinic operators confronted new, some said evolving, regulatory constraints. Complete one test, and another springs up to take its place. Complete the second test, and the third, and suddenly documents disappear into the black hole of the CBD. Then start over from the beginning.

In September 1975 WCHC was inspected for the fourth time. Twice more, clinic operators filed Certificate of Occupancy forms. Three months later, they received a letter reporting the results of the September inspection. In January 1976, the Cambridge Legal Department ruled that the clinic was improperly zoned and reminded WCHC that it had still not filed Certificate of Occupancy forms. Clinic representatives demanded a meeting. They wanted to know the grounds on which the department's ruling was based; and they wanted to assert a simple fact—that they had filed Certificate of Occupancy forms five times by now. The ruling was complicated, a city official admitted, because the term *clinic* was not specified in zoning regulations, and its absence created the possibility of multiple interpretations. Moreover, zoning for the area had been changed, from business to residential, during the period of their request. Collective members responded that a nearby clinic had had no problems clarifying its zoning status, and they demanded another meeting, this time with officials from City Hall and from CBD.

After the meeting, WCHC was granted a temporary Certificate of Occupancy as "a community center some of whose services are medical." A permanent Certificate of Occupancy was issued in June 1976, after a few building renovations had been completed. The same month, WCHC passed the commonwealth's safety inspection, and at this point, combat shifted to a new arena, the Massachusetts Department of Public Health (DPH). DPH had first inspected the clinic in November 1975, when a representative of the department's Health Care Standards and Regulations Division presented to collective members a detailed list of changes they would have to make to expect licensure. The representative warned the women that they were not permitted to call the clinic a health center, or to advertise health services, until the license had been granted. In March 1976, the inspector returned to WCHC and enumerated several more areas of concern, all of which had been apparent, and not remarked upon, at the time of the first inspection. She demanded a new round of changes.

In April collective members received the inspector's latest report. It cited them for violating the proscription against advertising by posting the clinic's name on the clinic's mailbox. The women were summoned to a meeting at DPH to answer this and other complaints. At the meeting, WCHC representatives aggressively defended the organization and won admission from DPH that none of the complaints came from women who had used clinic services. More difficulties emerged in July 1976 when the Massachusetts Department of Public Safety refused to authorize the clinic's final plans until zoning problems were cleared up. But the zoning dispute was ongoing, and WCHC was not setting the timetable.

In April 1977 the clinic filed an appeal with the Department of Public Safety. A new DPH official reinspected the clinic that month (the previous inspector had died) and informed collective members that some WCHC statements, copies of agreements, and responses to prior inspections had been lost. Because the clinic had copies of all materials and of mailing receipts, the official accepted their documentation. But on several important points, her inspection contradicted past inspections. In a letter to supporters, collective members reported that the official had "recommended that we withdraw our application and made several threatening remarks about closing us down" (WCHC 1977b).

It was at this moment that WCHC decided to go public about the endlessly repeating pattern of regulatory harassment. In a letter dated May 10, 1977, clinic operators detailed their experiences with local and state agencies during more than two years of efforts to secure state licensure. "We have acted in good faith . . . and . . . tried to comply with the regulatory agencies . . . We are no longer naively expecting positive results from our . . . compliance" (WCHC 1977b). They also kicked off a series of public forums and informational meetings about the history of lost records and applications, of contradictory inspection reports, of lengthy delays. The letter reaffirmed their goal: "ending the medical monopoly of health care and taking back control over our bodies." It also asserted that their experience was familiar to women's health organizations in other parts of the country, citing the examples of FWHCs in Tallahassee and Los Angeles.

Licensing protocols did not operate as advertised to protect public health, they charged. Rather, such protocols ensured that officials of the Commonwealth of Massachusetts would enjoy many, many opportunities to exercise discriminatory discretion against an oppositional group whose approach to health care undermined the power of mainstream medicine. "It has become clear to us in trying to meet the requirements that quality of care is not the issue," clinic representatives wrote. "In fact, quality of care provided at Women's Community Health has never been seriously disputed . . . We are a small, anti-profit organization without the financial resources and ready-made connections frequently employed to cut through the copious red tape licensure involves" (WCHC 1977a, 15).

Although they had long believed that antiabortion forces were behind their licensure woes, the relationship between "compulsory pregnancy advocates" (their term) and Massachusetts politicians became perfectly obvious in fall 1977 when Rep. Raymond Flynn repeated—in many public venues, with coverage in print and electronic media—false charges by antichoice groups that WCHC was an unlicensed and illegal abortion clinic. Strictly speaking, WCHC was providing abortions without a clinic license. But DPH policy allowed facilities to operate under the licenses of their physicians while they waited for licensure. And, of course, the process had already dragged on for a long time due to the hostility of CBD and DPH officials.

As a member of the legislature's Committee on Post Audit and Oversight, which had been investigating DPH records and activities related to abortion services, Flynn was in a position to do further damage. The committee asked the commonwealth's attorney general to rule on the question of whether health facilities should be allowed to provide abortions during the licensure process. Although the attorney general declined to issue a ruling, he pressured DPH to take action against unlicensed clinics. As a result of that pressure, DPH set a deadline by which WCHC must meet all requirements for licensure or be closed. The clinic responded in two ways. First, collective members conducted an intensive political campaign against the false charges and regulatory harassment. They organized a letter-writing blitz to demand that DPH allow the clinic to operate while licensure was pending. This effort proved so successful that the attorney general actually contacted the clinic to ask that the flood of letters be stopped, and the Post Audit Committee accused WCHC of harassing its members (WCHC 1979, 11). The collective also abandoned the attempt to gain licensure at its current location, opting to devote six months to intensive fund-raising for the move to a more suitable building. Negative publicity about WCHC made negotiations with prospective landlords more difficult.

Women's Community Health finally secured clinic licensure after two years—on April 25, 1978. In the center's fifth annual report, collective members drew the unavoidable conclusion: "red tape can be used for conscious harassment" (1979, 10). Although its long withheld license surely represented a victory for WCHC, the Post Audit Committee investigation of DPH policy led to change. Clinics would no longer be allowed to operate while application for licensure was under way. This looked like a fatal financial obstacle for small community or consumer groups that wanted to organize their own clinics, and there was more. DPH issued new reporting requirements that demanded information about every woman who had an abortion in Massachusetts, and about every physician who performed the procedure. Along with other abortion providers, WCHC objected to the new requirements because they violated the right of privacy and could compromise confidentiality, and because they would make it easy to compile and distribute lists of participating doctors, thus exposing them to public harassment. Although they succeeded in limiting the information they would be required to report, the clinic staff knew that the guidelines could be changed at any time, and they worried that the election of an antichoice governor (which happened that year) could lead to other battles about reporting requirements.

The struggle to obtain the clinic license involved the organization in considerable debt and the antiabortion movement flexed its muscles more and more insistently as neoconservatives advanced their political agenda. By summer 1981, a "bleak financial picture, combined with an equally bleak financial projection" (WCHC 1981, 1) forced the center's closure. In a letter to supporters, collective members referenced their "years of existence as a small business in an increasingly depressed economy," and their attempts "to create and maintain financial and staff stability as a low-volume, privately funded, non-profit feminist health center . . . In large part, we see the Health Center as a victim of the New Right and depression economics, and are enraged that so many years of good, hard, productive work still leaves us with no other option" (WCHC 1981, 2). WCHC was only one of the organizational victims of the increasing power of the New Right to influence state policy.

Dirty Money and Strings Attached

Feminist health activists did not enter lightly into decisions to seek state funds to operate their clinics. They understood that strings attached to government funding could undermine their autonomy and thwart their political ideals. But even though suspicions about the consequences of state funding were widespread, so, too, were financial pressures that inched the women's health centers toward those resources. Clinics always found it difficult to generate sufficient revenues from client fees, donations, and small-scale fundraising. Organizations that did not provide abortions—the most lucrative of the health services offered by feminist clinics—were most vulnerable to those pressures. Moreover, clinics that tailored their offerings toward lower-income women found fee-for-service an unreliable reimbursement model. Their clients did not command adequate individual or collective resources to support clinic staff, equipment, laboratory services, rent or mortgage payments, and insurance premiums.

So women's health centers looked to the state to fund some of their services, either through direct grants or through contracts with state and (often state-funded) nonprofit agencies. Many sought Medicaid reimbursement for health services, including abortions. Each strategy that supported public and third-party payments increased the clinics' dependence on the state, and although local impacts varied, different clinics confronted what was essentially the same problem: how to secure vital state resources without bowing to forces that threatened to co-opt the radical goals of the women's health movement.

The involvement of movement organizations with the state is part of a much larger trend in the 1960s and 1970s, and coincided with a dramatic expansion of the federal government's social welfare functions, especially as President

Johnson's Great Society programs responded to the contemporary upsurge in social activism. After World War II, the federal government had begun to increase its role in funding social services through subsidies to local and state welfare agencies and through grants to nonprofit organizations (Smith and Lipsky 1993, 50). Although these efforts paled in comparison with the GI Bill of Rights and related federal programs that scholars now see as crucial to the subsidization of a growing middle class in the postwar years (Brodkin 1998), there is no question that an expansion of the federal government's role in social welfare had begun even before the turbulence of the 1960s, when a series of legislative initiatives—declaration of the War on Poverty, passage in 1964 of the Economic Opportunity Act, and legislation that implemented Medicaid and Medicare—precipitously inflated expenditures for social welfare and health care. Between 1965 and 1969, federal spending for education, training, employment, social service, and health programs rose from just over $1.6 billion a year to $8.2 billion (Nathan, Doolittle and Associates 1987, 36). The pattern of an expanding federal social welfare role continued throughout the 1970s (Smith and Lipsky 1993), although Nixon's New Federalism departed in important ways from Johnson's Great Society agenda, and the severe recessions of that decade helped to fuel a growing conservative movement aimed at curbing big government.

But the story of expanding social services in the 1960s and 1970s is not simply a narrative of skyrocketing federal expenditures. It also tracks the rapid development of the nonprofit sector of the economy as theater of operations for the enlarged welfare state. In 1967 amendments to the Social Security Act (Title IV-A) encouraged states to enter into purchase of service agreements (contracts) with private agencies to provide services. By 1971 about one-quarter of state spending on social services went to nonprofit organizations; by 1976 the figure had doubled to almost 49 percent (Smith and Lipsky 1993, 55). This shift, of course, reverberated in the nonprofits, mightily complicating their heretofore, in some cases, oppositional relationships with the state.

Many traditional nonprofit agencies had roots in the early part of the century; many of the new nonprofits emerged in response to state legislation and funding in the wake of the mass movements of the 1950s through the 1970s. Some were government sponsored: Many community action agencies were created in association with the Office of Economic Opportunity, for example. But others sprang up from grassroots initiatives, conceived in the social movements of the period. The feminist clinics, health information and referral services, and advocacy organizations of the women's health movement, as we have seen, grew from grassroots.

Many feminist clinics sought and received state moneys in the form of grants and/or contracts from federal, state, or local agencies, as well as from private foundations. Most commonly, such funds came from Medicaid sources and from other allocations for family planning. But clinics took advantage of a range of funding opportunities from agencies as diverse as NIDA (National Institute of Drug Abuse), LEAA (Law Enforcement Assistance Act), CETA (Comprehensive Employment and Training Act), and from state and local programs funded by block grants, antipoverty programs, and county and state public health departments. Inevitably, the clinics differed in the degree to which they relied on such external funding and in their institutional responses to that funding.

For example, the Women's Health Services (WHS) was founded as a health information and referral service in the northeastern United States in the early 1970s. Lay health workers provided birth control, pregnancy, and abortion counseling; pregnancy testing; Pap smears; instruction in breast self-examination; and VD screening. Once members were able to recruit a physician (the father of one of the founders), they added gynecological exams, family planning, and post-abortion checkups. Like many other clinics across the country, WHS embraced an egalitarian ideology that emphasized social relations based on equality, women's autonomy, self-help, and collective action. In its early years the group struggled to make decisions collectively and to involve all volunteers in decision-making processes.

In 1975, the staff decided to seek external funds after they recognized two primary contradictions in their practice. First, their fees-for-services failed to generate adequate revenues and small-scale fundraising—events such as bake sales and benefit concerts—took time away from their health care service mission and from community education, and advocacy. Although WHS kept fees low, used a sliding scale, and permitted payment by promissory note, the clinic's funding structure limited clientele to those who could afford to pay and excluded Medicaid and Medicare recipients (unless they could pay for these services out-of-pocket). Until they could bill Medicaid for services, staff members believed, it would be almost impossible to attract large numbers of low-income women to the clinic. Second, they had begun to see that their reliance on an all-volunteer staff limited the services they could provide and, in effect, guaranteed that clinic workers would be skewed toward younger, white, middle-class women who could afford to volunteer their labor. To diversify staff by race and class, they would have to be able to pay salaries.

The decision to seek grants and contracts from the state was viewed among the staff as a choice between remaining pure, free from external pressures, or expanding in order to offer services and the opportunity of involvement in the center to working-class women. The choice was also conditioned by an understanding of the compelling health needs of women in the community. The community had unemployment and underemployment rates appreciably higher than average for the state; according to the 1980 census, the number of households with incomes below the poverty line (15 percent) was also higher than average, as were the number of families receiving public assistance (25 percent), and the number of census tracts deemed medically underserved.[2]

The first external funds allocated to WHS came through a small subcontract with a local agency to provide counseling services that clinic volunteers were already offering. The contract appeared to have few strings attached. It did, however, require that WHS name a director who would receive a salary to manage the contract. Until now, the group had functioned as a collective, avoiding hierarchical designations. Staff members agreed to appoint as director the one volunteer who expressed a desire for the job, but her title was to be regarded as existing on paper only. She would receive a salary to work full time; but she would have no greater power or responsibility than other workers.

With successful outreach and slow but steady growth in the numbers of women who contacted the center for services, its reputation grew. But growth brought problems. Increasingly, the small volunteer staff was unable to respond to the demand for services in a timely manner. Appointments for pregnancy tests and other procedures often had to be delayed up to a week, mimicking the practice of mainstream health and social service agencies. So WHS sought funding to hire additional paid staff. By the next year, the renewed and now larger subcontract allowed the creation of three new full- and part-time positions. More volunteers wanted the jobs now, and the group was forced to make choices among them.

The process of hiring paid employees from among those who had freely given their time to the center triggered a sense of difference among collective members. This distinction between paid staff and volunteers had practical as well as political consequences within the group. Paid staff necessarily knew more about the center's operations, and knowledge, of course, gave them more influence in decision making, particularly in administrative matters, including fund-raising. Although record keeping and contracts management was irreverently called "shit work," and was generally of less interest to volunteers who preferred to devote their more limited hours onsite to working directly with women, it soon became apparent that such information was itself empowering to those who commanded it. The pattern that emerged, a more specialized division of labor with attendant consequences for the social distribution of knowledge and influence, intensified over the next few years.

In 1976 WHS staff received notification that a federal site visit would take place the following week. The announcement from the social service agency that administered their subcontract came as a surprise, but the onsite inspection yielded high marks for the clinic in quality of services. It also mandated more extensive clinical and demographic record keeping. That meant additional administrative work, and administrative work was always burdensome. More worrying was the possibility that such records would compromise clinic policy of strict confidentiality for clients who sought sensitive services such as pregnancy testing, abortion counseling, birth control counseling and family planning, and post-abortion checks. Buoyed by positive feedback from the site visit, and indignant at the local human service agency for failing to inform them of their vulnerability to such intervention, WHS staff decided to seek their own grants and contracts.

The first of these was a grant written for a health education and training project to the local consortium responsible for administering funds from the U.S. Department of Labor for the Comprehensive Employment and Training Act program (CETA).[3] Late in 1977 WHS received just over $100,000 from CETA, funds earmarked for the employment and training of low-income persons: The grant was to subsidize salaries for fifteen women whose incomes made them eligible for Aid to Families with Dependent Children (AFDC) to work at WHS—conducting a survey of local health needs as well as providing an array of lay health and counseling services—for the following year. In a single move, WHS tripled the size of its paid staff and, for the first time in its history, hired workers who had not learned their way into the organization as volunteers.

Just before it won the CETA grant, WHS finally fulfilled the last requirement for billing Medicaid for clinical services (WHS did not have a doctor on the premises during most of its hours of operation, so it was obligated to secure a commitment from the local hospital to provide emergency backup). As of summer 1977, low-income women could seek services from the center under their Medicaid coverage. Because the paperwork associated with Medicaid billing and the CETA grant was daunting, WHS had to take another quantum leap forward in organizing its work assignments. Some de facto distinctions were already in place: Paid workers commanded more information about the center's operations than volunteers did, and the director, whose title had been merely a matter of form in 1975, exerted more power as the months passed and the center won more grants and contracts. But from now on, the division of labor and the distribution of information and influence were to be reconfigured.

In a slide toward hierarchy, regular staff was differentiated from CETA staff, a decision that was to be temporary. Regular staff decided not to include CETA workers in the center's weekly staff meeting. This was another first for WHS. No longer did the entire staff participate in collective decision making. CETA workers were given a measure of control over their immediate tasks, and they were slated for incorporation into the larger collective once they had completed the counselor training program (it took several months) and the survey of local health needs that was to be their principal responsibility, and once they had become familiar with collectivism, an ideology that was presumed to be foreign to them.

The period following the inauguration of the CETA project was one of unprecedented change and difficulty for the staff of WHS. A series of explosive conflicts divided workers, and there was increasing divergence between the center's egalitarian ideology and its everyday practice. Staff members registered their distress, talked of low morale, disenchantment, and the feeling of being overwhelmed and out of control (Morgen 1990). This took place as WHS developed and expanded its relationship with the state, and it is this period in the clinic's history that provides evidence of both the cooptive powers and processes of the state (Morgen 1986), and of the ways feminist activists can use state resources to contest and negotiate state pressures (Morgen 1990). An intensive examination of the experience of WHS suggests that the collective actively *resisted* the pressures that accompanied their growing dependence on the state. Cooptation is far too simple and definitive a description of the contradictory pushes and pulls of state funding and regulation on WHS and other clinics.

The Dynamics of Cooptation

The process of cooptation is less well understood than its social product: an organization, movement, or political group so fundamentally transformed that the (potential) challenge it poses to dominant power relations is significantly reduced. My analysis of cooptation is based on a theory of the state in advanced capitalism that defines the form and role of the state in terms of the reproduction of capitalist social relations and the mediation of relations between the ruling and ruled classes. The process of cooptation involves both direct and indirect pressures by powerful state forces, and accommodation and resistance to those pressures by the women who sought to maintain their oppositional organizations. Those responses—accommodation and resistance—are powerfully shaped by the dominant ideology and social relations that the state actively promotes.

The most obvious and powerful way in which the state influenced WHS was through selective funding of activities, channeling support toward direct service provision and away from community education, health advocacy, or other activist projects. In 1975, for example, the center was able to generate $10,000 to pay a counselor to provide services, but secured only $1,000 for community organizing efforts. Over time, in developing programs and activities, funding priorities quietly became organizational priorities—if not in spirit, in practice. Whenever the center sought to expand its activities, it was forced to go where the money was: in direct services such as counseling, family planning, drug education, and programs for battered women.

This observation is consistent with the analysis of scholars such as Piven and Cloward (1971, 1974), Wright (1975), and O'Connor (1973), who argue that a major, if covert, goal of state spending in this century has been to quiet unrest and to "cool out" social movements by diverting political activism into safer pursuits such as social service provision. As Wright argues, "the State . . . serves a vital legitimation function in capitalist society which helps to stabilize and reproduce the class structure as a whole. The legitimation function directs much state activity toward co-opting potential sources of popular discontent by attempting to transform political demands into economic demands" (1975, 28). This strategy guided the state's response to the Civil Rights movement (Allen 1970) and surfaced again in the mid-to-late 1970s in reaction to the growing feminist movement.

Not only did the state funding sources channel organizational activities toward service provision; they also tended to underwrite the very mode of service provision feminist health activists had sought to challenge—hierarchical, one-on-one, provider-client relationships. Because the community's need for services was always great, clinic staff continually felt the obligation to recruit new workers to provide those services. They no longer required that volunteers express commitment to feminist ideological principles and the alternative service organizational model; and, more important, they provided volunteers with a limited introduction to the political philosophy of the women's health movement.

So many of the routines that embodied feminist ideology in the center's early days—cervical self-examination, group attendance at feminist health conferences, the staff rap group, advocacy, and political activism—disappeared over the years. WHS had always emphasized the value of women, especially nonprofessional women, helping each other and its founding volunteer staff set out to provide information to women who would then be able to make informed decisions in groups that fostered support and solidarity. The clinic's counselor training program, the primary forum through which volunteers learned about the center's philosophy and operating procedures, changed dramatically over the years as staff gradually gave up political content in the sessions as they increasingly emphasized how-to instruction for their growing and diversifying services. The political context for the women's health services became attenuated. More and more, services were seen as ends in themselves.

As grants and contracts allocated money for one-on-one services, funding agencies built documentation of those individual contacts into their budgetary, record-keeping, and billing procedures. One contract, for example, paid WHS $12.50 per service unit (individual contact); another paid $400 per matrix unit (for services to one client over a six-month period). Although staff continued to organize some activities (birth control planning, for example) in group forums, the one-on-one provider-client model of services became more pervasive in practice and in theory as the center described its activities to funding agencies.

Self-help rhetoric gave way to an emphasis on paraprofessionalism. Over time, such language changes moved off the pages of grant proposals and into everyday discourse, and although the shifts were subtle, they were important. The center's earliest brochure referred to volunteers as "women helping women." By the late 1970s, WHS "paraprofessionals" served "clients." The same mechanism operated when the "staff rap group," which gave counselors the opportunity to share feelings and concerns about their work, was renamed "counseling supervision," and shifted gears to focus on discussions of difficult "cases" under the leadership of a psychologist. Furthermore, the political meaning of self-help was muted when it was portrayed as a cost-effective and successful strategy for health education rather than as a political tool for the collective empowerment of women.

The shift to paraprofessionalism dulled the edge of the critique of professionalism that had defined the foundational stories of the women's health movement. Now counselors occupied a position midway between health professionals and ordinary women, rather than standing for, and modeling through their own efforts, women's power and women's right to control their health care. This revision of the health collective's original radical model wasn't simply the result of direct state pressure. It was a gradual development, fueled also by the staff's commitment to meet the compelling, immediate needs of women in the community.

As a consequence of that commitment, the women's clinics sometimes made decisions that undermined their own political goals and ideals. The Feminist Women's Health Centers, for example, creators of the "participatory clinic," eventually found it necessary to drop this service mode in order to secure and maintain family planning funds when California agency officials cracked down on the use of nonprofessional health providers. And pressure from funding sources worked in indirect ways too. The state was able to count on the feminist clinics to provide extraordinary value for money. Typically, these oppositional organizations offered more services for each dollar awarded than mainstream health facilities because they could count on volunteer labor and on devoted employees who worked very long hours for very low wages.

Cooptive pressures were felt not only in the areas of political goals, service delivery, and staffing. They extended to organizational issues as well. As revenues from outside agencies multiplied between 1975 and 1979, the need for technical training and clerical and administrative work grew with them. Most of the center's funds were allocated on a contract rather than a direct-grant basis. (Direct grants, less common since the mid–1960s, furnish money for an agreed-upon program and often require only minimal follow-up in the form of a final report.) Contracts, on the other hand, often require periodic (quarterly or monthly) billing and documentation, time-consuming procedures that increase exponentially the work associated with a program. Moreover, because the billing and reporting forms are often complex, it can be difficult to rotate this responsibility among the staff. So state funding exacerbates the tendency toward task specialization and the specialization of service provision and administrative duties, two crucial features of bureaucracy. To the extent that these trends affected clinics such as WHS, it can be said that state funding promoted the process of bureaucratization, a process which some activists and theorists believe is antithetical to feminism (Ferguson 1984).

WHS typically received a series of small(er) grants and contracts from different agencies, each of which required a separate proposal, written to different specifications, and each of which enforced multiple billing and reporting protocols. In 1978, for example, WHS funding came from five different sources. Three staff members, the director and two clerical workers, devoted much of their time in administrative and clerical (that is, nonservice work) to securing these revenues and then documenting their use. This kind of specialization and separation of administrative/clerical from service delivery work would have been anathema in the early days of WHS, when task rotation and a commitment to an egalitarian social distribution of knowledge were viewed as critical for the effective functioning of the collective—and when clerical work was seen as meaningful only in the context of direct contact with clients.

Specialization is almost required, however, if small clinics such as WHS are to be successful at grantsmanship. Funding agencies often announce requests for proposals (RFPs) with relatively short lead times, and organizations whose skilled grant writers concentrate on research and proposal development have an advantage. But that advantage can be problematic. For example, in one instance a proposal for funds from the LEAA (Law Enforcement Assistance Act) raised objections from several WHS staff members who didn't want to work closely with an agency that strengthened police forces. But by the time they could voice their concerns in a staff meeting, the director had almost completed the application, giving her leverage with other staff who felt that, this late in its development, the proposal "might as well be sent in."

The institutionalization of a more specialized division of labor between administrative and service work, the increasing power of the director, and the sheer numbers of administrative tasks associated with the receipt of external funds—all these forces undermined collectivist practices at WHS. The structural scaffold of collective decision making—the weekly staff meeting at which consensus was sought on all political and operational issues in the center's early days—survived. But the new division of labor and the unequal distribution of knowledge among workers reflected real hierarchies solidifying within the collective: between the director and everyone else; between the regular and the CETA workers; between full- and part-time employees; and between paid staff and volunteers. The hierarchies themselves were not institutionalized, of course, as they are in most conventional agencies and workplaces. But they existed, and they shaped decision making, especially when decisions were contested.

In addition to fostering bureaucratic organizational features in grassroots collectivist groups, contract funding also creates an atmosphere of financial insecurity and dependency that mutes organizational autonomy and erodes oppositional practices. Contracts usually compensate for services after they have been provided. Because state agencies were notoriously late with reimbursements, WHS often found itself months behind schedule in receiving money from funding sources and, just as often, fell behind schedule with its own bills. Besides the obvious strain of not knowing whether the organization could meet its payroll, such insecurity wore against its autonomy in a variety of ways. In 1978, for example, one of its state funding sources owed WHS thousands of dollars for six months of contracted services. While it awaited payment, the center was forced to secure a short-term loan to cover payroll. During this interim period, a local women's community group that had organized to fight a controversial change in welfare regulations—a change instituted by the same agency that owed WHS money—asked the center for help. Some staff argued against becoming visible in this struggle, fearful that the agency might renege on its contract, or delay payment past the term of the bank loan.

As the clinic's dependence on external agencies increased, its political autonomy eroded. WHS fed an almost insatiable hunger for services, and it did so by hiring more and more workers. As funding for those paid positions became available, volunteers gave up their other jobs to work at the clinic. The number of staff who felt vulnerable to threats to their continued employment grew, and the organization, gradually but unmistakably shifted its orientation from social change to social service, as clinic staff designed activities to better suit the priorities of external funding agencies, and as they began to change their frame of reference to accommodate new interorganizational relationships. Whereas other feminist groups and health movement organizations had been the primary groups to which the WHS looked for guidance, support, and legitimation early in its history, its integration into the funding/social service network effectively mainstreamed the center. Now, staff were more likely to participate in in-service training sessions offered by other local social service agencies and less likely to attend feminist health conferences and workshops. And serving on the boards of those social service agencies began to seem as important as involvement with other grassroots organizations.

Such changing interorganizational relationships—with agencies to which WHS had once thought of itself as the alternative—moderated the center's oppositional spirit. Once again, the realities of state funding exerted a mighty influence. When the clinic received its first subcontracts, it had not been required to submit formal applications. However, when WHS started to compete on its own for federal and state grants and contracts, its success depended more than previously on positive relationships with local agencies. Proposals had to be accompanied by letters of support from other service providers, attesting to the legitimacy of the request for funds, the competence of WHS to carry out the proposed work, and/or the agency's commitment to cooperate with the clinic.

In fact, when WHS began in earnest to search for revenues through state grants and contracts, the director, a registered nurse who was hired in 1976, dedicated herself to improving the clinic's relationships with local health and social service agencies. Believing that WHS was seen as too radical by many, including the social welfare and health communities, she set out to accomplish what she called a systematic face lift. Although the staff did not explicitly endorse the muting of their political and oppositional stances, they did support the director's attempts to establish a more secure financial basis. She compared her interactions with local agencies with the more abrasive behavior of her predecessor. Advocacy, a crucial element of the alternative model, began to be perceived as an obstacle to the smooth operation—and the expansion—of center services.

It would be a gross distortion to suggest that the staff of WHS no longer saw the center as a feminist organization seeking to empower women. They surely did. But what became more apparent in the late 1970s was the change in all their relationships. Among themselves, with clients, and with other agencies, organizational survival and the need for women-controlled health service provision took precedence. WHS staff began to develop an insider strategy for change. Although this strategy may have introduced feminist ideas and alternative practices to other local agencies, it also diminished the intensity and oppositional nature of the center's advocacy activities. At one staff meeting, when a counselor reported the mistreatment of a client by another local agency, staff members agreed on the importance of maintaining a smooth relationship with the other agency. They decided to handle the criticism of the agency's practices "on an individual basis, talking to the particular case worker who made the mistake and not make a big deal of it."

The potential for conflict between the clinic's political ideals and goals and good working relationships with other agencies was most pronounced in instances when WHS depended on another institution for medical cooperation. In order to secure the important privilege of billing the state for Medicaid clients, the center was required to negotiate a contract with the local hospital to provide twenty-four-hour backup emergency services. Several months after the arrangement was finalized, the hospital announced that it was closing its prenatal and gynecology outpatient clinics. These clinics were the only alternative to private physician services available to women in the community (WHS did not offer prenatal or nonroutine gynecological care). Termination of the hospital clinics would force low-income women to pay more for services or to do without them. And it would deprive the women of some of the critical ancillary (social work) services that had been offered by the hospital clinics.

When a local community group organized to challenge the hospital's decision to close the clinics, WHS was invited to participate actively in the group. At first, the center took an active role. But after several months of angry meetings and demonstrations at the hospital, some staff members expressed concern that the clinic's visible presence on the picket line might alienate local obstetrician-gynecologists and jeopardize the arrangement with the hospital, on which their continuing ability to bill Medicaid depended. Others argued that the campaign was too important to abandon. Although WHS did not completely withdraw its support for this struggle, fewer staff actively participated, and the polarization of services and politics intensified.

The issue of such constraints on political action surfaced again when feminist health groups across the country mobilized to oppose the Hyde Amendment,[4] first passed in 1976, which restricted the use of federal Medicaid funds for abortions and struck at the heart of WHS politics. Again, a faction of staff members warned against a visible pro-choice stance. They claimed that the clinic was already seen as too political and predicted that radical positions on controversial issues might lead to the loss both of funding and of community support. That such a concern could be articulated by an organization that emerged from the women's health movement—whose raison d'être is women's right to control their reproductive lives and health—points to the ways in which dependence on state funding can wear down the political autonomy and will of an oppositional organization. At this point in the center's history, health advocacy and political action had been transformed into risks.

The state's control over critical resources and processes (financial, legal, regulatory) ultimately permitted it to influence the clinic's growth away from its original political goals and principles. But the process was not always overtly coercive. To be sure, some of the requirements attached to grants and contracts directly challenged alternative features of WHS's organizational structure (the naming of a director to ensure administrative and financial accountability) or its health service model (reimbursement only for services provided by physicians or other licensed professionals). Other forms of pressure were more subtle. By providing money to fund vitally needed services, but with resources well below what was necessary adequately to meet those needs, state agencies essentially put clinic staff in a position to feel overwhelmed by exigency. Funding sources did not have to come right out and prohibit cervical self-examination or staff rap groups or even advocacy and feminist political activities (although such direct intervention did come around the issue of abortion). Instead, the priorities of the state funding apparatus created the conditions under which particular activities and ideals were reinforced (women helping other women through direct caring, direct services) while others were either ignored (nonprofessional women's control of reproductive health care) or undermined (collectivist organizational structure and collective action).

This is how the state elicits the consent of those whom it rules. It shapes actions and beliefs through control of political and economic resources, institutions, and ideas. Cooptation thus transcends the simple operation of class power through economic and political means and moves onto the battleground of ideology. To the extent that a social or political movement can sustain an oppositional ideology that confronts the taken-for-granted or explicitly articulated values and assumptions of the dominant ideology, it can interfere with the organization of consent that bolsters hegemony. During this phase of the cooptation process, WHS did not strongly or actively sustain its oppositional ideology; feminism faded somewhat as staff gradually abandoned the routines and forums that embodied it. This does not mean that the staff explicitly disavowed feminist principles—the cooptive process can insinuate itself without insisting on notice. The clinic maintained its feminist rhetoric, even as staff members made compromises that had a long(er) term impact on their organizational autonomy and their ideological praxis. But the redefinition of their principles, the transformation of self-help into paraprofessionalism, for example, and the reconfiguring of work assignments changed the nature and the structure of the organization. The clinic now hewed to many of the values of the dominant ideology as they were expressed by the successful incorporation of state funding sources into their daily practices.

As our survey of clinics suggests, such changes were widespread as feminist clinics across the country struggled to provide services. In the years following the movement's first militant phase, most women's health organizations sought credibility with funding agencies by modifying decision-making procedures, administrative structures, and division of labor toward hierarchy and bureaucracy and away from radical politics. In the process, they came to more closely resemble the mainstream health care providers they had set out to replace, or at least to change (Selznick 1966; Zald and Ash 1966; Galper and Washburn 1976; Bush 1978; Newman 1980; Schechter 1982; Matthews 1994; Arnold 1995; Farrell 1995).

Even if the decision to seek state funding had never been taken, WHS was destined to become vulnerable to intense outside pressure in the late 1970s with the growing political power of the New Right. In 1978, the well-organized antiabortion movement won legislative victories in the state where the clinic is located, among them the requirement that all women's counseling and referral centers obtain clinic licenses from the state department of public health. To qualify for such a license, WHS would have to restrict procedures that were now performed by lay health workers; name a physician as medical director of the center (WHS hired doctors as consultants in family planning and routine gynecology but did not include them in decision making); and conform to costly building codes that would make it difficult to locate in a low-income neighborhood. Although it was dressed in the rhetoric of quality assurance, clinic licensure was a political provision that targeted alternative grassroots service organizations.

WHS fought and eventually won the battle against licensure, but not without cost. The struggle occupied clinic workers for much of 1978, and it was used repeatedly by the faction within the staff that wanted to focus on services against those who argued for advocacy and political activism. Once again, fears of alienating those agencies that would decide the licensure issue—the same agencies that WHS had originally seen itself as alternative to—guided the collective's actions. Despite the weight of evidence that routinization is inevitable if oppositional organizations are to sustain themselves, however, this wasn't the end of the story for WHS. Rather, after the period between 1974 and 1978, when co-optive pressures had their greatest influence on the center's operations, WHS reversed or modified its direction again, revitalizing its political goals and feminist connections. Even when an organization appears to have been co-opted, it is important to look closely, to see if there are other ways in which that organization retains or develops other goals or organizational features that engender an oppositional stance or actions.

Seeding Diversity, Revitalizing Feminism

Although the state has resources that allow, and a stake in fostering, the cooptation of oppositional social movement organizations, state funding can also help create conditions that reinforce oppositional/social change goals. This is what happened at WHS in the late 1970s. The center did get tangled up in the strings attached to outside funding, but staff members wove those encumbrances (and the real opportunities they offered) into a stronger organizational foundation that enabled them to sustain the center for more than two decades (continuing today) as a powerful base from which to advocate change in the community. The CETA grant (1977) planted the seeds of revitalization. A close examination of the impact of CETA funding reveals how WHS staff accommodated and resisted pressures that came with it; and shows how state funding can contribute to organizational revitalization.

When WHS staff first spoke with CETA officials in 1977, they learned that their chances for receiving a grant were better if their project was larger than the one they had originally proposed, and if they attached a survey component to their health education and training plans. After relatively brief reconsideration, staff incorporated these suggestions into the grant proposal. But both the increased size of the staff and the addition of a work project significantly different from regular staff assignments created enormous problems. The months following the inauguration of the CETA project, especially early in 1978, were particularly difficult ones. In planning and implementing the project, staff found themselves on a collision course with their familiar goals of collectivism and egalitarianism. That insistent, inescapable fact generated tension and left staff members demoralized. Nevertheless, and early on, regular staff—concerned about the impact of fifteen new workers on the already compromised collective process—decided not to involve CETA employees in the clinic's weekly staff meetings until they had finished the lengthy counselor training program and completed the community health needs survey that would be their principal responsibility (this would take three to six months of the twelve-month grant). CETA staff would meet on their own and would learn about the collective process in their own staff meetings. Otherwise, it was thought, they would be blown away by WHS decision-making procedures. For the first time in the center's history, a group of workers was excluded from the prerogatives of other collective members.

It was certainly true that most new staff members had not participated in a collective before; that had always been true of volunteers who worked at WHS. It was certainly true that the scale of the problem had never been so great. The CETA grant meant that fifteen newcomers must be introduced to an established organization of fewer than fifteen workers. It was certainly true that the new staff would spend time out of the building in the project's first months, canvassing the health needs and attitudes of low-income women. But none of these certain truths adequately explained the unprecedented decision to balkanize staff. Rather, racism and class prejudice underlay the regular staff's move to retain control of the clinic by creating two separate but unequal collectives.

The hirings made possible by the CETA grant changed the balance of class and color at WHS. More decidedly white and middle class before, the center now employed many poor women of color, few of whom had previous commitments either to WHS or to the label and politics of feminism. Now WHS had become a cross-class, multiracial, multiethnic organization, an organizational goal for years, but one that had been out of reach because limited funds had forced the center into a heavy reliance on volunteers. Race, class, and political heterogeneity now characterized a staff that had prided itself on its ideological commitments to collectivism and equality—and as any student of collectives knows, such organizations thrive when their members share fundamental values and beliefs and when they have clear, common goals (Mansbridge 1980; Rothschild-Whitt 1986).

We've seen that processes of participatory democracy were already eroding before the CETA project. Now the clinic formally institutionalized inequalities and differences within the staff. The bases of those inequalities had changed and were more easily identified. They did not express differences between individuals, the perceived need for specialization in fund-raising, grant-writing, or contract administration. Instead, the bases for inequality were race, class, and, to a lesser degree, political convictions. The problem that had no name during the early months of the project registered itself in an apparently endless series of troubles and tensions between members of the regular staff, and between the regular staff and the CETA workers.

CETA staff expressed resentment about many aspects of the center's operation, beginning with what they felt to be the stigmatizing label by which they were known. When regular staff imposed time cards and penalties in response to frequent and sometimes prolonged lateness of some of the new workers, CETA staff saw their action as expressions of racism and class prejudice. And gradually, the European American and middle-class staff began to understand the depth and consequences of the racism and class injuries that were endemic in the larger society and reproduced, sometimes unknowingly, in their own actions and attitudes. As the women of color and those who had struggled against class barriers grew more confident about themselves and more certain that they faced systematic oppression, not merely personal troubles, a more solid basis for trust and solidarity emerged among them and, slowly, in the group as a whole.

The process of change was set into motion by the intensification and growing collective awareness of the divergence between the clinic's ideals and its practices. Once that pattern was exposed, at first by the charges of the CETA staff, it became a wellspring for further conflict. More and more frequently, decisions were contested and the decision-making process became highly charged. (By this time, CETA workers participated in the weekly staff meetings.) Hidden power structures that had functioned in an apparently benign manner for two years or more—especially the greater influence of the director and the full-time paid staff—were unmasked as consensus became harder to reach in the face of widening differences among staff members. With more decisions being debated, there was more opportunity and reason to scrutinize the political implications of different courses of action. For the first time in several years, politics became thematic in staff meetings. Staff who were well versed in feminism and staff for whom feminism was new(er) were exposed to different political opinions and had to make decisions actively, rather than merely to assent to decisions already foreordained.

During this period there was a clear desire within the staff to find funds to retain all (or most) of the CETA staff after the grant ended. Nevertheless some of the collective's most heated political conflicts involved questions about grants and contracts, particularly when there were concerns that such external funds might compromise clinic ideology or practice. Staff members were divided, for example, over whether to apply for funding from the state Department of Public Health because new agency regulations intended to prohibit organizational support of abortion.

In another instance, the director and some staff members had agreed to hold signs for a local political candidate who had backed the center in recent efforts to get a building donated by the city for the clinic's use. Others objected to that public display of support because the candidate did not have a solid record on issues of concern to low-income women. Still others rejected the notion that WHS should engage in tit-for-tat exchanges of political favors. The conflict escalated. Supporters of the sign holding argued that it served the long-term interest of the center. The opposition angrily countered that the decision had not been brought to the full staff for endorsement. Although such fractious political disagreement was exhausting, it fostered a growing political sophistication in the staff and led to a leveling of the disproportionate power of the director and the regular paid staff.

By early 1979 hard work and creative budgeting permitted the clinic to hire or to project hiring many CETA staff members for (more) permanent positions. Some of these positions were in the health clinic; others were in projects that had grown from clinic services over the previous several years, including battered women's services, legal services for low-income families, and a small community organizing project. Because there was more state money available for domestic violence programs than for health services, some CETA staff members moved into new positions in that area. Organizational growth and programmatic change and the renewal of its commitment to collectivism led to the formation of a committee charged with the responsibility of creating a new organizational structure. The committee proposed a tripartite arrangement in which independent collectives ran the health clinic, the battered women's projects, and the legal services programs. Each unit was to have a representative on an administrative committee, which, with the director, would serve as the overarching policy-making body of the organization.

In the midst of these changes the director of WHS announced that she was going to leave the position she had held for five years. The process of the search for a new director reflected and reinforced the movement toward greater participation and control by the larger staff in center decision making. One faction was interested in finding a new director who had expertise in administration and grant writing. Another group sought someone who would articulate a more radical political vision for the center, who would reinvigorate community activism. After months of long and painful discussion, the staff finally hired a new director—a white, middle-class woman who combined extensive political experience (in feminist and antiracist organizations) with administrative and grant-writing expertise. With her direction and the staff's renewed commitment to their political objectives, the center was able to maintain external funding and to develop social action projects and forums for political discussion and internal self-education.

The organization's new self-description revised the conceptualization of those political objectives. "In trying to seek active community involvement, provide high quality services and programs, and function as a worker-controlled collective, the WHS is committed to growing as a feminist grassroots organization" (WHS n.d.). This new, overt, owned-up-to feminism is not, however, the same ideology that had given birth to the clinic. Rather, staff members were creating a conception of feminism that explicitly entailed recognizing and working with differences among women, especially race and class differences. About a year after the hiring of the new director, the center developed a pamphlet for International Women's Day that articulated a changing consciousness about racism and diversity:

> We have also realized that women's struggle for equality is closely connected with the struggles of other oppressed groups . . . Some of these struggles [that the WHS had been involved in that year] do not concern narrowly defined "women's issues" . . . That's because women cannot achieve equality or decent lives unless all working people get a better deal, nor will women be liberated unless racism is eliminated . . . The struggle for women's liberation includes all women struggling for equality and a better life as workers, as Black people, as Puerto Ricans, as lesbians, or as other oppressed groups.

The new director nurtured this new vision of feminism and the center's mission, and she also was clear about the importance of building leadership within the staff, particularly among women of color and white working-class women. When she decided to leave her job a few years later, the staff and board of WHS named two co-directors. One was a woman of color first hired under the CETA grant. For the first time in its history, the center would be led by a woman whose class (working class), race (black), and lifestyle (married, with children) approximated those of the majority of the women who lived in the community. By the time of her appointment, the decision-making process was more solidly collective. Although some task specialization continued, the staff had developed ways of coping with and circumventing these constraints in their purposeful recommitment to feminism.

What does the experience of WHS, admittedly an exception to the rule of routinization, tell us about the processes that condition the success of alternative health and social movement organizations? In 1977 and 1978, WHS was an organization that had lost important parts of its social movement identity and activity. The arc of organizational revitalization came as a gift—an unintentional one, of course—from the funding apparatus of the state, which unwittingly provided the resources that allowed this clinic (and many others) to hire a more diverse staff by race and class. Those women forced center staff quite consciously to redefine priorities and to rediscover political meaning in WHS plans and projects. Some of the strongest proponents of an activist orientation and a conception of feminism grounded in the experiences of women of color and poor women were originally hired through the CETA grant. Among these women were several who had considerable experience in political activism (community organizing), and who understood, as recipients, the limits of social services. State funds had enabled the center to hire the very women who would help to change the organization's direction. CETA staff outgrew the apparent stigma of that label. But even as state resources created the conditions that brought white, black, Latina, middle-class, and working-class women together, the social control functions of the state continued to exert strong pressures on the organization. The center staff was dependent on the state for their own livelihoods, for support of their alternative model of health services, and for the funds that underwrote the accessibility of these services for those in most need of services.

As the subtle and gradual effects of cooptation resulting from state funding were coupled with the more explicit and fundamental challenges to the clinic's political integrity—embodied in the strategy of the New Right to force licensure on feminist health providers—the balance between consent and coercion in the organization of hegemony was upset. As WHS staff faced clearly unacceptable compromises in the late 1970s and later, they were forced to consider the compromises they had already made to comply with the demands of state regulations. The political assaults on the clinic—from within over issues of race, class, and ideological direction, and from without by the New Right—created conditions that fostered a new feminist consciousness among staff members. I have argued that the effects of the political and economic power mobilized by the state to quell oppositional social movements are conditioned by the particular responses of those oppositional movements and by their ideological mechanisms. WHS exemplifies how the organization of consent can be interrupted both by a changing consciousness in social actors (a more developed political vision or political understanding of events) and by changes in the balance between consent and coercion.

Clearly, the state is neither simply friend nor foe. Supported and constrained by state resources and regulations, the women of WHS used those resources, at a particular historical moment, in ways that challenged and transformed dominant gender, race, and class ideologies and practices. But the contradictions that were embodied in relationships between feminist health organizations and the state changed and intensified during the 1980s as the New Right gained political power.

Chapter 8

The Three Rs

*Reagan, Retrenchment, and
Operation Rescue in the 1980s*

The changes that expanded opportunities for women of all races and for communities of color in the 1960s and 1970s triggered powerful political backlash in the 1980s. When the organizations that emerged from the women's health movement marked their tenth anniversaries, their celebrations were muted by the sense that they now confronted an economy in retrenchment and a national landscape more dominated by the New Right.

Although Reagan's resonance with many in the electorate found its theoretical justification in the mantra "getting government off the backs of the American people," women's health organizations felt the power of the state even more acutely after his election than they had in the 1970s. In fact, the New Right used the issues of abortion and family values as engines for transforming the power of backlash into political victories that eroded abortion rights, stepped up attacks on providers, and slashed state funding for programs associated with women's health (Petchesky 1990, 242).[1] But the news was not all bad for feminist health activists. Recognizing that complacency about abortion rights was ill advised, women revitalized the movement with fresh energies and developed new programs that widened its focus beyond issues of reproductive health.

The eighties actually began before the turn of the decade, when abortion foes, at work and growing since *Roe* vs. *Wade,* scored an important victory with passage of the Hyde Amendment (1977), which prohibited the use of federal Medicaid funds for most abortions. By 1979, no federal funds could be used for abortion or abortion-related services unless a woman's life was in danger.

At the same time, state legislatures across the country were passing laws that limited abortion rights and access, including the requirement of parental consent (for minors) and spousal consent or notification for all women who sought abortion, waiting periods, and restrictions on the use of the state's portion of Medicaid to pay for abortion (Petchesky 1990, 242). By 1988, only fourteen states still funded Medicaid abortions (Davis 1988, 44).

The big issue, though, was the combination of inflation and recession that had ravaged the economy. The average real wage of nonagricultural production workers had fallen by 4.3 percent between 1973 and 1979 and massive layoffs had displaced hundreds of thousands of workers (Albelda 1988, 19). To an electorate tired of recession and declining disposable incomes, President Carter promised cost control and condemned government waste and inefficiency (Bawden 1984). Although Carter's rhetoric anticipated the anti–big-government message of the Republicans and the New Right, his efforts to curtail government spending were mild compared with the dramatic cuts in social spending Reagan would implement when he took office in 1981. Wealth did not trickle down into clinics and other agencies that worked to improve the lives and health of women, people of color, and the poor under Reaganomics. The new president's policies produced drought for those organizations. With passage of the 1981 Omnibus Budget Reconciliation Act, the country experienced unprecedented cuts in domestic spending; they took shape through significant changes in welfare programs and through a dramatic decline in federal grants-in-aid to state and local governments.

The deepest cuts affected the many fixed-dollar programs that funded the delivery of education, health, employment, and social services by state and local governments and nonprofit agencies, and benefit programs that target the poor: AFDC, food stamps, child nutrition, housing assistance, and Medicaid (Nathan, Doolittle and Associates 1983; Coalition on Women and the Budget 1984; Palmer and Sawhill 1984). The toll on poor women and their families, and on the agencies and organizations that serve them—including the feminist clinics—was often terrible.

The Trickle-Down Effect of Federal Budget Cuts

Although President Ronald Reagan did not succeed in reducing the deficit or overall federal spending (both of which rose during his terms in office), his administration achieved its real goal: vastly to reduce the social welfare functions of government and federal efforts to support the gains of the women's, Civil Rights, and other grassroots movements of the previous decades. The able neoconservative strategist Richard Viguerie described this strategy accurately from the perspective of the growing New Right—a strategy to "defund the left" (1982). The left he is talking about is not the Communist Party U.S.A. or programs or groups associated with New Left or far left political organizations. Rather, this left is the institutional legacy of the many progressive movements of the 1960s and 1970s, including community and feminist health clinics and other community-based human service, educational, and health care organizations.

There is no question that neoconservative and New Right political ideologies gained currency in the 1980s; these principles gave birth to "antigovernment" policies that competed both with a declining liberalism and an ascendant neoliberalism aimed at restraining the growth of the state and restoring "market forces to areas of social life in which they have been displaced or altered by the state" (O'Connor, Orloff, and Shaver 1999, 53). Neoconservative and then neoliberal policies implemented during the 1980s were to slash federal spending for social programs; transfer responsibility for many of those programs to states and local governments; deregulate everything politically possible; reform and reduce taxes; reverse policies that had effected limited economic and political redistribution of power and resources to previously disenfranchised and "disadvantaged" (in federal lingo) groups.

Almost everyone knows that social spending was cut deeply during the 1980s, but there is less understanding of the effects of the cuts and the complex changes they set into motion. To comprehend those changes, we must first recognize the different routes through which federal funds are channeled into social spending: (1) directly by federal programs and agencies; (2) through grants-in-aid to states and localities, partners in implementing, and often funding, programs (for example, Medicaid); and (3) through support of nonprofit organizations that were often the vehicles for services and programs funded wholly or in part by state funds.

Feminist health clinics were not singled out for attention when the 1981 and subsequent federal budgets were passed. Rather, their losses and those of other community health organizations were part of a much greater devastation inflicted on states, municipalities, and the nonprofit sector as a whole. Implementation of the Omnibus Budget and Reconciliation Act of 1981 led to huge cuts in grants-in-aid programs to state and local governments and in means-tested programs for the poor (Palmer and Sawhill 1984). The new budget reduced federal grants to states and localities by $6.6 billion between 1981 and 1982, the first such decline in almost a quarter of a century (Nathan, Doolittle and Associates 1983, 2). In addition to reductions in aid, the federal government consolidated a wide variety of categorical grants (grants for specific programs) into block grant programs that handed states and localities less money and more discretion in how to spend it.

A summary of reductions in domestic spending by program area during Reagan's first term shows that grants-in-aid to state and local governments for preventive health programs declined by 22 percent; for health resources by 42 percent; for health services by 22 percent; for alcohol, drug abuse, and mental health by 34 percent; and for Medicaid by 7 percent (AFSCME 1984, 15). Cuts in funding for health care block grants averaged from 20 to 35 percent nationwide (Nathan, Doolittle and Associates 1983, 38). As deeply as cutbacks in the area of health care hurt, however, the worst savaging took place in the area of social services, including employment and training programs for the poor and the near poor (Palmer and Sawhill 1984). Cuts in federal grants-in-aid to states and municipalities, coupled with the effects of recession, brought about the worst financial conditions since the depression for state and local governments in the early 1980s (AFSCME 1984, 6).

In theory, reduced federal responsibility for social programs was to be compensated, at least partially, by state and local programs and by the private sector—particularly the nonprofit sector. But federal budget reductions hit these other sources of funds for community-based organizations hard, too. The nonprofit sector in the 1980s was heavily dependent on federal funds; federal dollars accounted for a significant percentage of the revenues of nonprofit social and health services. Dramatic cuts in federal spending in social welfare and community health service program areas, 42 and 43 percent respectively (Abramson and Salaman 1986), profoundly affected all the nonprofits, including the many community and women's health clinics founded in the 1960s and 1970s. The cruel irony is that nonprofits were supposed to take on greater responsibility for programs once in the domain of the federal government, even as the federal money that had supported the establishment and operation of many of these organizations diminished or disappeared.

By fiscal year 1984, real federal spending for programs relevant to nonprofit organizations was below 1980 levels, 3 percent below if one includes spending on Medicaid and Medicare, 15 percent below if these costly programs are excluded (Palmer and Sawhill 1984, 18). Cuts often came suddenly. Another Urban Institute study found that in one year, 1981–82, nonprofit service organizations lost almost 10 percent of their government support: "Agencies established under the aegis of the Great Society and those focusing services on the poor... [were] hit especially hard by the federal cutbacks" (Palmer and Sawhill 1984, 19).

So the spending cuts were drastic. But they tell only part of the story. With the consolidation of many categorical programs into block grants, some service areas lost far more than others, depending on their political appeal. For example, under the Social Services Block Grant, a greater share of spending continued for protective services (for example, child abuse programs) and adoption or foster care, at the expense of support for family planning and day care, programs that had been protected by categorical grants (Palmer and Sawhill 1984, 17). It took an enormous political mobilization to keep the Reagan administration from rolling the larger federal family planning program (Title X) into block grants in the early and mid–1980s, and although Title X remained a federal category, funding was slashed by 25 percent in the first round of the Reagan spending cuts (Coalition on Women and the Budget 1984, 21).

Many of the women's health clinics received some portion of their operating revenues from sources affected by these far-ranging cuts in federal social spending. Whether the money came from Title X or from other federal categorical grants, programs run by states or communities with funds from federal grants-in-aid, or contracts with state agencies or other nonprofit organizations, the supply of money to support health services and other programs contracted sharply. Family planning, maternal and child health, CETA, Medicaid, and domestic violence, teen pregnancy, community development, and mental health programs all suffered losses.[2]

Clinics such as the Berkeley Women's Health Collective and New Bedford Women's Health Services, both of which had steadily increased the money they received from state sources during the mid to late 1970s, faced financial insecurity coupled with new challenges and pressures as federal spending cuts began to take effect in the early 1980s. The July 1982 newsletter of the Berkeley Women's Health Collective anticipates the human costs of cuts in California's Medicaid program (Medi-Cal) and details the bad news of the end of the fiscal year for the clinic, which, as a consequence of a "crushing defeat on a new tax measure," would receive one-third of an expected $36,000 from the city's general funds. Staff members express their fear that these funds would evaporate next year, and they gave readers notice that they have been told to prepare for at least a 20 percent reduction in county moneys for the Medically Indigent Adults (MIA) program and more cuts in Medi-Cal funding (1982, 2), two critical sources of revenue for the collective. According to the clinic administrator most responsible for maintaining funding from state programs during the early 1980s, the BWHC had to function with "a constant sense of funds being cut off . . . [or] reduced," and although the actual cuts were sometimes less than had been feared, "there was a constant state of anxiety about the funding. That was the biggest problem."

In 1982 the California state legislature excluded "medically indigent adults" from Medi-Cal eligibility and handed off the burden of providing health care for this population to the counties. At the same time, legislators cut appropriations for MIAs by 70 percent. With one blow, they vastly increased the client load at many community clinics, including BWHC. But more patients did not translate into increased revenues. As a matter of routine practice, the state imposed long delays on payment to community clinics for the primary care they provided to MIAs. Between January and May of 1983, for instance, the collective received no reimbursement for services to between 60 and 75 percent of clients who qualified as medically indigent adults. The time gap between procedures and payments created huge financial problems, and, of course, prevented the clinic from paying its own bills. In a pattern repeated over and over again in clinics across the country, reimbursement policies threw the feminist clinics back on their first, slender support, labor-intensive local fund-raising. BWHC also faced a blizzard of new paperwork associated with the MIA funds. Even as problems with the new program began to be ironed out, the collective was informed that the governor planned further reductions in the budget for MIA health care and that the county might decide to channel funds away from community clinics and toward another set of providers.

When the new fiscal year began in July 1983, the BWHC newsletter tallied up statewide losses for the previous year and presented a grim forecast. Funds for Medi-Cal, community clinics, and MIA programs had been slashed by $121 million from the previous (already lean) year:

> Cuts in Family Planning, which were not even being considered before the governor's blue pencil took over, amount to $9.5 million, or one-quarter of the statewide family planning budget. 165,000 women this year would be denied services, resulting in 44,000 unwanted pregnancies . . . He [Governor Deukmejian] has attempted to curtail eligibility for Medi-Cal reimbursement for abortion in cases of rape, incest, danger to the life of the mother, or malformation of the foetus, even though the Supreme Court has ruled this action illegal many times . . . Further, he cut perinatal programs by $4,715,000. (BWHC 1983, 1)

As BWHC struggled to stand firm against the avalanche of financial challenges set off by neoconservative fiscal policies, the collective continued to expand programs. In August 1982, with a windfall grant of $10,000 from the Berkeley City Council (denied them several months before), collective members opened a satellite clinic especially for women of color at a church in a low-income neighborhood in South Berkeley. The space for the new clinic was donated, as was much of the equipment. The seed funding of this new program repeated a pattern. State protocols encouraged expansion of services; at the same time, they cut to the bone support for programs already in existence, a strategy calculated to deny the clinics their autonomy by making them dependent on continuing infusions of new state money. "It sounds really good to get government funding," BWHC's administrator observed, "and of course they should be funding these good programs. They fund you and then they start cutting and you are depending on the funds and pretty soon programs that were making it on their own cannot."

Social spending cuts drained staff time and energy as overburdened workers anticipated and worked to fight further cuts through fund-raising efforts and through participation in a statewide campaign by community clinics to defeat a public health block grant proposed by Governor Deukmejian. The grant, they argued, would have "severely undercut the perinatal, maternal and child health and other health programs which are currently under community control through community clinics" (BWHC 1983, 5). They managed to "block the block grant program" (their slogan). But they knew that they would have to fight the same battle again and again in years to come.

Like the Berkeley Women's Health Collective, other women's clinics across the country faced drastic shortfalls in revenue. For example, the New Bedford Women's Health Services (NBWHS) managed to survive the effects of the budget ax, but not without a dramatic downsizing of staff and activities. That clinic had successfully generated state money in the 1970s and very early 1980s to expand clinical services and community outreach and education programs, including developing programs for teens. The center landed several grants for its teen pregnancy, family planning, and sexuality programs, the biggest of which came from the state Department of Public Health. But as the director of development for the Women's Center noted, the availability of funding changed rapidly during the early and mid–1980s.

> The Department of Public Health came to us with new criteria and regulations [for our teenage sexuality project] . . . We lost that grant. They wanted the community health center, which we helped to build, to be where that money was . . . We've seen a real decline in funding for the health project. The staff dwindled over the years and there are only two full time now [in 1990]. Most of the rest are volunteers or paid on an hourly basis . . . We had some layoffs . . . and some people left for better paying positions. (Kelly 1990)

As state money dried up, NBWHS turned to patchwork funding from foundations and to more community-based fundraising. But foundations don't usually want to fund continuing services over the long haul, and their grants did not last many years. Because it is unrealistic to expect continuing support for programs, hard-pressed service providers often tried to develop new programs that were then difficult to sustain. The center launched an exciting program for teenage mothers and their mothers, for instance, with initial funding from a regional foundation. When that funding ran out, a local foundation carried the program for a short time. After that funding source had been exhausted, NBWHS initiated a program of health access and education issues with immigrants from the Cape Verde Islands. No matter how worthy each new program was, it was likely to take the place of an existing service and engage workers in high-intensity program building, rather than in high-quality program maintenance.

The clinic was also forced to recover more costs from fees, a course of action that always interferes with the goal of keeping health care affordable, and that usually leads to degradation of intensive counseling and health education services. In New Bedford, at about the same time NBWHS was forced to raise its own fees to make up for funding cuts, the community clinic initiated a walkin teen birth control project that used videos rather than counselors to provide information, lowering costs and compromising quality. The community clinic had already won family planning funds away from NBWHS. This new offering threatened the NBWHS even further.

Increasingly, the clinic turned to local and community-based fundraising, an effort that was specialized and professionalized in the 1980s and 1990s. In 1985, a longtime staff member of the NBWHS was hired to do development and fund-raising full time. By 1989 the Women's Center (which included the feminist health clinic) was raising $20,000 in memberships, up from $4,000 in 1985. The center's annual Men Who Cook event, which netted $4,000 in its first year, brought in $17,000 in 1989. Julie Kelly, the development director believes that reliance on the community for financial support had a silver lining. She said that it made NBWHS staff members feel like "part of the community, and [that the community was] more a part of us" (Kelly 1990). But private fundraising could not succeed in sustaining health services at the levels they reached in the late 1970s and early 1980s.

The funding woes confronting clinics such as the Berkeley Women's Health Collective and New Bedford Women's Health Services in the 1980s linked clinics across the country to the same hard political reality—state support for their services was ephemeral. Clinics that provided only family planning services or routine gynecological care faced the most serious financial problems. (Abortion services guaranteed more consistent and substantial revenues, even under assault by the New Right.) Our survey of health clinics and advocacy organizations indicated that fully 25 percent of respondents endured "serious" budget cuts during the 1980s. Two-thirds of these organizations were forced to lay off staff and to reduce non–revenue generating activities, such as education, outreach, or advocacy. Forty-three percent cut services; more than one-third reduced staff benefits; and one-third cut salaries.

Nevertheless, many of these organizations managed to survive. Most of my survey and interview data come from activists whose clinics succeeded in limping along during the Reagan years. But some clinics were forced to close. Others stayed open only by allowing themselves to be managed by mainstream health groups (such as county health departments) or to be bought out by physician-owner partnerships. The sharp reduction in available revenue for these community organizations did mean the end or significant change for some of the women's health movement clinics. And trouble didn't just come in the form of reduced revenues. The burgeoning power of the New Right and, especially, escalating assaults by the antiabortion movement posed colossal problems for feminist clinics, particularly those that provided abortion services.

Harassment and Violence against Abortion Providers

In March 1993 Dr. David Gunn was shot to death outside a Pensacola, Florida, clinic where he performed abortions. Five months later, Dr. Wayne Patterson, an abortion provider who had worked with Gunn, was murdered in Alabama. Soon afterward, Shelley Shannon wounded Dr. George Tiller outside a clinic in Wichita, Kansas. In July 1994, Paul Hill shot and killed Dr. James Bayard Britton and James Barrett, a clinic escort, at another Pensacola clinic. Barrett's wife, June, was also injured in the attack. In December 1994, John Salvi murdered Shannon Lowney and Leanne Nichols at two clinics in Brookline, Massachusetts. Salvi, who would kill himself in prison, was caught by Virginia police the next day. In the 1997 bombing of a clinic in Atlanta, a security guard was killed and another person was maimed. A year later Dr. Barnett Slepian was shot to death in the kitchen of his suburban Rochester, New York, home with his wife and children looking on. And this is only a partial list of incidents of violence against abortion providers in the United States.

The assassinations of abortion providers and clinic workers made headlines across the country and helped spur passage of the Freedom of Access to Clinic Entrances (FACE) Act in May 1994. FACE prohibited the use of force, threats, or physical obstruction to interfere with a person trying to enter or leave an abortion clinic. In July 1994, Attorney General Janet Reno ordered the creation of a Department of Justice task force to investigate possible criminal conspiracy within the most extreme wing of the antiabortion movement. But violence against abortion providers was not a new phenomenon for the 1990s, when it reached its full and logical flowering in an age of murder. Although no killings of clinic workers or physicians who performed abortions were reported until 1993, since the late 1970s antiabortion forces have made use of a range of terrorist tactics against people and property: arson, bombings, vandalism, stalking, and intimidation of staff and clients, physical assault, and blockades. Violence against abortion clinics first peaked in the mid–1980s; in the mid–

1990s, it peaked again. It took more than a decade, and the election of a pro-choice Democratic administration, before the federal government finally took official notice of the growing violence and extremism within the antiabortion movement and began to challenge it with new laws and vigorous enforcement policies.

Feminist clinics represent only a small percentage of abortion clinics nationwide. There are many Planned Parenthood and other nonprofit abortion clinics, as well as private, often for-profit clinics that provide abortions, and antiabortion groups have vandalized, set fire to, and bombed them regardless of their affiliations. What sets feminist clinics apart from these other targets of violence (other than their political missions, and often the way they provided services) is that they tend to command fewer financial resources and have fewer connections with police forces and representatives of local court systems, margins of difference that can make prevention of or recovery from violence all the more difficult.

An arson attack that destroyed a Planned Parenthood clinic in St. Paul, Minnesota, in 1977 is one of the first recorded acts of violence by antiabortion groups (Ms. 1995, 54). Women for Women Clinic of Cincinnati was bombed in 1978, the first reported bombing of an abortion facility. By 1982 the Army of God had firebombed an abortion clinic in Illinois and kidnapped a doctor and his wife and held them for more than a week. In 1983 three abortion clinics were bombed (Fugh-Berman 1985, 2). In 1984 violence against abortion clinics escalated dramatically. The toll: eighteen bombings, six cases of arson, six cases of attempted bombing or arson, twenty-three death threats, and nearly seventy clinic invasions with acts of vandalism (Ms. 1995, 55). The estimated cost of damage for the first two months of 1984 alone was $2 million, a figure that does not include the cost of security systems clinics were compelled to install (Fugh-Berman 1985, 2). In 1985, the numbers stayed high: four bombings, eight cases of arson, ten cases of attempted arson or bombing, and 127 other criminal acts (Ms. 1995, 55). According to the National Abortion Federation, the worst outbreaks of antiabortion violence from 1977 to 1936 occurred in Portland, Oregon; northern California, Los Angeles, and San Diego; Atlanta; Seattle; Philadelphia; Burlington, Vermont; Washington D.C., and northern Virginia (National Abortion Federation 1987, 4). Feminist health clinics, many affiliated with the Federation of Feminist Women's Health Centers, were located in each of these hot spots.

Of course, these are only the most violent of the forms of harassment abortion clinics and their clients had to endure. By the early 1980s, right-to-life groups had stepped up what they called sidewalk counseling in front of abortion clinics. They shouted at clients, called them baby killers, and shoved pictures of fetuses and bloody body parts in their faces (Davis 1988, 57). Demonstrators often invaded clinics, terrorizing clients and staff alike. The web site of the National Abortion Rights Action League (NARAL) reports that there have been more than 2,400 acts of violence against abortion providers since 1977, including bombings, death threats, kidnapping, and assaults, and another 44,400 acts of disruption, including bomb threats and harassing phone calls (NARAL 2000).

Violence against abortion clinics persisted through the middle and late 1980s, and in 1988 Joseph Scheidler of the Pro-Life Action League and Randall Terry, head of Operation Rescue, developed a new tactic: the clinic blockade. Operation Rescue quickly earned the highest profile among antiabortion groups. Its efforts to keep workers, doctors, and clients ("murderers" all, in Randall Terry's rhetorical world, although members of his organization professed concern for women who sought abortions) from entering the women's clinics sparked controversy everywhere and confrontations, some of them violent, in many cities. Women's health activists report unrelenting harassment by antiabortion zealots who assaulted them verbally and physically and damaged or destroyed their workplaces.

Clinic responses to our 1990 survey show clearly that the New Right, incarnated in antiabortion forces, exerted a powerful and negative influence on the movement. Almost 40 percent of respondents acknowledged that they had felt considerable pressure from the antiabortion movement. More than half the sample had had direct contact with Operation Rescue. Despite that organization's efforts to disrupt abortion services, though, feminist clinics, Planned Parenthood affiliates, and private facilities have continued to offer safe and legal pregnancy termination to the women of their communities. To protect itself and its clients, the women's health movement has developed an arsenal of measures to foil attacks by antiabortion groups, and feminist clinics have often pioneered grassroots and legal strategies to challenge Operation Rescue and related organizations. They established escort services to protect clients from blockades and verbal and sometimes physical harassment. They also turned to the courts for protection. The need to defend themselves, they say, only increased their resolve (and reinforced their pro-choice goals and activities).

The Portland Feminist Women's Health Center (PFWHC), long a target of antiabortion activity, exemplifies both the extent of harassment and the strategies of resistance many feminist clinics adopted. Originally founded in 1971 as the Southeast Women's Health Clinic, the organization changed its name and added abortion services in 1979. In a capsule history that appeared in each issue of its quarterly newsletter and was updated over the years, PFWHC details key events in its struggle with anti-abortion activists and its difficult relationships with police and the courts.

1985— "Advocates for Life" begins weekly pickets at the clinic, with groups occasionally as large as 150 people. Picketers harass patients and staff, and block access to the clinic.

1985—The FWHC receives a package mail bomb designed to maim or kill. A wave of vandalism hits the clinic: graffiti, damage to staff cars, and broken windows.

1986—The FWHC files a lawsuit against "Advocates for Life" and obtains an injunction restricting protests outside the clinic. It is the first to survive an appeal on free speech grounds, and thus paves the way for other clinics locally and across the country.

1989—"AFL" and "Operation Rescue" begin conducting blockades of the clinic doors on a regular basis.

1990—After a six-week trial, the jury finds members of "Advocates for Life" guilty of harassment and conspiracy. The FWHC received no financial compensation for legal expenses or economic damage inflicted on the clinic.

1990—The clinic moves to 1020 NE 2nd Ave. in Portland to get relief from anti-abortion picketers and blockades.

1992—The Feminist Women's Health Center opens a new clinic in Eugene. The clinic survives arson attack soon after opening (EPFWHC 1994, 2).

This summary can only begin to suggest the disruptive force of the attacks by antiabortion activists. Daily, weekly, monthly, and over the years, those attacks exhaust the emotional and financial resources of clinics and staff members. As Jude Hanzo, the director of the Portland Feminist Women's Health Center remembers, "It was terrible. Sometimes there were as many as 100 picketers, or 150, and they would be right up against our front door, blocking the door, harassing the patients. When they got in people's faces, screaming and yelling, it was really very bad" (Hanzo 1991). Over the next months, PFWHC continued to endure protests. The clinic's windows were boarded up now. Eventually, thanks to a small grant, staff members were able to strip the plywood off and put metal grates over the glass (window-breaking was one of the antiabortionists' favorite activities). When their lease ended in 1985, clinic administrators tried to move to a location that would offer workers and clients some protection from picketers, and where police might be willing to enforce existing ordinances. But whatever their personal feelings about the issue of abortion, landlords steered clear of PFWHC, understanding the potential for property damage and inconvenience to other tenants.

In 1986 the clinic filed suit against Advocates for Life (AFL), charging that the antis (a term used for antiabortion activists by the pro-choice and women's health movements) sought to deprive women of their civil rights (to abortion) and invoking the federal RICO (Racketeer Influenced and Corrupt Organizations) statute, which was designed to aid prosecutions against organized crime. The judge issued a preliminary injunction that pushed protesters back from the clinic door and prohibited them from impeding the passage of staff or patients. She also ruled that AFL members could not scream or shriek in ways that would impede the provision of health care services. Although AFL appealed the judge's decision on grounds of free speech guarantees, the U.S. Court of Appeals for the Ninth Circuit supported the judge's position. This was the first clinic-protection injunction to survive appeal based on free speech, and it paved the way for sister clinics to better secure their entrances. PFWHC's director believes that the violence of the picketers' actions and their willingness to block an ambulance that had been called to transfer a client to the hospital persuaded the judge, and then the appeals court, that the injunction was warranted (Hanzo 1991).

But within a week of the issuance of the preliminary injunction, the antis were back. Over and over again, PFWHC had to take them to court for contempt of the injunction. Eventually, some of the picketers disappeared and "the real outrageous behavior" diminished (Hanzo 1991). Nevertheless, clinic staff had to go back to court periodically to seek contempt of injunction rulings against particular individuals. The PFWHC director speculated that the injunction forestalled Operation Rescue's move against the clinic for a while (Hanzo 1991). Nevertheless, in 1989, Randall Terry's organization began blockades in full force.

The six-week trial of AFL did not occur until 1990, almost five years after the group had initiated protests in earnest against the clinic. And although PFWHC won the case, it received no financial compensation for legal expenses or economic loss beyond a small $4,000 damage award. In the meantime, the organization had received some compensation from the contempt injunctions. The clinic staff estimated the total at $20,000, including proceeds of a large fine levied on Priscilla Martin, a central actor in the long siege of the clinic.

The apparently endless assault by AFL caused serious harm. Clinic staff and clients suffered terrifying personal experiences. The effect on morale was significant. "Our morale, I mean I just cannot believe we psychologically survived all this. I just cannot believe it. People were so depressed . . . A lot of good people left . . . because it was just so depressing. You felt like you were just

barely hanging on and there was hardly anything you could do anymore"
(Hanzo 1991). Beyond emotional damage and high staff turnover, the clinic
suffered a drastic decline in revenues, from business lost during the protests
(up to 50 percent at times) and from increased outlays for security.

In 1990 the organization's luck changed. Staff members were able to rent
space in a downtown building with a large private parking lot (picketers could
no longer get close to their entrance without violating the law). The Portland
Convention Center was right across the street from the new location. Clinic
workers had every reason to expect more police protection there, and they
got it. For several years, as expenses outran revenues, PFWHC had been com-
pelled to slash salaries; impose layoffs; and cut outreach and education activities and some low-fee services. By 1990 staff suffered from extreme burnout
and the organization had come perilously close to bankruptcy. The director of
the clinic believes that PFWHC would have had to shut down within six months
if it had not moved to the new location.

Abortion clinics across the country shared many of the same experiences:
police often shirked responsibility for enforcement of laws against trespass and
assault, and elected and appointed officials sometimes dismissed pleas for help
from organizations whose work they disapproved. During the 1980s, the
Reagan and then Bush administrations essentially supported the aims and
winked at the tactics of antiabortion forces. From the Department of Justice
on down, it was very difficult to get relief for clinics under siege. When violence escalated in the mid–1980s, coalitions of abortion providers and pro-
choice activists sought to persuade the Department of Justice to define violence
against clinics as terrorism and to investigate national organizations that promoted such activities. But it wasn't until Bill Clinton was elected that an attorney general, Janet Reno, at last used federal resources against the most extreme
and violent sectors of the antichoice movement.

In Portland, the director of PFWHC remembers, she could not always count
on an aggressive police response to the clinic's requests for help. "Administratively, I would say, they wanted the problem to go away. Some people in positions of power were more willing to help than others . . . [The chief of police
in the mid–1980s] had a policy of not making arrests during big blockades. I
was trying to get them to change that policy and they arrested thirty-two people
at a blockade out on Foster [Street] in July of 1989. Then in October of 1989,
they didn't make any arrests at all" (Hanzo 1991). The refusal to make arrests
certainly didn't work against the blockades. AFL members were unlikely to
get tired and go away if the police left them alone. But the policy did add to
the terror staff members felt. "It scared the hell out of me," the director says.
"Things were just so out of control. It felt like at any time, there would be ex-

treme violence. It was very frightening. And the fact that they didn't make any arrests made it worse. [The police] just didn't seem to have the upper hand" (Hanzo 1991).

She is quick to point out that things changed when the clinic moved downtown, and she attributes that change, in part, to sympathetic press coverage of the first blockade. The *Oregonian,* Portland's major newspaper,

> found out that people were trapped in the building . . . all day [because of the protests] . . . and that all the police did was get our people in . . . and then they left . . . But it was moving here that has really [improved the situation] . . . Even though the chief of police might make a decision not to do arrests, they still let each precinct deal with it in their own way. So that when we came here, they made arrests right away. They'll help us. They helped us right away. We didn't even have a blockade the first Saturday we were here . . . The [antis] went into the parking lot, and then the police moved them out of there and said "no way you are going to do this". . . So part of it is a more supportive precinct and part of it is that the physical set up here is much easier for the police to cope with. (Hanzo 1991)

During its most difficult times, pro-choice advocates provided support and protection at PFWHC, which was able to count on a steady supply of escorts (volunteers who helped clients through the lines of picketers). They also held a yearly vigil at the clinic to call attention to what was happening. The clinic newsletter ran a stream of articles about the violence and fundraising always highlighted the financial and emotional costs of running a women's health clinic under battle rules.

After Clinton's election in 1992, there were important changes in federal policies concerning abortion. The gag rule, a statute that had prohibited any health facility from mentioning abortion as an option for pregnant women, was lifted, and bans on fetal tissue research and RU–486, the abortion pill, were overturned. As abortion foes saw their gains erode, they intensified violence against clinics. Their tactics already included arson, bombings, destruction of property, and intimidation of abortion providers. Now they expanded to include murder. How could the clinics defend against those who wanted to kill doctors and support personnel? As the director of development for the two-year-old Feminist Women's Health Center in Eugene, Oregon, reports in the clinic's newsletter (1994), there was only one answer to that question. "The Bureau of Alcohol, Tobacco and Firearms (ATF), FBI, and local police are all telling us to beef up our security immediately. Bringing our security up to necessary levels costs $4,000 a month. This amount of money is completely beyond our budget or expectations. There are no outside resources that cover this—no grants, no federal funds, no 'deep pockets' anywhere" (EPFWHC 1994, 2).

Murders in the rest of the country and renewed and vicious attacks in the Pacific Northwest and northern California naturally increased the clinic's sense of vulnerability; violence forced the installation of ruinously expensive security equipment and absorbed funds that might otherwise have been spent on services, outreach, and health education. In 1994 the Eugene FWHC tried to disseminate information, spread the outrage around. The center printed and distributed a poster that listed dates and locations of arson and bombings at clinics in the region and solicited information about the criminals. The list included arson attacks at the Feminist Women's Health Center in Redding, California, in 1989, 1990, and 1992; a bombing at a Planned Parenthood clinic in Olympia, Washington, in 1990; arson attacks at two Portland abortion clinics in 1992 and 1993; and an arson attack at the Eugene Feminist Women's Health Center soon after it opened in 1992. In addition to crimes against property, the antis targeted well-known pro-choice advocates. Advocates for Life picketed the home of the director of the Portland FWHC and filled her mailbox with postcards demanding that she "stop murdering kids," distributed fliers to her neighbors asking them to "let her know that you think she should not kill children for a living" (PFWHC 1995b, 2).

Even as the violence got worse there were some legal victories against the antiabortion movement. Shelley Shannon was convicted of attempted murder for shooting a physician and pointing a gun at a clinic nurse and sentenced to eleven years in prison. The following year, Shannon was sentenced to twenty years in federal prison after her conviction in a series of fire bombings and two butyric acid attacks at clinics in Oregon, Nevada, and California. In 1994, the United States Supreme Court dealt a major blow to Advocates for Life by letting stand punitive damage awards against them totaling $3.5 million. Now, momentum was with the pro-choice movement. In addition to the passage of the Freedom of Access to Clinic Entrances legislation, pro-choice advocates hoped to establish a buffer safety zone to protect doctors, patients, health care workers, and clinic facilities from violent attacks. In October 1995, the Portland Feminist Women's Health Center became a plaintiff in a nationwide class-action suit against antiabortion violence. Filed in federal district court in Portland, the lawsuit named Advocates for Life and American Coalition of Life Activists and fourteen individuals who argued for or condoned the use of violence against clinics and clinic workers by signing the "justifiable homicide" declaration or distributing the "deadly dozen" list of abortion providers (PFWHC 1995a, 1).

Antiabortion violence was not (is not) unique to Oregon or the Northwest.

Feminist clinics across the country have sustained extensive damage and revenue loss from the activities of abortion foes. The Atlanta Feminist Women's Health Center endured intense harassment and blockades by Operation Rescue for three months, especially during and just after the 1988 Democratic National Convention in that city. Lynne Randall, director of the center, reports that a clinic worker found two dead kittens on her front porch one morning with a note that read "Try killing something besides babies." Another clinic worker who was pregnant took early maternity leave because she feared that jostling and stress might lead to a miscarriage. In Atlanta, police made arrests—twelve hundred of them (Hairston 1990, 15, 16). The siege had serious repercussions on clinic services, programs, and finances, just as the AFL assaults had had on the Portland Feminist Women's Health Center. AIDS education work suffered. The clinic's property and then its liability insurance policies were canceled. "Nobody would say specifically [that] it was because of the antiabortion activity," Randall observes, "but everybody knows it is . . . Our insurance agent feels certain it was because of the presence and the exposure of the antis, that people were going to be pushed and shoved and there was more likelihood that somebody would fall down and sue" (18).

The newsletter of Emma Goldman Clinic in Iowa also reported devastating consequences of harassment:

> Businesses anticipate the intimidation tactics of the anti-choice minority when considering relationships with the clinic. Weighing their [the antis] loud opposition against the reasoned response of the pro-choice community, businesses sometimes make a decision inconsistent with the values of the majority to avoid confrontation. Recent examples include: Non-renewal of the Clinic's workers compensation policy resulting from "escalating violence" at clinics nationally; Restricted access to workplace giving because abortion is viewed as "divisive and polarizing" and Rejection of Clinic lease proposals by Quad City landlords fearing anti-choice backlash. (Cohen 1995, 1)

Such administrative difficulties don't make splashy news, like fire-bombings or protests (and, of course, anticlinic violence has been reported only sporadically and minimally by much of the media). But if clinics are unable to find landlords willing to rent space, or if they are forced to agree to above-market rents because of security issues, or if they are obliged to pay exorbitant insurance and workers' compensation premiums because they are considered high-risk enterprises, a category into which the antis put them, then the antis score victories.

Long struggles from antiabortion activism and continuing fiscal difficulties associated with those struggles put some feminist clinics out of business and saddled others with crushing debt. The Feminist Women's Health Center in Everett, Washington closed after it was firebombed three times in quick succession (Ginsburg 1989, 53). The Oakland Feminist Women's Health Center suffered financially from local harassment, and problems intensified after a fire destroyed its sister clinic in Los Angeles in 1985. Although clinic workers were certain that the LA fire was arson, investigators' findings were inconclusive. Because LAFWHC was not fully insured, the organization recovered far less than its total losses from the insurance company. So resources and staff from all the California FWHCs were diverted to Los Angeles. "Business wise we should have closed the clinic," said a FWHC staff member, "but as feminists we couldn't let a fire stop us, that is what they wanted. To re-open it, to spend money you don't have, it's not a smart business move." But it was a move that feminist organizations were forced to make.

News of fire bombings elsewhere made local landlords reluctant to rent to the Oakland FWHC when the organization sought to move after a long siege by protesters. Continually confronted by their own financial problems and by the obligation to provide resources and staff assistance when sister clinics were threatened, staff at the Oakland FWHC found that whenever they increased outreach or attempted to expand, it "just brought us more harassment." It became more and more difficult to attract and retain workers, one staff member admitted, because "our workplace felt like the center of a combat zone." The sense of being trapped in an endless war was everywhere in the clinic sector of the women's health movement. Eventually, both the Orange FWHC and the LAFWHC were taken over by private doctors.

Although the assault by the antiabortion movement has had undeniable financial, political, and emotional effects, the overall impact on many health clinics has been to reinforce their resolve to provide abortion services and to reenergize their political commitments. In Tallahassee, for example, the Feminist Women's Health Center withstood weekly pickets by antiabortion protesters, including one incident in which five adults (three were the clinic's codirectors) and one child, all supporters of the clinic, were arrested, "despite the fact," Brenda Joyner says, "that we did no violence, but had violence done to us—despite the fact that we broke no laws—we were still the ones arrested, not the anti-abortionists" (1990, 209). Joyner goes on to report that police used excessive force in making the arrests. She and her co-directors later discovered that the assistant chief of police and the state attorney general served together on the board of the Christian Action Council, the organization that had launched the attack on the clinic (209).

Incidents such as this one not only strengthen the determination of clinic staff; they also tend to build community support for the clinics. Surely this example of the law of unintended consequences helps explain why, according to our survey, representatives of the vast majority of feminist health organizations targeted by antiabortion groups believe their goals have actually been reinforced by the assaults they have endured. Indeed, the need to answer these assaults has led to the development of grassroots clinic defense strategies that have provided a new way for clinic supporters to become involved with the women's health movement and to demonstrate their commitment to reproductive choice. Serving as escorts for clients who must make their way through crowds of screaming protesters or acting as counterdemonstrators, women and men have used clinic defense and active pro-choice advocacy for reproductive choice as avenues for maintaining and building an oppositional consciousness within the larger women's health movement.

Changing State Policy, Growing Challenges

Violence against abortion clinics may be the most visible and abhorrent manifestation of the changing political climate in the country in the 1980s and since. But at the same time, women's health clinics had to contend with other threats to reproductive autonomy, threats that affected their day-to-day operations and their missions as advocacy and alternative service organizations. Many of these threats surfaced in state regulatory policies in the wake of elections at all levels of government of politicians beholden to an increasingly powerful antiabortion lobby.

A comprehensive account of the many legislative, legal, and administrative means used to limit women's reproductive freedoms, particularly their access to contraceptive and abortion services, is beyond the scope of this book (but see, for example, Fried 1990; Petchesky 1990). However, in addition to the cuts in funding for health, family planning, and abortion services, feminist health clinics faced a seemingly endless series of challenges as antiabortion political forces scored one key legislative victory after another. The first serious blow came in 1977 with passage of the Hyde Amendment, which prohibited the use of federal Medicaid funds to pay for abortions except when the life of the mother is at risk. Once the Hyde Amendment was secure, antiabortion activists took aim at state Medicaid regulations and succeeded in less than a decade (and in thirty-seven states), in prohibiting use of state-based Medicaid funds for abortion except for women whose lives are in danger or who are victims of rape or incest (regulations differ by state) (Fried 1990, 4). Needless to say, access to abortion was compromised for women who receive public assistance.

Clinics that provided abortions faced the choice of offering free or reduced-fee procedures (thus decreasing their revenues) and/or devoting time and energy to fund-raising to make up for lost income. In 1990, fifteen years after it opened, the Tallahassee Feminist Women's Health Center charged only fifty dollars more for an abortion than it had in 1975, this despite "huge increases in the expense of medical supplies, personnel, insurance and taxes" (Joyner, Grey, and Denenberg 1990, 1). Because Florida is one of the states that has not provided Medicaid coverage of abortion since 1978, the clinic devised reduced fees and payment plans for women who receive Medicaid or face other financial problems. The next round of restrictions came with the many laws passed in the late 1970s and 1980s that required parental notification or consent for abortions for minors, legislation popular among conservative politicians because it purported to be antichoice and pro-family.

Once Reagan took office, the notion of parental consent was expanded to the area of contraceptive services as well. Reagan used the strategy of executive regulation to and through the Department of Health and Human Services to require parental notification prior to delivery of contraceptive services or devices to unmarried teenagers. One feminist scholar who has studied state policy on reproductive rights calls this and related administrative actions "bureaucratic guerilla warfare that systematically harassed and intimidated abortion providers and restricted access, particularly for young unmarried women, to abortion and birth control services" (Petchesky 1990, 269). Pro-choice activists responded energetically to such attacks on women's reproductive freedom, mounting legal challenges, winning injunctions against regulations such as the gag rule and the squeal rule, and rebuilding the pro-choice movement, which had been relatively quiet since *Roe* vs. *Wade.*

Nevertheless, despite the incontrovertible fact that the majority of American citizens support the right to choose, the Reagan administration mapped out and pursued an effective obstructionist course. For example, the Department of Health and Human Services issued guidelines intended to segregate abortion facilities and services from other family planning activities in federally funded clinics and hospitals. Petchesky notes that guidelines, unlike regulations, require no public hearings or public comment prior to implementation (269). So at a time when family planning agencies were strapped for money, they were being told to organize services in a way that was both costly and inefficient. With the enactment of the squeal rule requiring family planning providers to notify both parents or the legal guardian of minors within ten days of issuing a prescription for birth control pills or devices, the administration capped its efforts to severely limit the flow of federal dollars into women's health organizations.

Feminist clinics responded to the new regulations and guidelines. In June 1982, the newsletter of the Berkeley Women's Health Collective warned that

"Proposed Family Planning Regulations Would Affect Teens," referring to the parental notification policy for services funded under federal Title X (family planning) programs. Again, clinics faced difficult choices. Should they forswear funds that came so encumbered by unacceptable regulations? Should they continue to operate as they had always done and risk losing funds if their failure to comply with regulations was proved? Should they try to develop creative strategies to circumvent the regulations and laws? In fact, most clinics chose the third option and found ways to provide services to teens and Medicaid recipients. But their jobs were made more difficult by oppressive policies promulgated from Washington, D.C. The need to bolster services with advocacy and political activity only increased as the eighties wore on.

In 1983 the antiabortion movement suffered a serious defeat when the Supreme Court, in *Akron Center for Reproductive Health* vs. *The City of Akron,* declared unconstitutional an array of restrictions on abortion imposed by state and local ordinances. Not long afterward, the antis sustained another disappointment: The Senate narrowly rejected a proposed constitutional amendment that would have banned abortion. These victories for pro-choice activists reverberated within antiabortion forces and strengthened the arguments of extremists. The antis still pursued legislative and legal strategies, but they adopted direct action tactics, too, blocked clinic access, engaged in verbal and physical harassment of abortion providers and clients, vandalized facilities, chained themselves to clinic doors (Ginsburg 1989, 51), and clothed their malicious intent under misleading organizational banners: Advocates for Life and Operation Rescue.

By 1989 the battle over abortion was still pitched, but a Supreme Court ruling, *Webster* vs. *Reproductive Health Services,* gave a new edge to antichoice advocates. In Webster, although the preamble asserts that "the life of each human being begins at birth," the Supreme Court nevertheless upheld numerous provisions of a Missouri law that prohibited the use of public facilities or public employees to perform or assist in the performance of abortions. The Webster decision kept feminist health and reproductive rights activists busy defending the basic right to abortion; and the Tallahassee Feminist Women's Health Center, which had struggled for years to build grassroots support for reproductive choice, had to redouble organizing efforts, not to expand, but simply to defend or win back gains supposedly guaranteed in *Roe* vs. *Wade* in 1973.

The struggle to protect women's reproductive rights by providing contested services such as family planning and abortion colored all aspects of the complex relationship between feminist clinics and the state, as regulation and oversight of these organizations penetrated into arenas not usually concerned with health care or family planning. The Chico Feminist Women's Health Center, for example, found itself embroiled in a five-and-a-half-year legal battle with the State of California Employment Development Department (EDD) over charges that clinic staff had engaged in conspiracy to commit employment fraud.

The case began early in the spring of 1983, when a former employee tipped EDD officials that FWHC workers were simultaneously collecting unemployment benefits and working full time at the clinic. An investigation was requested in May 1983, and an audit was conducted in February 1984, after which investigators seized many records, including confidential medical files of clients, during an eight-and-a-half-hour search of the clinic. Over the next four years the case took many twists and turns; charges, countercharges, and appeals were filed by both sides. In June 1986, for instance, the clinic sued the EDD, charging abuse of process, malicious prosecution, illegal search and seizure, and discrimination based on the health center's advocacy of abortion. Six months later, the district attorney replied by filing felony charges against the FWHC employees. It took almost two years, until November 1988, for a municipal court judge to dismiss the case on the grounds that the statute of limitations had run out before the charges were filed.

At issue in this complicated case was the question of whether the clinic broke the law by laying off workers and then allowing them to volunteer full time while they collected unemployment benefits. Center Director Shauna Heckert argued that the practice was neither unusual nor illegal. "As far as I know, it's an acknowledged practice of many nonprofits to lay off dedicated workers during tight fiscal times and rehire them later... We were very up front with local EDD employees. We'd tell them exactly what we were doing. EDD workers knew (to reach us at the center) if a job interview was available" (Abramson 1988, 8). While they were laid off and receiving unemployment benefits, workers could earn twenty-five dollars a week without incurring legal penalties. The Chico FWHC paid them that amount, as well as reimbursement for travel to other clinics and for out-of-pocket expenses. It was those additional expenses that concerned EDD and the district attorney's office. The state agency and the local prosecutor charged that clinic staff did not keep legitimate records of those expenses and argued that proof of fraud could be found in a surprising fact: Total reimbursement (including unemployment benefits) to each employee equaled almost exactly her regular salary.

FWHC staff believed that felony charges of employment fraud (that could have sent them to jail) constituted political harassment, and *Network News*, NWHN's newsletter, echoed their view when it noted that the investigation was begun shortly after the election of antichoice Governor George Deukmejian in 1983, and that felony charges were finally pressed the day after media coverage of FWHC's lawsuit questioning the legality of the state's investigation:

"these charges are an obvious attempt at retaliation for the suit and a continued political attack on women controlled clinics," *Network News* contended (Pearson 1987, 5).

The clinic's attorney argued that if the co-directors did commit a violation, it was a technical and unintentional one, but surely not an action that would justify a "major five year campaign against them" (Merin quoted in Abramson 1988, 8). The assumption that the case was an example of political harassment found support, attorney Merin said, in the state's offer to settle the charges administratively, but only if the defendants signed away their Fifth Amendment rights, leaving open the possibility that their statements might be used against them. On the day the charges were dismissed, Merin was quoted in the local newspaper as saying that he had known all along that the statute of limitations had expired and that "the state wasted a half a million dollars in this case, motivated by anti-abortionists and the refusal to recognize that they were wrong" (Merin quoted in Brooks 1988, B1).

From the perspective of the women whose lives were so disrupted by this lengthy, and ultimately unsuccessful, investigation of their organizational practices, practices they developed to keep their struggling clinics afloat against great odds, the investigation was a form of harassment. Nor was it an isolated instance, but another in a long series of difficulties they faced because of state regulation and antiabortion activism.

One of the goals of feminist theory has been to develop a penetrating analysis of the state, a difficult task given the complexity and changing nature of states. Even as feminist theoretical insights about the nature of the state and dynamics of state policies grew more sophisticated during the 1980s, the advanced capitalist states of Western Europe, the United States, and Australia were changing radically. Feminist activists (and scholars) had fundamentally to rethink what they had learned about the state in the context of fiscal crises, global restructuring, and the growing influence of conservative or anti-state ideology. The question no longer focused on whether a feminist health clinic should accept money from the state, knowing that one of the political goals of such funding was to coopt the movement. Now as state funds were slashed on every side, feminists had to find ways to sustain organizations that were meeting critical needs of women and serving as important public spaces identified with feminism. The choice was not whether but how to defend women's reproductive rights and the gains women had slowly achieved in controlling their own health care.

At the same time, new challenges confronted women's health activists. One of the most difficult of these was the powerful new set of problems unleashed by the AIDS epidemic. Between the first reporting of AIDS in 1981 and early political construction of the disease as a gay-only (or primarily) plague, the Reagan administration responded with "authoritarian moralism" rather than concern for public health (Eisenstein 1994, 139). It took a long time for the state to recognize that women were at risk for AIDS, but feminist activists soon understood that AIDS represented a threat not only to women's health, but also to the political gains the movement had secured for women (Banzhaf 1990; Corea 1992; Schneider and Stoller 1995; Hammonds 1996).

On the one hand, AIDS underscored how many of the problems women faced within the health care system remained entrenched even after more than a decade of sustained feminist health activism. Despite repeated movement claims that men and women experience health problems differently—heart disease, for instance—it was not until a decade after the first reported cases of AIDS that the CDC (Centers for Disease Control) protocols for HIV/AIDS were changed to include the specific opportunistic infections that afflict women. The old protocols, in practice, guaranteed that diagnosis of HIV/AIDS in women would be delayed; delay affected not only prognosis but also eligibility for experimental drug trials and SSI disability benefits. Moreover, AIDS prevention and treatment programs often fail for women because women lack power to protect themselves from infected partners and from the socioeconomic conditions that constitute an ideal medium for the spread of HIV/AIDS.

On the other hand, when the state did finally begin to put serious money into AIDS research and health services (only after long and valiant struggles by AIDS activists), it was hard to keep state money and policy focused on some of the other, far from conquered, public health issues for women—that is, maternal and child health, family planning, and breast and other cancers of women's reproductive systems. In an era of budget "restraint," the state's approach was to steal from Patty to fund Paula, rather than to expand the nation's commitment to public health and health care access for all.

In the wake of the rapid spread of AIDS, the feminist contention that women should have the power to control their reproductive lives and health care was tested by a long string of proposed and enacted regulations that limited (or attempted to limit) women's control of their bodies. Hortensia Amaro has argued that scientific and policy discussions about women and AIDS often focused on women as "vessels of infection" and "vectors of perinatal transmission" rather than as human beings facing serious illness (1990, 247). With calls to quarantine AIDS victims by politicians on the extreme right still echoing, many moderate politicians proposed routine testing of pregnant women and those seeking birth control. These proposals did not adequately protect women from inappropriate disclosure of test results and potential discrimination. A new legal status for fetal rights in the 1980s put women at risk of criminal charges for drug use during pregnancy, and potentially for child abuse or assault for passing HIV on to their babies. In an ironic twist, some advocated coercive measures to pressure HIV-positive pregnant women to abort fetuses that might be HIV positive.

Although it is true that rates of HIV infection rose for all women during the 1980s, and especially in the 1990s, AIDS has disproportionately affected poor women of color. In the United States, more than 50 percent of women who have AIDS are African Americans, and 21 percent are Latinas (Eisenstein 1994, 143). As AIDS began to spread rapidly within poor communities and, especially in communities of color, the "failures of the American health care system became increasingly evident even to conservative thinkers" (Rodriguez-Trias and Marte 1995, 301). The tragic demographics of AIDS infection revealed starkly how sexist, racist, and homophobic health care services and policy remained two decades after women, people of color, and gays/lesbians had fought so hard for social change.[3]

Women's health activism had never subsided since the early days of the movement, but new challenges during the 1980s fueled renewed activism. Powerful new actors had joined the struggle, including AIDS activists from the gay and lesbian communities and beyond. Some of the progress that had been made in increasing access to health care services and improving health status were stalled or reversed during the 1980s. Dramatically worsening economic conditions in low-income communities and cuts in social (including health care) programs intersected in rising rates of infant mortality, especially for African American women, and other evidence of declining health among the nations poor and disenfranchised (Roberts 1997). By the mid to late 1980s, new national health care organizations had been formed to address the particular needs of women of color. And in the wake of modest success in calling attention to the need for an aggressive national response to AIDS by the end of the decade, a new breed of women's health activists emerged concerned with the epidemic of breast cancer. These movements are politically and historically connected to the women's health movement.

Chapter 9

The Politics of Race and Class

Dreams of Diversity, Dilemmas of Difference

Like other sectors within contemporary feminism, the women's health movement has, from its earliest days, accommodated intense political and ideological struggles, none of them sharper or more consequential than those that cluster around racism and class. It is impossible to understand how the women's health movement changed from its founding days through the early 1990s and beyond without taking full account of the politics of race, ethnicity, and class. The external struggles that affected women-controlled clinics in the 1970s and 1980s produced difficult challenges, but the ways clinics responded to these difficulties was shaped, in part, by internal political struggles within these organizations, especially about race and class differences in women's needs, perspectives, and politics. Fault lines of race and class altered the workplace cultures and practices whose ideological divisions reveal a too-often neglected aspect of social movements—that they are sites not only of social action and political theory, but also of political passion.

North American feminists have commonly used a vocabulary of sisterhood to argue that women are universally subjugated and that gender is a collective identity with the potential to unite women politically. But women of color and poor women have long charged, as Sojourner Truth did in 1851 ("ar'nt I [an ex-slave] a woman?,"),[1] that the assumptions, ideologies, and activities of feminism fail to represent all women, and indeed that much feminist practice consolidates power among white and middle-class groups. But coalitions, alliances, and work relationships between working-class and middle-class women, and between European American women and women of color, have rarely been easy expressions of sisterhood. The explanation of why this is so lies at the heart of a body of critical scholarship that explores the roots of differences in power, privilege, and life experience among women differently socially located by race, ethnicity, and class (for example, Hull, Scott, and Smith 1982; Dill 1983; hooks 1984; Anzaldúa 1990a; Collins 1990; Bhavnani 2001). This scholarship problematizes and theoretically reconstructs race and ethnicity as fluid, multivalent, relational, and situated social constructions (Williams 1991; Brown 1992; Mohanty 1992; Frankenberg 1993). Even when we acknowledge that feminists may express or tolerate racism, homophobia, and inequitable class relations, we don't necessarily get any closer to the inclusive, multiracial, cross-class, diversity-rich organizations women's health activists imagined. Dreams of diversity often collided in the clinics with dilemmas over difference and led to protracted internal conflicts that played out against the backdrop of external political and economic assaults. The result: challenging, often emotionally wrenching, experiences, and, in many cases, significant organizational effects.

Sisterhood Is Powerful and Hard to Achieve across Class

Community Health Care for Women (CHCW) opened in the mid–1970s.[2] Most of the working-class staffers, constituents of a neighborhood association involved in local politics and seeking to establish an immunization clinic, were high-school graduates who held low-wage jobs and were raising children, some with, and others without, partners. The middle-class women, members of a socialist-feminist organization based in a neighboring community, were all college-educated. Many had worked in health care, as providers or as political activists. Few had children, although many were married or involved in long-term relationships. All believed that the women's liberation movement was too exclusively a project of the middle class and hoped to develop a cross-class women's health organization.

CHCW was one of only a few feminist clinics from these early days of the movement that made cross-class alliance one of their central principles, and it was unique in another way as well. It operated two separate enterprises under one roof, a mental health collective, staffed by professional women and offering fee-for-services counseling, and a health clinic much like those profiled in chapter 4, which defined itself as a collective; provided well-women services and abortion counseling and referrals (but not abortions); and commanded very limited financial resources. Once the health clinic began to receive external funds (in small amounts) and to conform to local and state regulations, it was forced to adopt some of the trappings of hierarchy by appointing a medical director (a psychiatrist who helped found the mental health collective) and a board of directors, most of whom were middle-class volunteers. In recognition of the different resources available to middle- and working-class women, CHCW reserved almost all its paid positions for working-class women. Some, but by no means all, of the middle-class members of the CHCW staff were also members of the mental health collective; the income they received from their fee-for-services counseling subsidized their volunteer activities at the health clinic.

The work of sustaining the organization was always difficult, as we have seen in the stories of sister clinics throughout this book. Conflicts over organizational policies and strategies came to a head in the late 1970s, when the mainly middle-class board of directors met secretly, fired CHCW's working-class staff, and closed the clinic for reorganization (workers were to receive three weeks of severance pay). Furious about the process and its conclusion, the paid staff organized a community meeting at which they labeled their firing a "coup" by middle-class women determined to deprive working-class employees, and the neighborhood, of community control of the clinic. By the meeting's end, the entire board of directors had resigned and the fired employees had been reinstated. CHCW functioned as a working-class enterprise for the next two years, until it could no longer sustain itself and had to close its doors permanently.

How did this alliance of working- and middle-class women committed to empowering working-class women as clients and staff reach the point at which class conflicts destroyed it?[3] To what extent were the divisions within the CHCW staff the result of class difference? How did class consciousness and identity affect the kinds of experiences clinic staff had on the job? Fifteen years after the firing and reinstatement of the paid staff, I talked with four of the principals: Margaret and Liz, who identified as middle class, and Betsy and Jesse, who identified as working class (these are all pseudonyms). Their memories suggest that despite good intentions and the articulation of institutional goals and practices designed to equalize power relations, class differences surfaced repeatedly in their relationships. And despite political aims and claims to the contrary, conflicts over working conditions and clinic policies often reproduced hegemonic class relations.

Soon after the crisis passed, three analyses appeared in the letters column of a community newspaper.[4] Betsy and four other women charged that the "middle class professional" women used "a dummy board that was never intended to have any real power" as a weapon of class privilege. Margaret, physician and medical director, observed: "My objection was not that [the clinic] was being run by working-class women, but that in my opinion it was being run very badly, and the fact that the staff was working class was no excuse." Jesse, a clinic founder who had resigned shortly before the firings because she believed that the actions of some working-class colleagues were ruining the organization, got more specific: "[The clinic] didn't become the utopian socialist feminist mini-society which proved that class was no obstacle for women working together. But the problem was not class, but a defect in our ways of handling situations. There was a lack of trust on the part of both community and professional women . . . There was a lack of solidarity in political objectives. We tried to pretend that we didn't need any rules."

Betsy Connor was eighteen when she first visited CHCW as a client, found a niche there, and trained as a lab volunteer. When a paid position became available, she quit her job as a waitress and went to work at the clinic. Betsy knew that she wanted a different life than she saw around her. Her working-class female identity, she reported, dictated clothes, makeup, and hairstyles that defined her as a "chick," scripted her into bar hopping with friends from high school, and predicted a dull workplace routine, regulated by the clock, like her father's. Life at the clinic subverted those rules. "During the day, I . . . wore flannel and sort of was a feminist and then, in the evening, I'd go out with my . . . friends and be a chick and a babe. It was very confusing to me" (Connor 1991).

Painfully aware that she lacked education, skills, and expectations in comparison with her middle-class coworkers, she nevertheless understood that clinic ideology valorized community women and that its political culture emphasized the equal worth of paid staff and volunteers. "We acted as if we were all equal," she said. "But in fact, they had a lot more advantages." Middle-class women had fewer struggles outside the workplace, Betsy believed. So when she and her coworkers began to feel that they were being monitored and judged as employees rather than as equals, her pain and anger spiked. She associated the transition from the perception of class differences to the experience of class conflict with the opening of the mental health counseling services facility within the clinic. (The counseling collective was an autonomous body. Its professionally trained women powerfully influenced the decisions of the health collective, but the arrangement wasn't reciprocal.) Betsy remembered how it felt to be told what to do by the middle-class professionals. "All of a sudden, the [counseling] collective decided they didn't like the colors [of the walls]. They wanted everything white . . . They wanted to not only be a separate group that helped us out, but they wanted to control the health [clinic]. Control the color the walls were painted. Control what we said on the phone . . . It just got to be, it was their clinic and we were workers." The collective had implemented a policy that compensated paid staff for hours they spent taking classes, an important benefit. But soon after she enrolled in a course, a committee was established "to check up on people," Betsy said.

I think the community women never felt like they were as good. And as much as we talked about it and hashed it out, in the end that's what it boiled down to. There were questions about whether we were really doing our jobs. There were questions about whether or not community women had the same commitment to the health project as the middle-class women . . . There was a belief [that] community women were only there for a paycheck . . . What they did was put all the community women in the paid positions. So of course it would appear that way to the naked eye.

Betsy's belief that she and her coworkers were not regarded as equals was confirmed when the board of directors fired them. "I think it came down to a real power struggle in the sense that they wanted control of the health project," she concluded.

Jesse Calas's analysis was different. A mother of four and lifelong resident of the community, she was attuned to the differences between her life experiences and those of the middle-class women with whom she worked, but she also shared important political beliefs with them and had, like them, actively opposed the war in Vietnam. When Jesse first heard the socialist feminists articulate their vision of a health center, she felt that their ideas were similar to hers. She remembered the year of meetings before the clinic was founded as exciting and sometimes stormy. Although some of the working-class women suspected the motives of the middle-class women from across the city, she noticed complementary strengths: "People who had skills to share would share them, and the women who had community expertise would share it, and working together . . . we would learn from each other" (Calas 1991). Jesse's assessment of her relationships with the middle-class members of the collective differed from Betsy's. She felt supported and believed that she gained important skills through her relationships with her professional coworkers. She took advantage of the education program the clinic provided for working-class staff and went back to college; over the years, she earned internship credits by working with the counseling collective.

Jesse acknowledged that disagreements within the staff were routinely defined by some working- and middle-class staffers as expressions of class difference. But in her opinion, these disagreements stemmed from differences in "politics" and what she called "work style and expectations." The clinic often hired former clients who lacked skills but needed work. Some of these women had problems (including alcoholism and the experience of domestic violence) that interfered with job performance. One staff member whose alcoholism resulted in frequent absenteeism, for example, was the subject of group discussions for six months. To the proposal to fire her, Jesse remembered, "other working-class women said absolutely no . . . we have to help her. I said, 'How?' 'Well, we don't know.' That was one of the issues I quit over."

Failure to address unsatisfactory job performance was an expression of paternalism, Jesse felt, and although she acknowledged that it was wrong to impose political views on community women, she believed that all clinic workers should share the clinic's political goals. Otherwise, she reasoned, the collective could not count on political commitment to motivate work discipline. In the absence of shared political commitment, other forms of work rules became necessary. But when work rules were proposed, class became what she called a "bogeyman," and polarization only grew.

Margaret Gordon's perspective was like Jesse's in crucial ways. She helped found the CHCW just after she finished her residency. When the clinic applied for licensure, Margaret was named medical director. She understood that the title was merely technical, supposedly only a matter of nomenclature. But impending financial crisis, the conviction that decision-making processes "had broken down completely" and that services were deteriorating fast forced the board to take drastic action and fire the clinic staff, Margaret said (Gordon 1991). Her own duty as medical director was plain: She was unwilling to accept "legal and moral responsibility for a situation over which I felt I had no control." Like Jesse, Margaret believed that the organization's failure to develop "basic points of political unity and to define our goals clearly" was to blame for ongoing crisis at CHCW.

Historically, a fear of conflict had led the collective to "sweep our differences under the rug," Margaret said: precisely because middle-class members were accused of being "insensitive" to working-class women and of using their "class privilege" to get their way when conflict did arise. And she pointed out that middle- and working-class women could be found on both sides of clinic disputes. She cited Jesse as an example of a working-class woman who rejected the view that a woman's class background and personal problems canceled out her responsibility to do her job well.

Margaret acknowledged how her class position, and especially her medical training, shaped her attitudes and actions. She admitted to having a "take-charge" attitude about the "power vacuum" at the clinic:

> We moved into this organization that I have to say was in great disarray when we arrived . . . We swept the floors, painted things. Part of that was the ideology that there shouldn't be an enormous division of labor along professional lines . . . But I think once you've been through an internship and residency and you move into a situation that is chaotic, you are accustomed to certain ways. Making structure, being work oriented, production oriented, not

particularly process oriented. I mean, I'm about as process oriented as they come for docs.

Margaret attributed the considerable power of the counseling collective not to class, but to an organizational reality. "If you kind of outlast everybody else, you got your way," she said; "so there were six of us [the counseling collective] and . . . we got our way." The professionals who had made a long-term commitment to the clinic sought to get organized when they painted the walls, searched for stable funding, proposed sliding-scale fees in place of free care, and completed paperwork and changed protocols that would enable them to bill Medicaid. Some members of the collective had a romanticized view of working-class women, Margaret believed. That made it difficult to develop reasonable standards for hiring and job performance. The decision to fire the staff and close the clinic was undemocratic, she admitted, but it was also unavoidable, a last, desperate attempt to save the organization.

Liz Rose, a middle-class woman who worked at the clinic for several years, left the organization about eighteen months before the mass firing. Her eight-page letter of resignation decries the actions of "professional women [who] were wrecking the clinic." She was troubled by "changes in the direction and tone of the [clinic] that . . . occurred slowly and subtly, not by mandate . . . but by unrecognized power manipulations" (Rose 1975). Liz argued that criticisms of working-class staff for not following work rules and time schedules arose out of a misunderstanding of how they functioned, particularly in outreach, community education, and community organizing: "Like pushing sex education in the schools . . . These are volatile issues and pretty risky for people who live here . . . And there was no appreciation of what that meant . . . All the groundwork and things the community women did to make us able to do what we did . . . [the professional women] didn't see that as work. It was invisible to them. It was the most narrow sense of responsibility and accountability. (Rose 1991)

Liz's understanding of the invisibility and the contributions of, and risks taken by, women from the community differed from Margaret's in important ways. Margaret's class privileges got in the way of her understanding both her own privilege and the ways the work of community women involved in the clinic differed from her own (and that of other professional) women both in substance and in meaning.

Her understanding of class deepened while she worked at the clinic, Liz said. "What was important about class was that different people have different amounts of control over their own lives, different amounts of power in society . . . and therefore different self-interests in the system." The middle-class women at the clinic "had blinders on," she observed, and class difference made it hard for working-class women to "go like a united group up against this united group of professionals . . . They have all these articulation skills and jargonize everything."

The problems were partly a result of organizational structure. Because the counseling collective functioned as a separate entity, the health clinic staff had no control over what it did. Moreover, any internal disagreements of the counseling collective were hidden from the working-class staff, while problems and divisions within the health collective were in full view of counseling collective members who were also members of the collective running the health clinic. For Liz, this imbalance of disclosure and distance, with the middle-class women protected and the community women exposed, mirrored the traditional professional-client relationship. "We had to do the same thing," one staff member said. "It wasn't like there weren't issues of accountability and responsibility [among us] . . . But we couldn't be open about them because they [members of the counseling collective] weren't open."

Liz resigned, she explained, because once the professionals, who wanted to "be their own bosses," took control of the work lives of community women, whom they regarded as incapable of sharing fully in the collective task of running the clinic, their class backgrounds had caught up with them. Given the degree to which class is mystified and dominant class relations are reproduced in everyday life in the United States, the breakdown of cross-class alliance at this clinic should not come as a surprise. Class relations in the United States are shaped and reproduced through housing and neighborhood patterns, education, the labor force, tax policies, and myriad other institutional and economic processes. Although middle- and working-class persons often work together, their opportunities differ. Routinely, middle-class people hold positions of authority over members of the working class, both in workplaces and beyond. Cross-class unity or understanding can be achieved only when those who benefit from prevailing class relations acknowledge and contest them, and when those subordinated by prevailing class relations have the resources, the will, and the support they need to initiate and guide change.

Absence of goodwill did not destroy the collective. Rather, structural barriers to egalitarian work relations combined with the different stakes and understandings of women from different social locations in the class structure to perpetuate conflict. Class, Betsy believed (and Liz agreed), meant that she had less influence in work decisions. When she was fired, she became the object, not the subject, of decision-making. Margaret and Jesse expressed frustration at the collective's refusal to fire staff that some believed were not doing a good job. Working-class solidarity, they observed, blocked hard personnel decisions and proved the weakness of the paid staff's political commitment to the clinic.

Although all four women mentioned a sense of diminished control over important decisions, they brought unequal resources to the decision-making process. This is where some of the structural barriers to creating egalitarian cross-class relations manifest themselves most clearly. Because the clinic had to conform to a web of state regulations governing health and nonprofit organizations, and because, as a community clinic, CHCW depended upon external funds, women with professional credentials or other class-related advantages (education, greater ease dealing with authority figures, and experience using the language of bureaucracy) accrued organizational power.

Theoretically, at least, the resources that gave structural advantage to middle-class women were balanced by equally valued resources of working-class women, and as long as there were few lines of fissure in the organization, the delicate balance of different skills and resources did represent equal, complementary contributions to the group. But community expertise was a vague concept, and once disagreements arose, the balance shifted, and power flowed to those who could articulate a position eloquently or attract money to the clinic. Moreover, the decision to reserve most of the paid positions for community women backfired when longtime volunteers and board members saw their own commitment in political terms (commitment) and attributed simple financial incentive to the work of the paid staff (working for pay). Once again, the class of women who were so often in a position to judge them (as teachers, nurses, doctors, social workers, prosecutors, judges, etc.) assumed the authority to measure the performance of the working-class employees. Conflicts between middle- and working-class women sharpened a problem endemic in other organizations that combine volunteer and paid labor, and the management-worker scenario that unfolded reproduced the dominant class relations of the larger society.

To this point I have used the terms *community women* and *working class* and *professional* and *middle class* as they were used by members of the collective, that is, relatively interchangeably. The vocabulary of class reveals ambiguities and problems that are embodied in the conflicts presented in this case. From the very beginning of meetings between the two founding groups, the term *community women* was used by, and in reference to, the working-class women. The term defined what CHCW presumed to be shared by the working-class women and what differentiated them from the middle-class women: being of or from the community. The term *community women* often substituted for *working class,* the use of which might suggest a higher degree of class consciousness or at least a greater ease with a politicized language of class. Encoded in the term *community women* is a recognition that these women had a higher stake in the community. This was both a reminder and a warning to middle-class outsiders to be cautious about imposing themselves where they did not belong.

On the other hand, the use of the term *professional* as code for middle class increased during the clinic's later years. Early documents are replete with the term *middle class,* but language referring to professionals is unusual, partly because the women's health movement sought to overturn the monopoly of professionalism in delivery of services. The term *professional* entered the vocabulary of the group as conflicts escalated, and particularly in reference to disputes between the counseling collective and CHCW. Liz's letter of resignation, for instance, dwells on the different interests of community women and professionals. The primary interest of the professionals, she argues, was to create "a place where they can work and make a comfortable income, be their own bosses, and preferably do work that doesn't make them feel guilty."

It was in the context of this evolving vocabulary of class that individuals came to understand their own class placement, cross-class relationships, and class politics within the clinic. The issue of class placement or identification is complex. Betsy talked freely of how she felt similar to and different from both her working-class family and friends and her middle-class coworkers. Jesse recognized that her class background situated her as a community woman, but she also shared key political experiences and ideals with most of the middle-class members of the staff. Margaret noted that her direct, take-charge attitude stemmed, in part, from her class background, but she also saw herself as giving up key class privileges and reorienting her class loyalties by choosing to work in a community health clinic rather than in a more lucrative or prestigious position. As one of only a few middle-class women to hold a paid position during the clinic's history, and as someone without professional training or credentials, Liz identified most strongly with the community women in the clinic. Her background, as well as her experiences, textured her understanding of class. Class "has always been an issue for me," she said. Growing up in one of the biggest houses in a relatively poor section of an economically diverse suburb, she often felt "at odds, either from one end or the other, in terms of class."

For Betsy, Jesse, Liz, and Margaret, class was more than a calculus of where they, as individuals, are positioned within a class structure. Class became meaningful as class identification and relations shaped power relations within the group and understandings of self in relation to others (in the group and in the larger society). Class identity emerged, solidified, and fragmented as individuals and groups perceived overlapping or divergent interests and felt understood, misunderstood, accepted, or judged by others. Moreover, although newsletters and other clinic documents expressed basic feminist and socialist principles, there was little sustained or systematic self-education provided for the staff or the larger community that would have created the foundation for a shared class politics, except in the broadest outlines. Such a process might have provided a forum for discussion of class differences and illuminated misunderstandings between middle- and working-class coworkers. But obstacles to such an effort included the middle-class women's awareness that it would be wrong to impose a political vision on their working-class coworkers; the demanding everyday reality of running a health clinic in a community with significant and unmet health needs; and, as time passed and conflicts escalated, fear of fanning the flames of disharmony.

My point here is to suggest that when Jesse and Margaret argued that the absence of a shared political vision was the real source of the collective's problems, they had grounds for their position. Part of the problem was the difficulty of cross-class communication. Honest, constructive discussion rarely followed divisive conflicts. One of the founders of the collective described a pattern: "It would be unfair to us to say that we were totally unconscious of class differences before we opened the [clinic]—if nothing else, we were terrified of talking to working class people because we so objectified those class differences" (CHCW 1973, 6). The result: "We did not know how to talk about those differences in a useful way and ended up . . . by only feeling guilty for who we were" (CHCW 1973, 6). At the same time, the language and style of their middle-class coworkers, especially their polished, articulate, "jargonizing" talk, intimidated and silenced many of the working-class women.

Class differences, divisions, and conflict played a significant role in the dissolution of the alliance that had created and maintained the clinic for more than five years. Both middle- and working-class women brought a healthy dose of distrust to their relationships. Although the middle-class cofounders and members of the collective genuinely sought to implement a socialist, working-class-oriented politics, they also wanted to maintain control: "We had a defined set of politics we wanted to communicate," a clinic history declares; "we did want the clinic to be eventually community controlled but we wanted that control to be by women who agreed with our politics" (CHCW 1973, 6). The desire to maintain control, to run the clinic according to their vision, was behind some of the actions professional women took to save the clinic. The directors fired the paid staff because they had convinced themselves that the clinic's future depended on the suspension of community control, at least long enough to replace current working-class staff members. From the perspective of (most of) the working-class staff, this was just one more example of hegemonic class relations in action. (Though, obviously, this would not have been their language.)

As long as class (and race, ethnicity, and other power relations) structure the resources, opportunities, and textures of relationships among women, work organizations that aim to subvert or transform dominant power relations need sustained forums in which workers learn from each other and communicate directly about their different perspectives. But the process of transforming hegemonic power relations requires more than better communication across class. It requires that those who bring class or racial privilege into an organizational context be open to hearing and changing how that class or racial privilege operates to silence, marginalize, and overwhelm others. More significantly, it requires structural change within organizations and within the larger society. Social movement organizations will have to go beyond promotion of diversity to respect the multiple perspectives of those who occupy different social locations and to change organizational practices that obstruct the development of truly diverse and democratic organizations.

Key aspects of identities (including class, race, ethnicity, gender, and sexuality) are contested, affirmed, and/or reshaped by large-scale historical processes that produce differences of power, privilege, and meaning. It is in the interest of strong alliances and coalitions that groups develop ways of talking and acting that contribute to the redistribution of power and resources in both the short and the long run. That means that everyone involved has to change. But because scholars, activists, and other women do not fully understand how class works in everyday life, and because class privilege is hard to give up, difficulties in forging cross-class relationships and alliances in workplaces and political communities continue to plague feminist and other progressive organizations.

A Tale of Two Clinics: Struggles Over Race and Racism

The particular political landscape of the United States during the 1970s and 1980s, especially in progressive social movements, foregrounded racial and ethnic diversity as the goal of, and the most intractable source of division within, feminist organizations. Once women of color articulated their compelling critiques of racism in the women's movement, feminists across the country began to talk about, and in some cases to act, on their dreams of creating multiracial clinics. But failure by many white women really to understand racism and the privileges of whiteness as they were embedded in social relations and political ideologies meant that women of color routinely experienced both subtle and not-so-subtle racism in health movement organizations (Frankenberg 1993).

An illustrative case is that of Women's Health Services (WHS), a feminist clinic that used state resources specifically from the Comprehensive Employment and Training Act (CETA), to hire fifteen low-income women, about one-third of whom were women of color.[5] Diversification by race and class was a major goal of the CETA project, but implementation was vexed and torturous over the next two years or so, a period of dramatically accelerated growth in the center's programs, staff, services, and budget. If the collective measured success by statistical measures—revenue, number of clients, range of services—then surely the clinic was increasingly successful during this period. But difference reverberated here just as it did at CHCW, as the WHS registered a growing divergence between collectivist feminist ideology and everyday practice, with the erosion of egalitarian social relations and estrangement from the political goals of the larger social movement that had spawned the center in the first place.

The training program for new CETA staff members emphasized information about women's reproductive health, feminism, and specific skills both to carry out the counseling and health work of the clinic and to implement a community survey that had been funded as a major activity of the project. Woven throughout the training were messages about social relations of equality and the centrality of gender as a common bond between women. The facilitators of the training talked about the importance of a diverse staff, emphasizing their hope that women would feel comfortable coming to a health clinic where they could relate to "other women like themselves," they said. But there was little discussion of the profound effects of race, ethnicity, and class on women's lives, and their experience in their new workplace belied the ideology of sisterhood for CETA employees.

Stigmatized even by the term *CETA staff,* the workers were effectively excluded from the collective decision-making process (the staff meeting), a measure designed to be temporary while they were engaged in the community survey, rather than in the routine health work that the regular staff were doing. A series of conflicts and crises ensued and the CETA staff were subject to what they perceived to be increasingly authoritarian treatment by the regular staff. The distance between the dream of diversity and its reality was so great that change had to come. Three incidents capture the essence of the painful but enriching process that transformed organizational politics for clinic workers as they sought to construct a collective identity that encompassed gender commonality and race and class differences.

In 1978, about six months after the CETA project began, the U.S. Department of Labor (the agency that administered CETA) appointed a middle-class white woman who had been associated with the clinic for years to plan and coordinate a "Low-Income Women's Conference" for the city. "Cynthia" (not her real name) scheduled several planning meetings with CETA staff, and she often used the inclusive term *we* when she talked about the goals and opportunities the conference offered low-income women: "It's a great opportunity for us to tell them how we feel about their policies," she said.[6] At one meeting, Cynthia mentioned, rather proudly, a fight she was waging with the Department of Labor over the automatic deduction of five dollars (for lunch) from the fifteen-dollar stipend low-income women were to receive for attending the conference. "You won't have to buy lunch," Cynthia told the women. "Bring a sack lunch, and the catering will be happening anyhow. Let's let the men pay their five dollars. You bring your sack lunches, and I'm sure there will be plenty of leftovers, and for sure we can go up after a while and have some coffee."

Cynthia's words ignited a firestorm. "I'm going to pay for my lunch like everyone else," one African American woman asserted. "I've been eating leftovers all my life," another declared, "and I don't have to eat them at this conference." Once Cynthia left the room, others exploded in anger at the suggestion that they should be content with—instead of embarrassed by—plenty of leftovers. "Women like her don't have a clue about the lives of low-income women," an African American CETA staff member said. "This kind of thing always happens when women like that get involved," she added, and she elaborated what she meant by "women like that." Referring to a series of events that demonstrated the greater power of white middle-class women within the organization and their racist and class-biased actions, she pointed out the selection of representatives to an international women's conference in Mexico the year before. "They did nothing to involve anyone other than white middle-class women," she said. "Look at the delegates—one token black and she is middle class. All those women had been in airplanes and to conferences. It would have been an excellent opportunity for poor or black women to have gone to that conference and have it paid for, but no, those women had to go."

Cynthia could say *we* as often as she liked, but the working-class women and women of color spurned her assertion that gender was the central social relationship among clinic workers. Middle-class white staffers draw lines that divide members of the collective into unequally privileged groups, they insisted. By their refusal to set themselves apart as the leftovers group at the Department of Labor's conference on low-income women, the working-class white women, and women of color acknowledged their alienation and contested their exclusion at the same time. Race- and class-based differences were out in the open now. The collective would not now be able to take gender bonds for granted.

Several months later, word reached the center that the Department of Labor planned to allocate several million dollars to grassroots organizations in the city as an experimental alternative to CETA. The clinic formed an ad hoc community coalition to assemble a package of proposals involving "minorities" (U.S. Department of Labor language), and clinic staff, who were beginning to realize that incorporating women of color into "their" organization was more complex than they had originally envisioned, proposed that women of color who worked at the center should meet on their own to determine priorities and plans.

This meeting was the first in the organization's history exclusively for women of color, who now felt empowered to talk. A Puerto Rican woman spoke of feeling uncomfortable and nervous with white women. An African American woman, recalling an experience she had once had with a white counselor, suggested that autonomous consciousness-raising groups be organized for minority women. She had hated the consciousness-raising group that was part of their clinic training because she did not trust the white, middle-class facilitators: "Now she wanted to get into my mind, pick my brain, find out how a woman like me feels, and I wasn't going to let her know, a white lady, sitting all dressed up and nice, no way." In the community, the women of color agreed, the feminist clinic was regarded as a white middle-class women's institution. The Puerto Rican woman remarked that "Spanish women in this community have either not heard of the [clinic] or if they have they have heard really bad things. They think it's a place to come for bullshit."

Despite their distrust of white women, though, many of the women of color felt that they had grown enormously through their involvement with the clinic. Again and again they returned to a single theme, expressed by one employee, as "a changing sense of myself as a woman since being here." As they considered program proposals that would help other women and their families, they thought about ways to offer the experiences that were changing them—learning about their bodies, sharing and working with other women, recognizing sexism—to others. They wanted to find strategies for overcoming deeply rooted race- and class-based distrust so that women of color and poor women could participate in and benefit from an organization that was perceived to be controlled by middle-class white women.

Gender was an important part of the collective identity and concern of the women of color, but their gender consciousness was race and class specific, filtered through their experiences as poor people of color. In the four-month interval between the leftovers incident and the women-of-color-only meeting, the regular staff had begun to grasp that difference, too, as one middle-class member of the collective observed. "Even though we always said we had respect for our clients as women and treated them as equals, it's different having your main contact with minority women being with them as clients and with them as fellow staff. Your relationship with clients is short term and really defined through a helping relationship. Working together, though, black, Hispanic, and white women—we really have to respect and understand the differences in our lives and values, not just say we do."

Some months after this groundbreaking meeting, the texture of social relations within the staff had changed substantially, and the group as a whole recognized the need to project their new understandings about the intersections of gender, race, and class. The center's board of directors decided to host a summer fair to celebrate the growth of the women's center (the clinic's umbrella organization) and its anticipated move to its own building (donated by the city) and appointed a committee to plan the event. Staff members were invited to participate, but no one got involved until April, just two months before the fair was to be held, when a white middle-class collective member attended a meeting of the fair committee and returned to her colleagues concerned about plans for the event.

She believed the conference as planned would undermine the "hard work of changing that image [as a middle-class organization] we have been about over the past couple of years." The clinic staff now included about half the ex-CETA workers (hired through different grants). They called for a meeting with the fair committee to discuss four concerns: the absence of childcare for the fair; its location in the community arts center; preregistration requirements; and the titles and content of the proposed workshops.

Women of color and poor and working-class white women would be discouraged from attending the fair if they had to preregister, health collective members argued; if there were no arrangements made for childcare; or if the fair was held in the arts center, a venue clearly associated with the white middle class. Moreover, staff members believed, proposed workshops—particularly those that focused on spirituality and career planning—reflected ignorance of the needs and concerns of most women. "We feel that the content of the workshops draws barriers between women. A workshop on spirituality which focuses on the nonreligious kinds of spirituality denies the fact that for most working-class women in this community, religion and spirituality are linked, and turns off those women rather than reaching out to them to expand their ideas about spiritual matters. Worse, calling a workshop 'career planning' in a community where most women have real limited job options makes it clear that you are really addressing professional white middle-class women."

Another staff member expressed her fear that the fair would alienate many women: "We are afraid it will set up a different relationship with our clients, one that is uncomfortable. We think they will come to the fair and see the membership (of the larger Women's Center the health project was part of) as a group of people completely different from themselves. They could easily see the [clinic] serving low-income women by doling out services, without seeing it as a place they could work into, [where they] feel they belonged." In a heated discussion, board members protested that the staff appeared to be censoring activities of concern to "a group of women who have been involved with the center for a long time but who are not interested in or in need of the *services* of the center." A staff member retorted, "We do see the fair as geared to a particular group of women, and we ourselves feel we cannot relate to it and don't want it labeled as representing the clinic." Another added, "it is one thing to schedule one speaker or event that is geared to the specific interests of a small group of women. It's another thing when the event is to symbolize who we are as an organization."

The staff succeeded in having the fair postponed until they could work out some of these difficulties; in fact, the event was never held. But the controversy surrounding it marked a turning point in the clinic's history, with the staff as a whole articulating a conception of gender that did not favor the experiences, priorities, needs, or values of the most powerful groups of women in the organization. Although there was still much struggle ahead, more explicit and painful conflicts over race and class issues, from this point on, the reality of differences and divisions among women was at least as influential in the group's political consciousness as was presumed "sisterhood." This understanding grew and led to changes in the articulation of the organization's mission and activities. This can be seen in a pamphlet the group produced for International Women's Day in 1980, which states explicitly:

> Women's struggle for equality is closely connected with the struggles of other oppressed groups . . . Some of these struggles [referring to activities the organization participated in during the previous year] do not concern narrowly defined "women's issues" . . . That is because women cannot achieve equality or decent lives until all working people get a better deal, nor will women be liberated until racism is eliminated. The struggle for women's liberation includes all women, including women struggling for equality and a better life as workers, as Black people, as Puerto Ricans, as lesbians, or other oppressed groups. (WHS 1980)

When the clinic staff first wrote the proposal to use CETA funds to diversify their staff, they at least implicitly believed that sisterhood provided a sufficient foundation from which to practice egalitarian social relations. Within the context of their political commitment to women, they faced the challenge of revising their assumptions about shared sisterhood and either dealing with their own racism and class privileges (the white and middle-class women) or their distrust and suspicions of white and middle-class women (the women of color and the working-class women). This case study confirms that progressive social movement organizations—intentionally organized to foster egalitarian social relations and structures—must explicitly confront underlying racism and class biases that are daily reinforced by the dominant society. It also demonstrates that once this process begins, very significant changes can take place in the power relations between individuals and groups. In this case, staff of a previously predominantly white clinic shifted their emphasis from an assumption of shared sisterhood to the recognition that bonds between women are textured by their different experiences. With that recognition, they moved from desire for diversity to the hard work of constructing a collective identity and organizational goals and actions that encompassed differences and changed power relations between groups of women. In the process, sisterhood became less an assertion of commonality than a basis for alliances and for shared commitments to empower women.[7]

In both the case of the CHCW and the WHS (the two clinic case studies just discussed), the nature of and main impetus for struggles over race and class were shaped in large part by the racial and class demographics of these organizations. But the politics of difference did not always play out simply, or even primarily, as a consequence of who or which racial groups were represented in a particular organization. Racial and class politics in the larger communities also plays a significant role. Moreover, the politics of difference arose in response to issues that were being debated movement-wide, as women of color challenged feminism to account for racism, some from positions within predominantly white organizations, others from locations within left, civil rights, Black Nationalist, Latino, tribal, Native American, and Asian American groups.

Many of the women I interviewed were veterans of other movements that had grappled with (and sometimes splintered over) issues of race and class, so debates about difference were familiar to them. And print resources that circulated widely within the movement—books, pamphlets, journals, newsletters, transcriptions of speeches at conferences—also influenced the nature of political struggle in individual organizations (for example, Beale 1970; Cade 1970; LaRue 1970; Ladner 1971; Moraga and Anzaldúa 1981; Davis 1981; Hull, Scott, and Smith 1982; Giddings 1984; hooks 1984; Lorde 1984; Combahee River Collective 1983; Smith 1993).

Nevertheless, debates within health movement organizations about the primacy of race, ethnicity, class, and sexuality in the formation of women's identities rarely took abstract form.[8] Struggles around difference typically erupted over specific issues: the language of an organizational mission statement; development of services that targeted particular groups of women (a clinic shift devoted to lesbian health care, or a satellite site located in a neighborhood of color); support for political coalitions or causes (endorsement of HEW guidelines against sterilization abuse of women of color); and finally, and probably most frequently, decisions about hiring and firing.

Ciel Benedetto, director of the Santa Cruz Women's Health Center (SCWHC) from the mid–1980s through 2000, explains why personnel matters sparked such controversy within the clinic sector of the women's health movement. "There are two issues. One is affirmative action and that has to do with law and ethics. And the other has to do with cultural diversity and richness. You know, what kind of work environment do you want to have. What kind of face do you literally want to show to the world . . . When you don't have that many job openings each hiring then becomes important because it's going to define [the workplace] for a very long time" (Benedetto 1992).

Benedetto, the working-class daughter of immigrants from Italy and England, kept her distance from SCWHC in its early years because she perceived it as an all-white and all middle-class organization. "I didn't want to put my politics there . . . You know when really who is present represents a very limited view of the world. So . . . it was not necessarily like I was against this place or felt anything negative about it. When I looked at it from the outside, it was . . . there is not much for me there" (1992).

But by March 1982, when the clinic newsletter published "The Challenge of Change," things had changed. "Over the past year, the Santa Cruz Women's Health Collective has begun to confront its racism," staff member Laura Giges began. She described the process: First comes acceptance that "each of us internalizes [the] racism of our society on many levels and this racism is ingrained in all of our assumptions, values and judgments." Next we acknowledge "the privilege that white women have—such as the ability to choose when and if to challenge the status quo of racial inequality." Then we admit that our efforts to confront racism are "shaking some of our basic structures, creating conflict, frustration, [and] pain," along with "excitement, and new visions" (Giges 1982, 114–115).

Giges argued that earlier discussions of racism and affirmative action at SCWHC yielded "little translation into change" because of collective reluctance by middle-class white staff members to give up control over the clinic. In summer 1981, however, SCWHC entered a different phase. The clinic hired two bilingual, bicultural Latina health counselors; initiated a program to provide mobile health services from a van in the Latino community; and participated in a full-day retreat that "set a goal to have paid staff be at least 50 percent women of color, with current staff willing to give up jobs, if need be, to reach this goal" (Giges 1982).

Staff members agreed on a timetable of one year, but the necessary anticipated resignations of middle-class workers was a bitter pill to swallow, and debates about the transformation of the clinic into a cross-class, multiracial organization continued over several months. Increasingly, women of color on staff felt "disgusted" and "alienated," not only with what they identified as the racism of their white, middle-class co-workers, but also with the way the process of collective decision making seemed to cut into the more important (to them) service mission of providing health care: "They did not have the time in their lives to talk for hours and make no decisions," especially when "their input was [being] ignored." "We were naive in believing that we could achieve diversity without affecting how we work and how decisions get made . . . We began to let go of the feelings that we knew what was right for the SCWHC. As the 'we' of the SCWHC was changing, new ways of working together would emerge" (Giges 1982, 123–124).

"Basically the collective was transforming itself out of existence because the systems that were in place did not work . . . trying to hold all these new people and mix them with old people within the construct of a collective just did not work" (Benedetto 1992). SCWHC was to have a new structure along with a more diverse staff and board of directors, to move away from pure collectivity, with its long meetings, consensus decision making, and egalitarian staff roles, and toward hierarchy. But for "a group of women who had sort of grown up together and formulated their own socialist feminist ways of looking at the world and defining what's important," Benedetto explains (1992), the process of letting go was excruciating.

Nevertheless, she defends SCWHC's decision. "After three years or more of struggling on a theoretical basis, these women at the time had the courage to say: we are going to do something" (Benedetto 1992). Almost two decades later, she surmises that the clinic's radical policy may in fact have violated the letter (though not the intent) of some labor laws, and certainly wouldn't survive scrutiny in the "post–Proposition 209" period (Benedetto 2000a, 36).[9] But, she points out, the health clinic is still in operation, one of very few to endure for more than a quarter century, and at century's end, more than 70 percent of its clients are low income, many of them women of color. The obvious inference? Re-creating the collective in the image of the women it served increased its effectiveness and extended its life. By the late 1980s, changes in goals, leadership, and staff of the clinic had generated a new mission statement.

> [The clinic] is a democratically managed, private, non-profit primary health care and health education center operated by and for women and their

families. We are dedicated to the provision of client centered, affordable, accessible, quality and culturally sensitive services. As feminists, part of our mission is the empowerment of women and the eradication of race, class, gender oppression, homophobia and all other forms of institutionalized oppression. It is our intention to offer needed services to people of all races, classes, religions, physical abilities, cultures, ages and sexual preferences. (SCWHC 1988)

The moment when the women of SCWHC "summoned the courage to not only condemn racism in the larger society and in the women's movement, but confronted the organization's internal racism and culture of exclusion" (Benedetto 2000b, 130) was one of the most remarkable in its history, Benedetto says. "[A]ll social and revolutionary change" comes with "mistakes . . . and pain. [But] the struggles born of those bold actions strengthened and matured the organization and, in part, made the SCWHC what it is today" (Benedetto 2000b, 130–131).

These several examples of feminist clinics' struggles over race and class demonstrate both the affective intensity and the important organizational effects that internal political division, especially about difference, created within the women's health movement. The learning curve about difference, but especially about race, was a steep one for many women, especially white women, in feminist organizations over the last quarter century. And struggles over difference, especially over racism and class, were painful and left lasting scars on those who lived the struggles in organizations they cared about deeply. Confronting racism, the injuries of class, and homophobia in the lived reality of building, sustaining, and changing organizations ignited feelings of fear, anger, betrayal, and sometimes pride and hope.

In 1981 Cherrie Moraga, tired of seeing the cost of struggles over racism borne so painfully on the backs of women of color, published a poem, the title of which served as the title of her influential book "This Bridge Called My Back" (Moraga and Anzaldúa 1981). However, the costs of contesting racism and class privilege were often disproportionately borne by women of color. Some stayed in predominantly white feminist organizations, working slowly to build multicultural organizations. Others left these organizations, some to found or participate in the new women of color health organizations organized in the 1980s and 1990s.

Over time the staff and boards of clinics across the country began to learn the same lessons: if they were to have a multiracial staff that also included low-income women, they would have to recruit for paid positions women who had not previously been clinic volunteers; they would have to reevaluate and be prepared to change their organizational structure, mission statements, and services and activities; they would have to examine their race or class privileges (if they were white and/or middle class) and weather and learn from political confrontations over power, control, and ideology.

The legacy (and continuing reality) of years of political struggle in clinics and other movement organizations was changing ideologies, goals, and racial demographics in women's health movement organizations. Longtime activist Helen Rodriguez-Trias assesses the distance the movement has come: "It took a quarter century of struggles, studies, publications, teaching and learning, organizing, discussion and disagreement to create and mature a women's health movement that is now beginning to recognize diversities as sources of strength" (1997b, xii).[10] Rodriguez-Trias is clear that the goal of building a multicultural movement is in process, not completed. Exclusionary practices and political struggle continue to be part of the experience of feminist activism, as well as theory. There remains much ground to be covered before the dreams of diversity are a reality.

The Best of Times, the Worst of Times: Passion, Politics, and Political-Economy

Research on social movements, even new social movement research, often misses the mark by failing to examine the political passion that helps to explain why the lived experience of social movement involvement is so compelling and intense. Clearly, struggles over race and class within feminist clinics exemplify what Dickens meant in saying of revolutionary times that "it was the best of times, it was the worst of times." So often, participating in a social movement blends headiness, excitement, ardor, disillusionment, anger, and pain. The preceding analysis of race and class struggles in feminist health organizations is important for what it reveals about the tenacity and depth of racism and class division in progressive movements for change. And there is more to learn about social movements from this investigation. Specifically, understanding social movement experience entails recognizing how political passions and complex feelings animate and are part of the social relations and organizational dynamics of movements, including the women's health movement.

In foregrounding the political struggles over race and class as an example, but by no means the only example, of the affective dimension of social movement experience, I do not mean to suggest that these struggles emerged primarily from the emotional or psychological realm of human experience. Quite the reverse. Unjust and inequitable power relations are embodied in the thoughts, feelings, and actions of individuals, but they are mightily structured by the political, economic, and social institutions of society. Just because someone is politically committed to, or part of an organization intent on, ending injustice does not mean that their consciousness and actions will seamlessly follow from progressive political ideals. Just as political passion can help individuals and organizations weather what is hard about being in a social movement, so other emotions can complicate, even subvert, the translation of political ideals into actions. Social movement organizations are excellent incubators of a wide range of emotions, some that nourish powerful bonds among members and between individuals and the organizations they build and others that can lead to despair, alienation, and suffering.

The analysis of the affective dimension of social movement experience is more than simply acknowledging that women and men who are politically active have feelings and are motivated and sustained by political passion. Rather, the affective dimension of social movement experience, what I have called "the politics of feelings" (Morgen 1983), is affected by historical and political-economic processes and helps to shape and catalyze political commitments, ideas, and actions.[11] Put simply, political activists are motivated by political ideologies, but they are also driven by political commitments and feelings that include anger and other emotions rooted in the experiences of oppression and injustice. Activists are neither simply "conscious, cognitive actors" or "unconscious, emotional actors" (to borrow from Hochschild's critique of research that neglects feelings); they are "sentient actors with conscious feeling" (Hochschild 1975). Until scholars who study social movements attend to the emotional aspect of social movement experience, the subjectivities of political activists will be incompletely understood, undermining our understanding of agency.

My interviews with women's health activists were punctuated with deep feeling, even when stories were told about events, in some cases, years after they happened. These women recalled the intensity of their experiences, good and bad. For example, more than fifteen years after the clinic closed, one staff member at Women's Community Health told me: "I got so much out of working there . . . I mean, talk about . . . personal empowerment—I learned everything I know about working from working at the health center." Another member of the same clinic recollected more tortured experiences, especially the last months before CHW was forced into bankruptcy. "I'd already seen a fair amount of personal tragedy . . . and a lot of growth and a lot of empowerment. [But] it was just too hard to stay there . . . People were so tired, and people left, and your best friend from last year was telling you she couldn't take it anymore, and [that she was leaving] would be the most incredible desertion."

Many factors contributed to this kind of emotional intensity in feminist workplaces. Women health workers were constantly engaged with clients themselves in crisis (often because of an unwanted pregnancy, domestic violence, illness, financial problems, and more). Workers faced pressures from external forces and internal divisions at the same time. By opting for participatory democratic processes that are time-consuming, emotionally charged, and difficult to maintain even under the best of conditions, the health collectives committed themselves, ideologically and practically, to taking seriously the subjectivities of their members. And conflicts were rampant: about race and class, about the priority of service provision or working to change mainstream health care, about whether a source of needed funds would compromise the organization's politics, about whether collectivist practices were working, and more, much more. So it should be no surprise that feminist clinics were and are intense, rewarding, draining workplaces.

Decisions to join and leave these organizations were frequently motivated by political passions and other feelings. The director of a clinic that endured long-term financial difficulties and protracted political struggle finally decided life in this organization had become too emotionally costly for her:

> Because I'm afraid I'll be scapegoated at the meeting, my presence would serve only the purpose of creating further tension and stress . . . I don't believe given what's coming down the road because of the governor's budget cuts that [the clinic] will survive without serious change. I wish you all the luck in resolving the issues [the clinic] must come to terms with . . . Any plan will fail if the group continues to assume the worst of and expects to be screwed by and refuses to work with each other. . . I've put my heart and soul in here. I love the place . . . and shed a lot of tears over having to leave this way. . . but . . . I can no longer work in a group that lacks a sense of process, compassion, and cooperation.[12]

Across the country, in one feminist clinic after another, different versions of the same story unfolded as the "sense of process, compassion, and cooperation," the ideal with which these enterprises had begun, eroded or was overshadowed, sometimes only temporarily, by intense internal division and conflict. Gloria Anzaldúa gives a name to this kind of internal conflict: "entreguerras, a kind of civil war among intimates, an in-class, in-race, in-house fighting" (1990b, 144). Anzaldúa is talking about conflict among Latinas, but this concept is useful for talking about other kinds of intraorganizational strife. She combines the analysis of history, political economy, and experience to comprehend how colonial and imperial processes have "indoctrinated [women in] the old imperialist ways of conquering and dominating, adopting a way of confrontation based on differences while standing on the ground of ethnic superiority" (1990, 142). This kind of analysis is all too rare. Feminist theory must elaborate these processes if it is ever to capture what power relations feel like and how resistance and domination work in political organizations.

As difficult as the conflicts, the external assaults, the financial pressures, and the overwhelming needs of clients were, for many, involvement in the women's health movement was a high point in their lives, a richly rewarding experience. Of the women I interviewed, many talked about forming friendships from their days in the movement that endured into their present lives; others remembered the heady feeling of changing society, being part of making a difference as an experience they cherish always. The following quote from a woman involved in a clinic that has endured its share of dramatic ups and downs speaks for many others in the movement:

> You could actually have you know political work, personal fulfillment and service all happen at the same time. That's how it should be . . . And to really make a difference on so many different levels . . . In the health collective we were able to support each other tremendously . . . We got to have training for our lives while we were getting that incredible support. That we were able to do, have, you know, direct hands-on experience . . . That you could do all that in the same experience . . . What an amazing thing . . . Having the convergence of many different factors in history that made that possible . . . And the tears and the pain in that context was more acceptable to me than when I have that same kind of pain and strife at my job here [her current job, not at the health collective] or in other places. Because there was like a womblike quality in which all that happened. That even though it was very terrible and painful, it didn't take away what was wonderful.

Too often, the stories of social movements are told without enough attention to what the experience of being part of that movement meant to and felt like to those who participated in the movement. I don't believe we can understand the agency of political actors without recognizing that politics is lived, believed, felt, and acted on all at once. Incorporating the experience of social movement involvement into analyses and theories about social movements may be difficult, but it adds a great deal to what we can learn about politics, social transformation, and political subjectivities.

The story that began with women taking their bodies and health care into their own hands in the late 1960s unfolded over the next quarter century and continues today. Many of the individuals whose political energies helped to build, sustain, and change this movement are no longer actively involved in its organizations, and a good many of the movement's organizations are no longer in business or have changed markedly from their founding years. The movement has contended with powerful enemies, and while it has not yet been able to achieve all its goals, there is no question that women's health care today is different, is in fact *better* than it was before tens of thousands of women took it upon themselves to make a difference. For years the Boston Women's Health Book Collective told their own story in their publications under the heading "A Good Story." Their story, like the many others I have recounted and analyzed in this book, are good stories—stories about democracy, difference, struggle, and empowerment. Movements such as the women's health movement continue to contest injustice and work toward social transformation. Their stories need to be told and retold. These days we need many more such stories.

Afterword

The Movement in the 1990s

Accomplishments and Continuing Challenges

The magnitude of change in women's health services and policy and in women's consciousness about health and health care over the past quarter century is nothing short of stunning. In the early years of the movement, women organized to demand reproductive choice; more information about their bodies and health; expanded individual and collective roles in health care decision making; demedicalization of birthing and other routine reproductive experiences; more female health providers, especially physicians; protection from unnecessary and coercive medical treatment; respectful, dignified health services; and access to affordable health care that does not stigmatize women on the basis of gender, race, sexuality, class, first language, or age. Today, the movement continues to be a strong voice for the right of all women to know, to choose, to be active in health care decision making and policy. It is more diverse now because of the leadership and commitments of women of color and because its reach has expanded beyond reproductive health.

Thirty years after the founders of the Boston Women's Health Book Collective, Jane, self-help gynecology, grassroots and national health advocacy organizations, and feminist clinics envisioned a revolution in women's health, many of their revolutionary ideas and practices have become so much a part of "the fabric of women's health care in this country," Eagan argues, that it is no longer apparent how radical those changes really are (1994, 26). Although there are fewer feminist health clinics today than there were twenty-five years ago, they do still exist, and they continue to provide excellent community-based health care as well as continuing innovation in health services. The basic shape of the health care pyramid remains unaltered, with few women, especially women of color, at the top, where the most critical decisions are made and salaries are highest (Olesen 1997, 408). But there are more women, including women of color, in medical schools and in medical practice, and female physicians, health researchers, health care managers and administrators, and members of medical and nursing faculties are making a difference (Weisman 1998). Information about women's health is more widely available than ever before—in books, pamphlets, videos, and on the web. Materials produced by the movement or by groups or individuals influenced by the movement encode a political critique that aims to raise women's consciousness about the politics of women's health and often targets the health needs and perspectives of particular groups of women (for example, White 1990; Villarosa 1994; Solarz 1999).

Women's health activists have scored important gains in health policy, and they have kept abortion legal (despite inroads by the extremely powerful and well-funded antichoice movement, which has made it much more difficult for poor women, teenagers, and women who live in rural areas to have pregnancies terminated). Hospitals must now secure informed consent for procedures ranging from sterilization to breast biopsies to Caesarian sections, and regulations about what constitutes informed consent have helped protect women from sterilization abuse, medical experimentation, and unnecessary medical procedures. Much to the chagrin of pharmaceutical companies, the right to know has been extended through FDA requirements for patient package inserts that provide more information about the side effects and contraindications of prescription drugs, including oral contraceptives and hormone replacement therapies (Norsigian 1996).

During the 1990s, a series of health policy victories emerged from the movement's relatively new focus on biomedical research (Seaman and Wood 2000). The biggest and most visible of these victories is the allocation of more federal dollars to research on women's health. The adoption of new policies at the FDA and at the National Institutes of Health (NIH) to promote greater gender equity in health research marks another milestone for advocacy organizations (Narrigan et al. 1997; Weisman 1998; Laurence and Weinhouse 1997). The National Women's Health Network, the National Black Women's Health Project, and many other groups worked hard on this issue during the 1980s and 1990s (in 1987 the NIH Women's Health Advisory Committee admitted that only 13.5 percent of the organization's funds were spent on women's health issues). But it wasn't until 1990 that "political inquiry and public criticism propelled NIH to change" (Narrigan et al. 1997, 564). That year, NIH established the Office of Research on Women's Health and mandated inclusion of women in all research grants. In 1991 Dr. Bernadine Healy became the first woman director of the NIH. Soon afterward, she announced the launch of the Women's Health Initiative (WHI), a $625 million, fourteen-year study that focuses on cardiovascular disease, breast cancer, and osteoporosis in 160,000 women.

The political pressure that led to changes at NIH came from a broad coalition of women's health movement organizations; women's professional organizations in public health and medicine; and women in Congress who introduced legislative measures designed to foster change in health policy and health research. Some in the women's health movement have objected to the Women's Health Initiative, pointing to continuing inequities in federal health research funding and the narrowness of the biomedical paradigm that undergirds the study (Ruzek, Olesen and Clarke 1997; Norsigian 1996; Laurence and Weinhouse 1997),[1] and some in the biomedical research community have also criticized the initiative (Weisman 1998). But it is indisputable that this huge undertaking represents a victory for a movement that has sought to transform the entrenched infrastructure of medical research.

On the other hand, many serious issues identified by feminist health activists decades ago remain problems today, foremost among them the continuing lack of affordable, accessible respectful health care for poor women, especially those without insurance coverage. Judy Norsigian, a founding member of the Boston Women's Health Book Collective, assesses the overall impact of the movement: "Although the WHM has had a significant impact on the consciousness of many, most medical institutions remain largely unchanged. Many of the inequities that stirred feminists to action in the early 1970s continue to exist. Poverty, the single most important factor affecting health and well-being, continues to affect a growing percentage of the population" (1996, 93).

Women who lack health insurance may have trouble accessing any health care at all, let alone services that are empowering and respectful. Hospitals and free-standing birthing centers may offer a homey atmosphere and family-friendly policies, but many low-income women cannot get prenatal care, infant mortality rates for women of color remain higher than for Euro-American women, and labor and delivery remain highly medicalized in most hospital settings. Abortion is still legal, but the Hyde Amendment still prohibits Medicaid funding for abortions and the Supreme Court has permitted a host of restrictions on women's reproductive choices. Women command more information about birth-control methods, but Norplant and Depo-Provera, methods with serious documented side effects, are still more likely to be prescribed to poor women than to others. Women of color continue to experience higher morbidity and/or mortality rates from many different diseases as well as from violence. Nevertheless, activists among them have raised the visibility of health issues affecting communities of color and spurred the establishment by President Clinton of the Initiative to Eliminate Racial and Ethnic Disparities in Health in 1998, "a program designed to promote racial and ethnic equity in six areas by 2010: cancer screening and mammography, cardiovascular disease, diabetes, HIV, immunizations and infant mortality" (National Black Women's Health Project 2001).

Despite these real gains by the movement, other powerful political-economic forces have produced changes in the U.S. health care system, and the growing influence over the past ten to fifteen years of managed care has forced clinics that survived into the 1990s to adapt to new regulatory and financial constraints (Weisman 1998, 183–187). The growing numbers of uninsured persons and those who are insured by managed care plans, combined with the insatiability of the health care industry in its pursuit of customers, has produced a curious paradox for women, Judy Norsigian observes: "Women are at significant risk for overtreatment when we have insurance . . . and are under greater risk of undertreatment when we have no form of medical coverage. Access to appropriate care remains an unattained goal for many women regardless of their insurance status" (1994, 112). Mainstream women's health services have enjoyed explosive growth since the 1980s. These private physician or hospital-owned or sponsored practices are often geared toward affluent women, those women whom Dr. Bernadine Healy characterizes as today's more active and effective consumers of health care (Healy 1995, 89). The language of empowered consumers, very much a part of the neoliberal agenda, contributes to a depoliticization of health care advocacy and translates discourse about power into the language of the marketplace.[2] As telling as it is commonplace, it suggests and reinscribes the commodification of women's health.

In the 1980s, feminist health activists took on two issues that were emphatically *not* about well-women's health: AIDS and breast cancer. It quickly became clear that breast cancer and AIDS activism would have to involve new types of and targets for organizing and advocacy. Because so little was known about the etiology or best treatments for these epidemic (and often catastrophic) diseases, expanded health research with consumer input became an important priority; advocacy, always a primary activity of women's health movement organizations, moved away from its grassroots beginnings during the 1990s and adopted what Ruzek and Becker call a professional orientation, with Congress and the scientific establishment as its principal audiences (1999).

A second catalyst for this strategic shift in advocacy was the effort by the Democratic Party to restructure health care in the United States. The political struggle over reform was so significant, and for a short time appeared so promising, that it concentrated the energies of many health movement activists. A new coalition of more than one hundred national, state, and local organizations, the Campaign for Women's Health, served as a voice for women in the debate over health care reform. Its director, Ann Kasper, a long-time feminist health activist who once served on the board of the National Women's Health Network, believes that even though restructuring efforts collapsed, the campaign helped change the national conversation about health care by linking women's health concerns with the larger goal of reform (Weisman 1998, 210–214).

Carol Weisman's work (1998) is an important resource for information about the movement in the 1990s. She examines five periods of women's health activism—the 1830s, the late nineteenth century and the progressive era, the 1960s, the 1970s, and the 1990s—and suggests that "the recurring episodes of multi-issue women's health activism could be viewed as waves in a women's health 'megamovement.' This 'megamovement' is a series of movement episodes in which women's health and body concerns have emerged into public discourse and evoked collective action by successive generations of activists intent on changing some aspect of women's health care or policy" (1998, 29).

My analysis of the women's health movement over the past three decades differs from Weisman's in a crucial way. She suggests that the episode of activism in the 1990s represents a separate stage in the development of the movement after a period of what she calls "relative quiescence during the 1980s" (1998, 77). But, as I have shown in preceding chapters, the women's health movement in the 1980s was both active and embattled, buffeted from without by the medical establishment, the state, and the New Right and torn from within by struggles over race, class, and political direction. Much of what Weisman documents so well about the movement in the 1990s makes more sense if the 1960s through the 1990s is viewed as continuous, rather than episodic, and as politically realistic and adaptive, even as it retained its transformative intent.

It is difficult to disentangle the crowded cast of characters and the dynamic interrelationships between them and political-economic forces on the changing terrain of women's health. The grassroots feminist health movement helped to birth its own alternative organizations and its own publications, but its influence spread far beyond those boundaries to a global territory where, in concert with the larger women's and racial justice movements, it has transformed the way women think and feel about their bodies, reproductive rights, sexualities, and health care. The movement also helped open doors for a new generation of women health providers, administrators, and researchers who have now had their own collective impact on the politics of women's health care. The question, then, is no longer, where does the authentic radical voice for women's health come from? Now we must ask, how do the various constituencies that seek a more just and equitable health care system work together?

The movement's future as an effective political force depends on its ability to answer this question. There is no shortage of critical challenges for women's health movement organizations and activists in the United States and around the world as globalization and the ascendancy of neoliberal social policies affect health care systems everywhere: the increasing impoverishment of women in all countries; welfare reform in the United States; the growing income gap between the nations of the North and the South and between the wealthy and the middle and working classes in the United States; the continuing problem of violence; the effective denial of reproductive rights to poor women who cannot afford to pay for them; the specter of a Supreme Court that might overturn *Roe* vs. *Wade;* enduring racism resulting in racial and ethnic disparities in health status and access to primary health care; the escalating epidemic of cancer with increasing evidence of its environmental causes; the anticipated health effects of genetically modified organisms. These issues cry out for a movement that is politically sophisticated, racially and class inclusive, vibrant, adaptable, and willing to nourish alliances with other movements and organizations that envision a more just and equitable society. To date, the women's health movement has succeeded in demonstrating that improvements in women's health care depend not just on technological advances in medicine, but on social policies and practices that eradicate poverty, sexism, racism, homophobia, and other forms of discrimination and injustice. Given that insight, there is a long road ahead.

Appendix 1

Persons Interviewed

Interviews with Women Cited by Name

Luz Alvarez Martinez, May 20, 1990, Oakland, Calif.

Byllye Avery, May 8, 1990, Boston, Mass.

Ciel Benedetto, February 21, 1992, Santa Cruz, Calif.

Pat Cody, November 11, 1990, Berkeley, Calif.

Belita Cowan, June 1990, Washington, D.C.

Carol Downer, September 30, 1990, New York, N.Y.

Barbara Ehrenreich, April 11, 1997, Eugene, Oreg.

Mary Jane Gray, M.D., July 13, 1999, Corvallis, Oreg.

Jude Hanzo, January 27, 1991, Portland, Oreg.

Julie Kelly, September 1990, New Bedford, Mass.

Judy Norsigian, January 3, 1991, Boston, Mass.

Cindy Pearson, June 1990, Washington, D.C.

Cheri Pies, November 11, 1990, Berkeley, Calif.

Helen Rodriguez-Trias, February 8, 1997, Eugene, Oreg.

Julia Scott, June 1990, Washington, D.C.

Interviews with Women Not Identified

In some cases the organizational affiliation of those interviewed (either by the actual name of the organization or the pseudonym used in the text) is identified; in other cases a pseudonym is used.

Berkeley Women's Health Collective: Five staff interviewed in Berkeley, California, May 20, May 21, and November 10, 1991. Of these, one is Terry Brock, M.D. (pseudonym).

Concord Feminist Health Center: Group interview with six staff, December 1990.

Emma Goldman Clinic for Women: Two staff interviewed, June 28, 1995, Eugene, Oregon.

Women's Community Health: Four staff interviewed, one on September 5, 1990, and a group interview with three staff on November 19, 1990.

Feminist Women's Health Centers: Three staff members of different clinics interviewed in May and June 1991.

National Black Women's Health Project: One member interviewed May 22, 1991; one staff member interviewed November 1994.

Community Health Care for Women (pseudonym): Jesse Calas (pseudonym), January 3, 1991; Betsy Connor (pseudonym), January 3, 1991; Liz Rose (pseudonym), June 12, 1991; Margaret Gordon, M.D. (pseudonym), June 12, 1991.

Women's Health Services (pseudonym): Four staff interviewed 1977–79.

Appendix 2
Clinics and Organizations Surveyed

Federation of Feminist Women's Health Centers, Los Angeles, Calif.
Westside Women's Health Center, Santa Monica, Calif.
Buena Vista Women's Services, San Francisco, Calif.
Lyon Martin Women's Health Clinic, San Francisco, Calif.
Women's Clinic, San Francisco, Calif.
Women's Choice Clinic, Oakland, Calif.
Women's Choice Clinic, Santa Rosa, Calif.
Haight Ashbury Women's Free Medical Clinic, San Francisco, Calif.
Santa Cruz Women's Health Center, Santa Cruz, Calif.
T.H.E. Clinic for Women, Los Angeles, Calif.
Womancare, San Diego, Calif.
Women's Community Clinic, San Jose, Calif.
Women's Health Service Clinic, Colorado Springs, Colo.
Women's Health Services, New Haven, Conn.
Feminist Women's Health Center, Tallahassee, Fla.
Birth Center of Tallahassee, Tallahassee, Fla.
Childbirth Alternatives Network, Winterville, Ga.
Chicago Women's Health Center, Chicago, Ill.
Women's Health Resources at Illinois, Chicago, Ill.
Women Organized for Reproductive Choice/Chicago Women's AIDS Project, Chicago, Ill.
Emma Goldman Clinic for Women, Iowa City, Iowa
Southern Coastal Family Planning, Portland, Maine

Mabel Wadsworth Women's Health Center, Bangor, Maine
Maryland Women's Health Coalition, Baltimore, Md.
New Bedford Women's Health Services, New Bedford, Mass.
Women's Health Clinic, Provincetown, Mass.
Women's Health Care Association, Minneapolis, Minn.
Minnesota Indian Women's Resource Center, Minneapolis, Minn.
Women's Self-Help Center, St. Louis, Mo.
Blue Mountain Women's Clinic, Missoula, Mont.
Women's Place, Missoula, Mont.
Concord Feminist Health Center, Concord, N.H.
St. Mark's Lesbian Health Collective, New York, N.Y.
Fertility Awareness Center, New York, N.Y.
Womancap, New York, N.Y.
Women's Health Center, Cortland, N.Y.
Maternity Center Association, New York, N.Y.
Portland Feminist Women's Health Center, Portland, Oreg.
Southeast Women's Health Clinic, Portland, Oreg.
Allentown Women's Center, Allentown, Penn.
Elizabeth Blackwell Health Center, Philadelphia, Penn.
Black Women's Health Services, Pittsburgh, Penn.
Rhode Island Women's Health Collective, Providence, R.I.
Southern Vermont Women's Health Center, Rutland, Vt.
Vermont Women's Health Center, Burlington, Vt.
Aradia Women's Health Center, Seattle, Wash.
45th Street Community Health Clinic, Seattle, Wash.
Women's Health Center of West Virginia, Charlestown, W.Va.
Bread and Roses Women's Health Center, Milwaukee, Wis.

We also received questionnaires from women's health advocacy organizations that were analyzed but are not part of this sample, which is drawn mainly from service-providing organizations.

Notes

Two   Foundational Stories and Movement Making

1. Lorraine Rothman developed this method and dubbed the instrument a "del-em" device, which could easily be constructed from materials accessible to anyone.
2. Mary Howell was a physician and author of the book *Why Would a Girl Go into Medicine? Medical Education in the United States: A Guide for Women* (1973).
3. Some of these included Suzanne Arms's (1975) *Immaculate Deception: A New Look at Childbirth in America*; Paula Weideger's (1975) *Menstruation and Menopause*; Rose Kushner's (1975) *Breast Cancer: A Personal and Investigative Report*; Adrienne Rich's (1976) *Of Woman Born*; Linda Gordon's (1976) *Woman's Body, Woman's Right*; Claudia Dreifus's (1977) *Seizing Our Bodies: The Politics of Women's Health*; Gena Corea's (1977) *Women's Health Care: The Hidden Malpractice*; and later the first two scholarly works on the women's health movement: Sheryl Ruzek's (1978) *The Women's Health Movement* and Helen Marieskind's (1980) *Women in the Health System*. Other print resources also helped connect activists in more than one thousand organizations—information and abortion and health care referral groups, alternative gynecology and abortion clinics, and health advocacy and health policy groups—that constituted the women's health movement by the mid-1970s. *The New Women's Survival Catalog* (Grimstad and Rennie 1973) devoted twenty-two pages to women's health, listing clinics, newsletters, and other periodicals. *Circle One: Self Health Handbook* (Ziegler and Campbell 1973), published by a feminist health group in Colorado Springs, circulated widely within the movement. I've already mentioned the first appearances of *The Monthly Extract: An Irregular Periodical* (1972) and Belita Cowan's *herself* (1972). In 1974, *HealthRight*, a quarterly based in New York, started publication of articles on women's health and on the working conditions of women in health care, especially nonprofessional women (*HealthRight* was published by an organization of the same name that was closely associated with HealthPAC, the community health advocacy group of which Barbara Ehrenreich was a member. It focused on capitalism and race in its analysis of women's health issues).

   Soon after its formation, the National Women's Health Network began to distribute its newsletter, *Network News*, which reported on policy advocacy activities in Washington, D.C., tracked women's health organizations in other parts of the country, and offered in-depth analysis of a wide variety of women's health issues. The Coalition for the Medical Rights of Women (CMRW) published a pamphlet on sterilization abuse in the mid–1970s (CMRW 1984), and feminist health clinics traded pamphlets on topics such as lesbian health care, contraceptive safety, the pelvic exam and nonpharmaceutical remedies for vaginal infections. Both Belita Cowan, in Ann Arbor, and Sheryl Burt Ruzek, in the California Bay Area, compiled and distributed bibliographies of the past-proliferating publications of the women's health movement. Ruzek, a sociologist, and Helen I. Marieskind, whose academic focus was public health, wrote doctoral dissertations that later became the first scholarly books on the women's health movement—Ruzek's *The Women's Health Movement* (1978) and Marieskind's *Women in the Health System: Patients, Providers, Programs* (1980)—which seeded a vital and growing research base of scholarship on women's health that fed women's studies programs in colleges and universities over the next two decades.

Three   On Their Own

1. Mission statements of organizations with long histories change over time and are strongly influenced by a changing political climate and by the racial and class identities and commitments of members and staff. The New Bedford Women's Health Services did not always identify as a multiracial organization; in fact, long struggles over racism within the organization predated the development of a more racially inclusive mission and program.
2. For example, as late as the 1992 edition of *Our Bodies, Ourselves*, written within two years of the National Black Women's Health Project Book authored by Linda Villarosa, *Body and Soul: The Black Women's Guide to Physical Health and Emotional Well-Being* (1994), self-help is first described in reference to women becoming knowledgeable about the appearance of their sexual organs and especially with their vagina and cervix (BWHBC 1992, 241). Self-help groups are identified as important sources of "courage and information," especially about birth control, fertility awareness, menopause, breast cancer, DES, and cervical self-examination (672). While a later section acknowledges that "people have always banded together to help one another deal with everyday problems. Self-help means discussing feelings and experiences, supporting each other to learn together; finding out what we *do* know, what we do *not* know, what we *want* to know; demystifying health professionals 'expertise' and our own bodies; making choices based on our own valid experiences and knowledge" (702).
3. This does not mean that the NBWHP rejected cervical self-examination, menstrual extraction, or other self-help practices more identified with the white women's health movement, though these were not regular features of NBWHP self-help groups. For example, the February 1994 issue of *Vital Signs* on reproductive freedom includes articles on both menstrual extraction and cervical self-examination. But clearly, self-help connotes some very different meanings as it is used by the NBWHP and by many predominantly white women's health movement groups.

4. There are a number of other Latina organizations about which I have only limited information, including the National Latina Institute for Reproductive Health. The Pro-Choice Public Education Project web site describes it as a "new and up and coming organization. It strives to enhance the quality of life for Latinas nation-wide, focusing on reproductive health through advocacy, networking, public policy, information, education and communication."

5. *The Women of Color Health Data Book* (Leigh and Lindquist 1998, 4).

6. There are organizations that I have not highlighted in this chapter for lack of sufficient information and because my goal is less to be comprehensive, and more to understand the varying origins and trajectories of these organizations and their relationships with each other and the organizations of what they would call the white women's health movement.

Four Into Our Own Hands

1. It may be confusing to distinguish between the pro-choice or pro-abortion movement and the women's health movement. This is so particularly since my research confirms a theme that is repeated in other work on the movement—that abortion services, including pregnancy testing, abortion counseling, and the provision of abortions have been a significant part of the services of many women's health clinics. In fact, the pro-choice movement tends to be seen as an advocacy movement focused on building public support for reproductive choice, lobbying for abortion and other reproductive rights, supporting legislative and judicial work in support of abortion, and responding to actions by the antiabortion movement in the courts and beyond. Moreover, organizations such as Planned Parenthood that do provide abortions are seen as squarely within the pro-choice movement. However, many feminist health activists wanted to see very different kinds of abortion services than were available from Planned Parenthood, an organization many saw as an ally in the context of reproductive choice work, but as an organization providing abortion services in ways that came closer to conventional medicine than feminist versions of abortion services (Joffe, 1986). Moreover, the history of Planned Parenthood is inextricably bound up with population control policies, policies that, far from being designed to empower women with greater control over their bodies, instead sought to limit population growth, often at the expense of the health of women and without their fully informed consent.

2. Petchesky and others are correct in analyzing the actual rights women won in *Roe* vs. *Wade,* which did not, in principle, give women the right to reproductive self-determination (1990), but rather legalized abortion and gave physicians the right to provide abortions they and their patients determined were justified. In fact, in practice, women did win the right to choose abortion as long as they could afford to pay for the service. See, for example, Fried (1990) and Roberts (1997) for a discussion of the post *Roe* vs. *Wade* struggles over abortion, and especially the ways race and class differences among women effectively gave some women (read: white, middle class, urban, those with access to health insurance or Medicaid—until the Hyde Amendment) more abortion rights than others.

3. In fact, the most common formerly prescription medications for vaginitis became

available over the counter a few years after the women's health movement pioneered the use of these home remedies as drug companies sought to compete with these inexpensive, and often successful, remedies.

4. To the contemporary reader much of this may sound like mainstream medicine. To the extent that this is true, it is because of changes in abortion and women's reproductive health services deeply influenced by the women's health movement. But in the 1970s these service features were bold and different from mainstream medical practices and protocols.

5. I chose these particular clinics because they were among those for which I had the richest data and because they represent much of the diversity of organizational experience I uncovered in my research. I do not claim to have studied any one clinic over its entire organizational life course. Instead, my goal is to shine a light on a few of the hybrid politicized workplaces of the women's health movement and examine how they changed as the political actors around them, the New Right, the state, and their primary target, the health care establishment, changed. Surely some of the women who worked in the clinics profiled here will wish that I had emphasized other things, will be sure that I omitted crucial incidents, will hunger for more analysis of other time periods. But although I cannot capture the richness and complexity of their personal and organizational lives, these snapshots are meant to bring the experience of involvement in feminist clinics in the 1970s and 1980s to life, to exemplify how groups of women embodied their ideals and re-imagined health care against the backdrop of a hostile and resistant political and economic environment.

6. Information about the Berkeley Women's Health Collective is derived from interviews with four women whose involvement with the clinic spans the period from the clinic's founding through the late 1970s, and one woman who was involved in the early 1980s. I also interviewed a woman who was involved with a feminist health advocacy organization in Berkeley during the 1970s who shared her outsider/insider recollections about the clinic. Three of these women shared organizational documents with me, including copies of newsletters, a "clinic herstory" and correspondence, including the letter of resignation by one of the women I interviewed. I also used a published written narrative by Julia McKinney Barfoot (1973).

7. Salaries remained very low throughout the 1970s and well into the 1980s. One of the women I interviewed said that she could only survive on the low salary by getting Food Stamps and MediCal, California's Medicaid program. By the latter 1970s salaries were at about $500/month and by the early 1980s at about $900/month.

8. Information about the Concord Feminist Health Center is from a group interview with six staff members of the clinic in December 1990, the survey Alice Julier and I conducted of feminist health clinics in 1990, from documentary evidence staff members shared with me, including issues of *WomenWise*, the clinic newsletter, and from Bruce (1981), an article published about the clinic in the scholarly journal *Studies in Family Planning.*

9. Information about the Emma Goldman Clinic for Women comes from four sources: interviews with two of the founding members of the clinic, who each worked there for several years in the mid–1970s; the 1990 survey of health clinics; organizational documents, including the edition of the clinic's newsletter *Emma's Periodical,* published in commemoration of the twentieth anniversary of the clinic; and an eighty-minute documentary video *From One Place to Another: Emma Goldman Clinic*

Stories, produced by Lee Ann Erickson (1996) that includes interview material from twenty-two women who worked at the clinic at some point between its founding and 1996.

10. I interviewed four women who were members of WCHC during much of its history. One of these was a group interview with three of the women who had gathered at the request of a woman I contacted in her kitchen for this purpose. In addition, I have extensive documentary evidence about the clinic these women provided to me, including a history covering the period March 1975–April 1977; an article by staff members Sommers, Bell, Wolhandler, and Stein published in the feminist journal *Quest* in 1977; annual reports for 1975, 1976, 1977, and 1979; an article published by Bell about the pelvic teaching group in 1989; and articles in Boston and Cambridge newspapers covering the clinic's closing.

11. My information about the Federation of Feminist Health Clinics and the individual FWHCs I discuss in this section comes from interviews with Carol Downer and three other women who worked at one or another of the California FWHCs during the 1970s and 1980s; answers to the survey by four FWHCs; and documents that range from published materials on the FWHC in Ruzek (1978) to articles written about the FWHCs and the Federation by Downer (1974), Hornstein (1974a, 1974b), Abramson (1988), and other articles and books about the women's health movement.

Five   Against the Odds

1. Planned Parenthood clinics have not been included in the discussion of feminist clinics here. However, many staff members of these clinics are feminists and many Planned Parenthood clinics have been subject to assaults by the anti-abortion movement. For a study of these clinics, see Joffe 1986.

2. A faculty grant from the University of Massachusetts helped defray the costs of copying, mailing, coding, and analyzing the survey. Some feminist health organizations that did not reply to the survey still existed in 1990, I am confident that our fifty respondents comprise the majority and represent the range of those women's health movement clinics in 1990. A significant number of questionnaires were returned by the U.S. Postal Service marked "addressee unknown," confirming a widespread impression among health activists that many of the movement's organizations did not survive the economic and social dislocations of the late 1970s and the 1980s. We made an attempt to determine whether the organization still existed, even though we did not receive a response by calling directory assistance in the city or town where the organization was located. It was difficult to differentiate between feminist health groups affiliated with the movement and the new crop of women's health services that were developed by physicians, hospitals, and other mainstream health organizations in the 1980s. The proliferation of such organizations demonstrates the dramatic impact of the women's health movement in the two previous decades. Many of these second-generation women's clinics have no affiliation with the women's health movement. Nor do they share the goals of feminist health advocacy. Instead, they represent a successful (profit-driven) response by the mainstream medical establishment to the alteration of women's consciousness of and expectations about health care (Kay 1989), a change accomplished by the women's health movement.

We made an effort to use the information we had about different organizations to exclude these mainstream women's facilities from our sample, but the boundaries between them and the feminist clinics are not always clear, particularly on paper. As we distributed the questionnaire, we chose to err on the side of inclusiveness rather than risk the exclusion of feminist health care providers. As a result, 28 percent of the organizations in our final sample do not claim to be women controlled.

3. I carried out this research over much of the 1990s with limited external financial support for this research. The interviews with members of clinics and other health movement organizations were done over the course of a decade as I was able to contact and then interview these women in person. Because I had no funding for this research, I interviewed respondents as I was able to combine a visit to them with other professional or personal travel—for example to professional meetings or communities where I was invited to give a lecture. I also traveled to clinics relatively close to where I lived in both the northeastern and northwestern United States.

Six   The Changer and the Changed

1. See Joffe's excellent book, *Doctors of Conscience*, for a discussion of physicians who provided illegal abortions before 1973.
2. For more about CESA and CARASA, see Shapiro 1985; Davis 1988; Petchesky 1990.
3. The history of this organization is very interesting. For more about it see Regina Markell Morantz-Sanchez's excellent history *Sympathy and Science: Women Physicians in American Medicine* (1985). She describes the change in this organization from one associated with a relatively militant feminism to one that had a "distinctly negative image" among women physicians. She quotes one physician who said it "seemed like an old ladies tea party" (1985, 338).
4. It was routine practice at the time to move directly from biopsy to mastectomy in one operation, without consulting the patient or discussing options if a biopsy showed the presence of a malignancy.
5. My own research preceded the period of intense breast cancer activism within the women's health movement, and I do not claim to be expert in this area. However, there is a growing scholarship about breast cancer activism including Batt 1994; Leopold 1999; Klawiter 1999.
6. See, for example, Marco, Hollingworth, and Durham 1987; Batt 1994; Brady 1991.

Seven   Neither Friend nor Foe

1. I am relying on WCHC documents and interviews with former staff for this narrative. I have not checked the narrative with the agencies discussed here, and I have no reason to distrust the story as told by the documents, particularly given my familiarity with somewhat similar experiences of other clinics in Massachusetts and other parts of the country.
2. Because I am not identifying the name of this community, I will not reference these census data, except to indicate that this data comes from the census data for this city.
3. For more information about CETA, see Morgen and Weigt (2001).
4. The impact of the Hyde Amendment cannot be overstated. This legislation was one

of the first victories of the antiabortion movement and was precedent-setting policy that eroded the responsibility of the state for poor women's reproductive rights. While states could opt to use the state Medicaid match funds to assist poor women who wanted abortions (and some states did), poor women did face severe hardship for years because of this piece of legislation. It also created a wedge within the movement between groups that actively opposed the Hyde Amendment and worked to contest it and those that did not. Later, when National Black Women's Health Project members talked about racism in the women's health movement they referred to struggles over the import of the Hyde Amendment as a moment of political rupture between women of color and (many) white women's organizations.

Eight   The Three Rs

1. The long struggle against reproductive freedom, and particularly against women's right to abortion, began as soon as the ink was dry on the 1973 Supreme Court decision in *Roe* vs. *Wade*. I will not detail here the battle against abortion that was launched first by the well-organized Catholic Church and that has continued even until today by religious, and especially Catholic and Protestant, fundamentalist groups, as well as by conservative and New Right political organizations. But within nine months of the *Roe* vs. *Wade* decision 188 bills to restrict abortion had been introduced in forty-one states (Davis 1988, 55), and by the mid–1970s antiabortion organizing was widespread (Petchesky 1990; Luker 1984; Fried 1990).
2. For a more detailed examination of how the "defund the Left" strategy affected even a state program such as the Department of Labor's Comprehensive Employment and Training Act jobs programs for low-income people, see Morgen and Weigt (2001).
3. For the most part my research on the women's health movement concerns the period of 1969 to 1990, and therefore my discussion of AIDS is far less detailed than it might be if I had set my sights on a rigorous analysis of the movement in the post–1990 era. Given my decision to restrict my focus to that period, my discussion here is limited, meant mainly to suggest some important issues and dilemmas that were foreshadowed by but not fully developed during the period I am examining.

Nine   The Politics of Race and Class

1. Sojourner Truth, whose real name was Isabella Baumfree, delivered the speech that this question is drawn from in Akron, Ohio, at a women's rights gathering in 1851. Apparently there is controversy over aspects of this speech, which is being reexamined by historian Nell Painter (Guy-Sheftall 1993, 35).
2. This is a pseudonym. Because I am using a pseudonym here, I will refer to clinic and community documents that will not be referenced fully in order to maintain the confidentiality that was promised to each of the four women I interviewed.
3. For a longer and more complete version of this case study, see Morgen 1997.
4. Because I promised confidentiality to these four women, I cannot reference the community newspaper, which would then give away the name of the clinic and of these individuals. But the article is from a feminist community paper from the late 1970s.
5. For more detail about these struggles, see Morgen 1986, 1988a, 1990. As in the pre-

vious example, citations from documents and interviews here will be incomplete in order to protect the confidentiality of the clinic and its members.

6. I was involved in this clinic for more than two years; much of my description of these events is drawn from field notes taken during a period of intensive participant observation.

7. There are some other case studies of race and class conflicts within feminist organizations. See, for example, Scott 1998, 2000.

8. A number of women I interviewed referred, though not extensively, to struggles over sexuality in women's health movement organizations. Debates about homophobia, conflicts between straights and lesbians, are well documented in the larger feminist movement (Echols 1989), for example. Whether or not the lack of information about struggles over sexuality in this book stems from my own failure to specifically address this issue or to what was primary on the radar screen of the women I interviewed, I am not sure. Perhaps the following quote from a collective member of an important feminist health clinic dating back to the early 1970s may shed some light on the difference between struggles over sexualities and race and class. "[The collective] was diverse in terms of sexuality—gay, straight and bisexual . . . It was a really nice experience for most people; there was a lot of fluidity in what people were doing [sexually] and there was a lot of discussion and it was a reasonably nice environment. [She gave an example from collaborative work on sex education.] It was a very positive thing for people to validate all the diversity in our sexual orientation. And I remember that issues was hugely in the foreground of what people were dealing with in the health collective. And there were some tensions between . . . the issue about separatism and there was tension about people who were kind of one end of being lesbians and separatists, and their feelings about straight women in the collective . . . but mainly it was okay."

9. Proposition 209, the California Civil Rights Initiative (better known as the initiative to strike down affirmative action) was passed in November 1996. Prop. 209 made it illegal for the state of California to "grant preferential treatment" on the basis of race, sex, color, ethnicity, or national origin.

10. For example, this foreword to an impressive anthology by Sheryl Ruzek, Virgnia Olesen, and Adele Clark (1997) is organized around the theme of differences among women in their health and their perspectives on health services and policies. There is more diversity represented in other movement or movement-related publications. The Boston Women's Book Collective 1984 and then 1992 editions of *The New Our Bodies, Ourselves* were more comprehensive than previous editions in its coverage of the specific issues of women of color in the United States and international health issues than in past editions (Boston Women's Health Book Collective 1984, 1992). Books by and about the health of women of color have become more available, reaching farther into diverse communities of women (White 1990; Bair and Cayleff 1993; Chin 1993; Villarosa 1994). Even mainstream organizations such as the National Institutes of Health have organized conferences and released publications focusing on the health of women of color. While there remains much ground to be covered, the direction appears to be one of facing the challenge of diversity and coming closer to the reality of a movement that is more inclusive.

11. Although social science has focused on emotions in particular arenas of experience, in the family, for example, or in friendship groups, it has practically ignored, until

quite recently, the emotional discourses and experience of work or social movements. Now, interest in emotions as a dimension of all forms of social life is growing (Lutz and White 1986), and recent studies have expanded, politicized, and historicized our understanding of the social construction of feelings. Lutz and Abu-Lughod (1990), for example, situate emotional discourse within power relations in concrete historical instances; and with other feminist scholars, they have offered us new theoretical insights about how profoundly emotion is conditioned by, and is itself a dimension of, the dynamics and reproduction of hegemonic power relations (Hochschild 1979, 1983; Lutz 1988; Lutz and Abu-Lughod 1990; Taylor 1995). In chapter 3, I offered a brief description of the feminist health clinic as workplace, highlighting the importance assigned to feelings in organizational deliberations and in the invention of daily work protocols. Many clinics encouraged caring and its visible signs: hugs, kisses, even tears. Those expressions of feeling were not merely decorative; they were important parts of feminist work culture. The analysis of women's work cultures has been a project of feminist anthropologists, sociologists, and historians who investigate the ways women create networks, values, relationships, and social spaces that contest the wholesale control of work within mainstream workplaces (Bookman 1977; Benson 1978; Melosh 1982; Lamphere 1987; Zavella 1987; Sacks 1988). This research conceives of work culture as a relatively autonomous sphere of action on the job, a realm of informal, customary values and rules that mediate the formal authority structure of workplaces and distance workers from its impact. Most of this research focuses on workplaces that are organized from the top down—factories, hospitals, or department stores—and tightly controlled by management. I argue that the work cultures constructed in women's health organizations were different. In general, they embodied active contestation of bureaucracy and hierarchy, opposition to the valorization of rationality in public life, and the dream of sisterhood. Most clinic workplaces sought to foster sensitivity to individual needs and feelings and to take process seriously, to acknowledge that how things get done is as important as what gets done. (For a more extended analysis see Morgen 1995.)

12. Again, to maintain confidentiality I will not name the clinic and therefore provide information about this document, which was a letter of resignation submitted to the collective. She provided me with a copy of this letter when I interviewed her.

Afterword   The Movement in the 1990s

1. Medical journalists Leslie Laurence and Beth Weinhouse begin their preface to a 1997 book with a sobering assessment of the limits of change at the federal level. "In September 1996, five years after women's health muscled its way into the national agenda," 150 medical researchers attended "a little-publicized meeting in Philadelphia to assess the state of women's health research and chart a course for the 21st century." Their conclusion? "But while women's health hasn't retreated, the sobering conclusion of the meeting was that it hadn't sufficiently advanced either" (1997, ix). They also discuss what they consider to be a powerful backlash to these reforms from drug company executives, physicians, and medical school deans.

2. I first developed this argument, which I develop more fully in Morgen (1988b) in my analysis of a heated struggle between a group of low-income women and a hospital that closed the prenatal and gynecology clinics that offered the only affordable

source of care for poor women in a particular community. For an even more compelling and recent analysis of the language and strategy of a discourse about medical consumerism see Maskovsky (2000). Another example of the same depoliticized language is the reference to women's clinics, especially those owned and operated by mainstream physicians and hospitals as providing "women-centered," rather than "women-controlled" health care.

References

Abramovitz, Mimi. 1988. *Regulating the Lives of Women: Social Welfare Policy Reform from Colonial Times to the Present*. Boston: South End Press.

Abramson, Alan, and Lester Salaman. 1986. *The Nonprofit Sector and the New Federal Budget*. Washington, D.C.: Urban Institute Press.

Abramson, Hilary. 1988. "Feminists versus the State." *The Sacramento Bee Magazine* (May 1): 7–8, 15.

Acker, Joan. 1990. "Hierarchies, Jobs, Bodies: A Theory of Gendered Organizations." *Gender and Society* 4 (2): 139–158.

———. 1995. "Feminist Goals in Organizing Processes." In *Feminist Organizations: Harvest of the Women's Movement*, edited by Myra Marx Ferree and Patricia Yancey Martin. Philadelphia: Temple University Press.

Ahrens, Lois. 1980. "Battered Women's Refuges: Feminist Cooperatives vs. Social Service Institutions." *Radical America* 14, no. 3 (May/June): 41–47.

Ahron, Jonina, and Felicia Ward. 1989. "When and Where We Enter." *Vital Signs* 6, no. 1 (February): 4–5.

Albelda, Randy. 1988. *Mink Coats Don't Trickle Down: The Economic Attack on Women and People of Color*. Boston: South End Press, Center for Popular Economics.

Allen, Robert. 1970. *Black Awakening in Capitalist America: An Analytic History*. New York: Doubleday.

Alonso, Ana Maria. 1988. "The Effects of Truth: Re-Presentation of the Past and the Imagining of Community." *Journal of Historical Sociology* 1 (1): 33–57.

Alvarez Martinez, Luz. 1991. Interview with author, May 20, Oakland, Calif.

Amaro, Hortensia. 1990. "Women's Reproductive Rights in the Age of AIDS." In *From Abortion to Reproductive Freedom: Transforming a Movement*, edited by Marlene Gerber Fried. Boston: South End Press.

American Federation of State County and Municipal Employees (AFSCME). 1984. *The State, the People and the Reagan Years*. Washington, D.C.: AFSCME.

Anzaldúa, Gloria., ed. 1990a. *Making Face, Making Soul: Haciendo Caras: Creative and Critical Perspectives by Women of Color*. San Francisco: Aunt Lute Foundation.

———. 1990b. "En Rapport, In Opposition: Cobrando Cuentas a las Nuestras." In *Making Face, Making Soul/ Haciendo Caras: Creative and Critical Perspectives by Women of Color,* edited by Gloria Anzaldúa. San Francisco: Aunt Lute Foundation.

Apple, Rima. 1990. *Women, Health and Medicine in America: A Historical Handbook.* New York: Garland.

Arms, Suzanne. 1975. *Immaculate Deception: A New Look at Childbirth in America.* Boston: Houghton Mifflin.

Arnold, Gretchen. 1995. "Dilemmas of Feminist Coalitions: Collective Identity and Strategic Effectiveness in the Battered Women's Movement." In *Feminist Organizations: Harvest of the Women's Movement,* edited by Myra Marx Ferree and Patricia Yancey Martin. Philadelphia: Temple University Press.

Asetoyer, Charon. 1990. "First There Was Smallpox." In *Women, Aids and Activism,* by Act Up New York Women and Aids Group. Boston: South End Press.

———. 1994. "From the Ground Up." *The Women's Review of Books* 11, no. 10–11 (July): 22.

Avery, Byllye. 1982. "Black Women's Health Project: Network Launches New Project." *Network News* 7, no. 1 (February).

———. 1990a. "A Question of Survival/ A Conspiracy of Silence: Abortion and Black Women's Health." In *From Abortion to Reproductive Freedom: Transforming a Movement,* edited by Marlene Gerber Fried. Boston: South End Press.

———. 1990b. "A Message to Members." *Vital Signs* (fall): 3.

———. 1991. Interview with author, May 8, Boston, Mass.

Baehr, Ninia. 1990. *Abortion without Apology: A Radical History for the 1990's.* Boston: South End Press.

Bair, Barbara, and Susan E. Cayleff, eds. 1993. *Wings of Gauze: Women of Color and the Experience of Health and Illness.* Detroit, Mich.: Wayne State University Press.

Banzhaf, Marion. 1990. *Women, AIDS, and Activism.* Boston: South End Press.

Barfoot, Julia McKinney. 1973. "Free Care for Women by Women: The Berkeley Women's Health Collective." In *Getting Clear: Body Work for Women,* by Ann Kent Rush. New York: Random House, and Berkeley, Calif.: Booksword.

Barnett, Bernice McNair. 1995. "Black Women's Collectivist Movement Organizations: Their Struggles during the 'Doldrums.'" In *Feminist Organizations: Harvest of the Women's Movement,* edited by Myra Marx Ferree and Patricia Yancey Martin. Philadelphia: Temple University Press.

Bart, Pauline. 1987. "Seizing the Means of Reproduction: An Illegal Feminist Abortion Collective—How and Why It Worked." *Qualitative Sociology* 10 (4): 339–357.

Batt, Sharon. 1994. *Patient No More: The Politics of Breast Cancer.* London: Scarlet Press.

Bawden, D., ed. 1984. *The Social Contract Revisited: Aims and Outcomes of President Reagan's Social Welfare Policy.* Washington, D.C.: Urban Institute Press.

Beale, Frances. 1970. "Double Jeopardy: To Be Black and Female." In *Sisterhood Is Powerful: An Anthology of Writings from the Women's Liberation Movement,* edited by Robin Morgan. New York: Random House.

Bell, Susan. 1989. "Political Gynecology: Gynecological Imperialism and the Politics of Self-Help." In *Healing Technology,* edited by Katherine Strother Ratcliff. Ann Arbor: University of Michigan Press.

Bellah, Robert et al. 1985. *Habits of the Heart: Individualism and Commitment in American Life.* New York: Harper and Row.

Benderly, Jill. 1990. "Does Corporate Giant Fill Health Care Needs Like Feminist Clinic?" *New Directions for Women* 19, no. 1 (January/February): 1, 13.

Benedetto, Ciel. 1992. Interview with author, February 21, Santa Cruz, Calif.

———. 2000a. *Ciel Benedetto: A History of the Santa Cruz Women's Health Center, 1985–2000*, edited by Irene Reti and Randall Jarrell. Santa Cruz: University of California, University Library.

———. 2000b. "Our Center, Ourselves: 25 Years and Counting: A Celebratory Reflection on the History of the Santa Cruz Women's Health Center (SCWHC)." In *A History of the Santa Cruz Women's Health Center.*

Benjamin, Beth Cooper. 1995. "Mary Howell: Breaking Ground for Women in Medicine." *Network News* (September/October): 1, 6.

Benson, Sue Porter. 1983. "The Customers Ain't God?: The Work Culture of Department Store Saleswomen, 1890–1940." In *Working Class America: Essays on Labor, Community and American Society*, edited by Michael Frisch and Daniel Walkowitz. Urbana: University of Illinois Press.

Berglas, Nancy. 1995. "The First FDA Protest: The Network's First Action." *The Network News* (November/December): 1, 4–5.

Berkeley Women's Health Collective (BWHC). 1971. Unpublished document.

———. 1976. Unpublished document.

———. 1977. Unpublished document.

———. 1982. Newsletter (June).

———. 1982. Newsletter (July).

———. 1983. Newsletter (July/August).

Bhavnani, Kum-Kum, ed. 2001. *Feminism and "Race."* Oxford, U.K.: Oxford University Press.

Bickel, Janet, and Phyllis Kopriva. 1993. "A Statistical Perspective on Gender in Medicine." *Journal of the American Medical Women's Association* 48 (5): 141–144.

Bloom, Amy. 1995. "The Pill Hearings: Alice Wolfson Breaks the Silence." *Network News* (January/February): 1, 3.

Bloom, Amy, and Ellen Parsons. 1994. "25th Anniversary of *The Doctor's Case Against the Pill*." *Network News* (November/December): 1, 3.

Bookman, Ann. 1977. "The Process of Political Socialization among Women and Immigrant Workers: A Case Study of Unionization in the Electronics Industry." Ph.D. diss., Harvard University, Cambridge, Mass.

Boston Women's Health Book Collective (BWHBC). 1971. *Our Bodies, Ourselves: A Book by and for Women*. Boston: New England Free Press.

———. 1973. *Our Bodies, Ourselves: A Book by and for Women*. New York: Simon and Schuster.

———. 1975. "A Good Story." Unpublished document.

———. 1978. *Ourselves and Our Children: A Book by and for Parents*. New York: Random House.

———. 1979. *Our Bodies, Ourselves: A Book by and for Women*. New York: Simon and Schuster.

———. 1984. *The New Our Bodies, Ourselves*. New York: Simon and Schuster.

———. 1987. *Ourselves, Growing Older: Women Aging with Knowledge and Power*. New York: Simon and Schuster.

———. 1990. "The Twentieth Anniversary Celebration of *Our Bodies, Ourselves*." *Women of Power* 18: 8–9.

————. 1992a. *The New Our Bodies, Ourselves: A Book by and for Women, Updated and Expanded for the '90s*. New York: Simon and Schuster.

————. 1992b. "When Yogurt Was Illegal." *Ms.* 3 (1): 38–40.

————. 1995. *Boston Women's Health Book Collective Newsletter*.

Brady, Judith, ed. 1991. *1 in 3: Women with Cancer Confront an Epidemic*. Pittsburgh: Cleis Press.

Breines, Wini. 1989. *Community and Organization in the New Left: The Great Refusal*. New Brunswick, N.J.: Rutgers University Press.

Brock, Terry [pseud.]. 1991. Interview with author, May 21.

Brodkin, Karen. 1998. *How Jews Became White Folks and What That Says about Race in America*. New Brunswick, N.J.: Rutgers University Press.

Brooks, Clark. 1988. "Clinic's Charges Dropped." *Sacramento Bee*, November 2, B1.

Brown, Elsa Barkley. 1992. "What Has Happened Here: The Politics of Difference in Women's History and Feminist Politics." *Feminist Studies* 18: 295–312.

Bruce, Judith. 1981. "Women-Oriented Health Care: New Hampshire Feminist Health Center." *Studies in Family Planning* 12, no. 10 (October): 353–363.

Budu-Watkins, Akua, and Byllye Y. Avery. 1995. National Black Women's Health Project. Letter to Members, November 17.

Buechler, Steven. 1990. *Women's Movements in the United States: Women's Suffrage, Equal Rights, and Beyond*. New Brunswick, N.J.: Rutgers University Press.

Burchell, Clay. 1974. Discussion of "The Challenge of the Women's Movement to American Gynecology." *American Journal of Obstetrics and Gynecology* 120 (5): 664.

Bush, Diane. 1978. "The Routinization of Social Movement Organizations: China as a Deviant Case." *Sociology Quarterly* 19, no. 2 (spring): 203–217.

Butler, Edith. 1984. "NHFHC Celebrates Tenth Anniversary." *Women Wise* (fall): 2–3.

Butler, Judith, and Joan Scott, eds. 1992. *Feminists Theorize the Political*. New York: Routledge.

Byrd, W. Michael, and Linda Clayton. 2001. *An American Health Dilemma: A Medical History of African Americans and the Problem of Race*. Vol. 1. New York: Routledge.

Cade, Toni. 1970. *The Black Woman: An Anthology*. New York: Signet Books, New American Library.

Campbell, Mary [Mary Howell, pseud]. 1973. *Why Would a Girl Go into Medicine? Medical Education in the U.S.: A Guide for Women*. Old Westbury, N.Y.: Feminist Press.

Carroll, Bernice. 1979. "Political Science, Part I: American Politics and Political Behavior." *Signs* 5: 289–306.

Carroll, LaNedra. 1980. "Doctors Yield to Women's Health Center." *Tallahassee Democrat*, January 15, 1, 6A.

Cavanagh, Denis. 1974. Discussion of "The Challenge of the Women's Movement to American Gynecology." *American Journal of Obstetrics and Gynecology* 120 (5): 664–665.

Chalker, Rebecca, and Carol Downer. 1992. *A Woman's Book of Choices: Abortion, Menstrual Extraction, RU–486*. New York: Four Walls Eight Windows.

Cherniak, Donna, and Allan Feingold. 1974. *Birth Control Handbook*. Montreal, Canada: Montreal Health Press.

Chesler, Phylis. 1972. *Women and Madness*. Garden City, N.Y.: Doubleday.

Chicago Women with Health Right. 1975. "A View from the Loop: The Women's Health Movement in Chicago." *HealthRight* 2 (fall): 3–4.

Chico Feminist Women's Health Center. 1981. "Hospital Inspections." Women's Health Movement Papers, compiled by the Federation of Feminist Women's Health Center. Los Angeles: FFWHC.

Chung, Mary. 1996. "'Coming Together, Moving Strong: Mobilizing and Asian Women's Health Movement,' Opening Session." In *Coming Together, Moving Strong: Mobilizing and Asian Women's Health Movement: Proceedings from the First National Asian Women's Health Conference*, edited by Afton Hirohama and Priya Jagannathan. NAWHO.

Clarke, Adele E., and Virginia L. Olesen, eds. 1999. *Revisioning Women, Health, and Healing: Feminist, Cultural, and Technoscience Perspectives*. New York: Routledge.

Coalition for the Medical Rights of Women (CMRW). 1984. *Second Opinion*. San Francisco: CMRW.

Coalition on Women and the Budget. 1984. *Inequality of Sacrifice: The Impact of the Reagan Budget on Women*. Washington, D.C.: The Coalition.

Cody, Pat. 1990. Interview with author, November 11, Berkeley, Calif.

Cohen, Marilyn. 1995. "Letter," n.d.

Collins, Patricia Hill. 1990. *Black Feminist Thought: Knowledge, Consciousness, and the Politics of Empowerment*. New York: Routledge, Chapman & Hall.

Combahee River Collective. 1983. "The Combahee River Collective Statement." In *Home Girls: A Black Feminist Anthology*, edited by Barbara Smith. Latham, N.Y.: Kitchen Table, Women of Color Press.

Community Health Care for Women (CHCW) [pseud.]. 1973. Unpublished Document.

Concord Feminist Health Center (CFHC). 1989. "A Brief History of the Concord Feminist Health Center." Unpublished document.

———. n.d. Brochure.

Corea, Gena. 1977. *Women's Health Care: The Hidden Malpractice*. New York: William Morrow.

———. 1992. *The Invisible Epidemic: The Story of Women and Aids*. New York: HarperCollins.

Cousineau, Michael Rio. 1987. "Organizational Transformation of Community Clinics in Two California Counties: Their Commitments to Social Change." Thesis, UCLA School of Public Health.

Cowan, Belita. 1991. Interview with author, June, Washington, D.C.

Dan, Alice, ed. 1994. *Reframing Women's Health: Multidisciplinary Research and Practice*. Thousand Oaks, Calif.: Sage Publications.

Davis, Angela Y. 1981. *Women, Race, and Class*. New York: Vintage.

———. 1989. *Women, Culture, and Politics*. New York: Random House.

———. 1990. "Sick and Tired of Being Sick and Tired: The Politics of Black Women's Health." In *The Black Women's Health Book*, edited by Evelyn C. White. Seattle, Wash.: Seal Press.

Davis, Flora. 1991. *Moving the Mountain: The Women's Movement in America since 1960*. New York: Simon and Schuster.

Davis, Susan E., ed. 1988. *Women under Attack: Victories, Backlash, and the Fight for Reproductive Freedom*. Boston: South End Press. Pamphlet no. 7.

DeFine, Michael Sullivan. 1997. "A History of Governmentally Coerced Sterilization: The Plight of Native American Women." Retrieved from the Women of Color web site: http://www.hsph.harvard.edu/organization/healthnet/WoC.

Dill, Bonnie Thornton. 1983. "Race, Class and Gender: Prospects for an All-Inclusive Sisterhood." *Feminist Studies* 9: 131–149.

Downer, Carol. 1974. "What Makes the Feminist Women's Health Center 'Feminist'?" *Monthly Extract* 3 (March/April): 10–11.

———. 1990. Interview with author, September 30, New York.

———. n.d. "Self Help." Federation of Feminist Women's Health Center.

Downey, Alice. 1979. "Never on Thursday!: Why NHFC Is Closed on Thursday." *Women Wise* 2, no. 3 (fall): 1–2.

Doyal, Leslie. 1995. *What Makes Women Sick: Gender and the Political Economy of Health.* Piscataway, N.J.: Rutgers University Press.

Dreifus, Claudia, ed. 1977. *Seizing Our Bodies: The Politics of Women's Health.* New York: Vintage.

Drexler, Madeline. 1989. "Collective Wisdom: The Boston Women's Health Book Collective." *Boston Globe Magazine,* September 10, 64–65.

Eagan, Andrea Borrof. 1994. "The Women's Health Movement and Its Lasting Impact." In *An Unfinished Revolution: Women and Health Care in America,* ed. Emily Friedman. New York: United Hospital Fund of New York.

Echols, Alice. 1989. *Daring to Be Bad: Radical Feminism in America, 1967–1975.* Minneapolis: Minnesota University Press.

Edwards, Margot. 1984. *Reclaiming Birth: History and Heroines of American Childbirth Reform.* Trumansburg, N.Y.: Crossing Press.

Ehrenreich, Barbara. 1998. Interview with author, April 11, Eugene, Oreg.

Ehrenreich, Barbara, and Deirdre English. 1973a. *Witches, Midwives, and Nurses: A History of Women Healers.* Old Westbury, N.Y.: Feminist Press.

———. 1973b. *Complaints and Disorders: The Sexual Politics of Sickness.* Glass Mountain Pamphlet, no. 2. Old Westbury, N.Y.: Feminist Press.

———. 1978. *For Her Own Good: 150 Years of the Experts Advice to Women.* New York: Anchor Press, Doubleday.

Eisenstein, Hester. 1995. "The Australian Democratic Experiment: A Feminist Case for Bureaucracy." In *Feminist Organizations: Harvest of the Women's Movement,* edited by Myra Marx Ferree and Patricia Yancey Martin. Philadelphia: Temple University Press.

Eisenstein, Zillah. 1994. *The Color of Gender: Reimaging Democracy.* Berkeley: University of California Press.

Elze, Diane. 1988a. "Underground Abortion Remembered: Part I." *Sojourner: The Women's Forum* 13, no. 8 (April). Reprinted in *Abortion,* ed. Janet Podell (New York: Wilson Co.), 1990.

———. 1988b. "Underground Abortion Remembered: Part II." *Sojourner: The Women's Forum* 13, no. 9 (May): 12–14.

Emma Goldman Clinic. 1993. "Happy Twentieth Birthday, Emma." *Emma's Periodical* 4, no. 2 (summer): 1, 8, 10–11.

———. 1996. "Sand's Farewell to Emma." *Emma's Journal: Newsletter of the Emma Goldman Clinic* 7, no. 1 (March): 1–2.

Erickson, Lee Ann. 1996. *From One Place to Another: Emma Goldman Clinic Stories.* Produced by Lee Ann Erickson, directed by Lee Ann Erickson and Camille Seaman, 80 minutes. Video recording .

Eugene and Portland Feminist Women's Health Center (EPFWHC). 1994. Newsletter (winter).

Evans, Sara. 1979. *Personal Politics: The Roots of Women's Liberalism: The Civil Rights Movement and the New Left.* New York: Random House.

FAAR. 1977. "Watch Women Harassed." May/June.

Farber, Shelley. 1976. *The Women's Health Movement.* New York: Praeger.

Farrell, Amy. 1995. "Like a Tarantula on a Banana Boat: Ms. Magazine, 1972–1989." In *Feminist Organizations: Harvest of the Women's Movement,* edited by Myra Marx Ferree and Patricia Yancey Martin. Philadelphia: Temple University Press.

Federation of Feminist Women's Health Centers (FFWHC). 1981a. "Taking the Mystery Out of a Medical Visit." *How to Stay Out of the Gynecologist's Office.* Culver City, Calif.: Peace Press.

———. 1981b. *A New View of a Woman's Body: A Fully Illustrated Guide.* New York: Touchstone Books, Simon and Schuster.

———. 1981c. *Women's Health Movement Papers.* Los Angeles: FFWHC.

Fee, Elizabeth. 1977. "Women and Health Care: A Comparison of Theories." In *Seizing Our Bodies,* edited by C. Dreifus. New York: Vintage Press.

———, ed. 1983. *Women and Health: The Politics of Sex in Medicine.* Farmingdale, N.Y.: Baywood Publishing Co.

Ferguson, Kathy. 1984. *The Feminist Case against Bureaucracy.* Philadelphia: Temple University Press.

Ferree, Myra Marx, and Patricia Yancey Martin, eds. 1995. *Feminist Organizations: Harvest of the Women's Movement.* Philadelphia: Temple University Press.

First Annual Women-Controlled Health Projects Conference. 1974. Statement. November 18.

Fishel, Elizabeth. 1973. "The Women's Self Help Movement, or Is Happiness Knowing Your Own Cervix?" *Ramparts* (November): 29–31, 56–59.

Foucault, Michel. 1980. *The History of Sexuality: An Introduction.* New York: Vintage.

Fox, Kenneth, et al. 1982. *Crisis in the Public Sector: A Reader.* New York: Monthly Review Press, Union for Radical Political Economics.

Frankenberg, Ruth. 1993. *White Women, Race Matters: The Social Construction of Whiteness.* Minneapolis: University of Minnesota Press.

Frankfort, Ellen. 1972. *Vaginal Politics.* New York: Quadrangle Books.

Franzway, Suzanne, Diane Court, and Robert W. Connell. 1989. *Staking a Claim: Feminism, Bureaucracy, and the State.* Boston: Unwin Hyman.

Freeman, Jo. 1972. "The Tyranny of Structurelessness." In *Radical Feminism,* ed. Anne Koedtz, Ellen Levine, and Anita Rapone. New York: Quadrangle/New York Times Book Co.

Freeman, Mark. 1995. *Rewriting the Self: History, Memory, Narrative.* London and New York: Routledge.

Fried, Marlene Gerber, ed. 1990. *From Abortion to Reproductive Freedom: Transforming a Movement.* Boston: South End Press.

Fugh-Berman, Adriane. 1985. "Bombing of Abortion Clinics Escalates." *Network News* (January/February).

Galper, Miriam, and Carolyn Washburn. 1976. "A Woman's Self-Help Program in Action." *Social Policy* 6 (5): 46–52.

Gary-Smith, Sharon. 1989. "Self-Help: Our Past, Present and Future." *Vital Signs* 6, no. 1 (February): 6–7.

Gelb, Joyce. 1995. "Feminist Organizations' Success and the Politics of Engagement."

In *Feminist Organizations: Harvest of the Women's Movement*, edited by Myra Marx Ferree and Patricia Yancey Martin. Philadelphia: Temple University Press.

Gelb, Joyce, and Marion Lief Palley, eds. 1987. *Women and Public Policies*. Rev. ed. Princeton, N.J.: Princeton University Press.

Giddings, Paula. 1984. *When and Where I Enter: The Impact of Black Women on Race and Sex in America*. New York: Morrow.

Giges, Laura. 1982. "The Challenges of Change." In *Ciel Benedetto: A History of the Santa Cruz Women's Health Center, 1985–2000*, ed. Irene Refi and Randall Jarrell. Santa Cruz, Calif.: University of California Library Collection.

Gillis, John R. 1994. "Memory and Identity: The History of a Relationship." In *Commemorations: The Politics of National Identity*, edited by John Gillis. Princeton, N.J.: Princeton University Press.

Ginsburg, Faye D. 1989. *Contested Lives: The Abortion Debate in an American Community*. Berkeley: University of California Press.

Glennon, Lynda. 1979. *Women and Dualism*. New York: Longman.

Gordon, Linda. 1976. *Women's Body, Woman's Right: A Social History of Birth Control in America*. New York: Grossman Publishers.

Gordon, Margaret [pseud.]. 1991. Interview with author, June 12.

Gray, Mary Jane. 1999. Interview with author, Corvallis, Oreg.

Gray, Mary Jane, and Judith Tyson. 1976. "Evolution of a Woman's Clinic: An Alternative System of Medical Care." *American Journal of Obstetrics and Gynecology* 126 (7): 760–768.

Grewal, Inderpal, and Caren Kaplan, eds. 1994. *Scattered Hegemonies: Postmodernity and Transnational Feminist Practices*. Minneapolis: University of Minnesota Press.

Grimstad, Kirsten, and Susan Rennie, eds. 1973. *The Woman's Survival Catalog*. New York: Coward, McCann & Geoghegan/ Berkeley Publishing Corp.

Guy-Sheftall, Beverly. 1993. *Words of Fire: An Anthology of African-American Feminist Thought*. New York: New Press.

Haire, Doris. 1972. "The Cultural Warping of Childbirth." *Special Report*. International Childbirth Education Associates.

Hairston, Julie. 1990. "Killing Kittens, Bombing Clinics." *Southern Exposure* 18 (2): 14–19.

Hammonds, Evelynn. 1986. "Missing Persons: African American Women, AIDS and the History of Disease." *Radical America* 20 (6): 7–23.

Hanzo, Jude. 1991. Interview with author, January 27, Portland, Oreg.

Hartmann, Betsy. 1995. *Reproductive Rights and Wrongs: The Global Politics of Population Control*. Boston: South End Press.

Hasper, Dido. 1981. "Feminist Women's Health Centers: Interview with Dido Hasper." In *Women's Culture: The Women's Renaissance of the Seventies*, edited by Gayle Kimball. Metuchen, N.J.: Scarecrow Press.

Healy, Bernadine. 1995. Editorial. *Journal of Women's Health* 4 (6): 589.

Hearn, Frances. 1978. "Rationality and Bureaucracy: Maoist Contributions to a Marxist Theory of Bureaucracy." *Sociological Quarterly* 19, no. 1 (winter): 37–54.

Higginbotham, Elizabeth, and Mary Romero, eds. 1997. *Women and Work: Race, Ethnicity, and Class*. Thousand Oaks, Calif.: Sage Publications.

Hine, Darlene Clark, ed. 1985. *Black Women in the Nursing Profession: A Documentary History*. New York: Garland.

————. 1989. *Black Women in White: Racial Conflict and Cooperation in the Nursing Profession, 1890–1950.* Bloomington: Indiana University Press.

Hirsch, Lolly, and Jeanne Hirsch. 1972. *Monthly Extract: An Irregular Periodical* 1 (1): 1.

————. 1973. *Monthly Extract: An Irregular Periodical* 1 (4): 1.

Hochschild, Arlie R. 1975. "The Sociology of Feeling and Emotion: Selected Possibilities." In *Another Voice,* edited by Marcia Millman and Rosabeth Kanter. New York: Anchor.

————. 1979. "Emotion Work, Feeling Rules and Social Structure." *American Journal of Sociology* 85 (3): 551–75.

————. 1983. *The Managed Heart: Commercialization of Human Feeling.* Berkeley: University of California Press.

hooks, bell. 1984. *Feminist Theory: From Margin to Center.* Boston: South End.

Hornstein, Frances. 1974a. "An Interview on Women's Health Politics, Part 2." *Quest* 1 (2): 75–80.

————. 1974b. "An Interview on Women's Health Politics, Part 1." *Quest* 1 (1): 27–36.

Howell, Mary. 1975. "A Women's Health School?" *Social Policy* 6 (September/October): 50–53.

Hull, Gloria, Patricia Bell Scott, and Barbara Smith, eds. 1982. *All the Women Are White, All the Blacks Are Men, But Some of Us Are Brave: Black Women's Studies.* Old Westbury, N.Y.: Feminist Press.

Hyde, Cheryl. 1991. "Did the New Right Radicalize the Women's Movement? A Study of Change in Feminist Social Movement Organizations, 1977–1987." Ph.D. diss., University of Michigan, Ann Arbor.

————. 1992. "The Ideational System of Social Movement Agencies." In *Human Services as Complex Organizations,* edited by Yeheskel Hasenfeld. Newbury Park, Calif.: Sage.

————. 1995. "Feminist Social Movement Organizations Survive the New Right." In *Feminist Organizations: Harvest of the Women's Movement,* edited by Myra Marx Ferree and Patricia Yancey Martin. Philadelphia: Temple University Press.

Jaggar, Alison. 1989. "Love and Knowledge: Emotion in Feminist Epistemology." In *Gender/Body/Knowledge: Feminist Reconstructions of Being and Knowing,* edited by Alison Jaggar and Susan Bordo. New Brunswick, N.J.: Rutgers University Press.

Jane. 1990. "Just Call Jane." *The Fight for Reproductive Freedom: A Newsletter for Student Activists* 4, no. 2 (winter): 1, 2, 4, 6.

Joffe, Carole. 1986. *The Regulation of Sexuality: Experiences of Family Planning Workers.* Philadelphia: Temple University Press.

————. 1995. *Doctors of Conscience: The Struggle to Provide Abortion before and after Roe v. Wade.* Boston: Beacon Press.

Jones, Charles, ed. 1998. *The Black Panther Party (Reconsidered).* Baltimore: Black Classic Press.

Jones, Georgeanna. 1974. Discussion of "The Challenge of the Women's Movement to American Gynecology." Edited by Barbara Kaiser and Irwin Kaiser. *American Journal of Obstetrics and Gynecology* 120 (5): 665.

Joyner, Brenda. 1990. "Fight Back to Save Women's Lives." In *From Abortion to Reproductive Freedom: Transforming a Movement,* edited by Marlene Gerber Fried. Boston: South End Press.

Joyner, Brenda, Linda Grey, and Risa Denenberg. 1990. "Dear Friends Letter." Unpublished document. November 3.

Kaiser, Barbara L., and Irwin H. Kaiser. 1974. "The Challenge of the Women's Health Movement to American Gynecology." *American Journal of Obstetrics and Gynecology* 120 (5): 652–661.

Kanter, Rosabeth Moss. 1972. *Commitment and Community.* Cambridge, Mass.: Harvard University Press.

Kaplan, Laura. 1995. *The Story of Jane.* New York: Pantheon Books.

Kay, Bonnie. 1989. "The Commodification of Women's Health: The New Women's Health Centers." *Health/PAC Bulletin* (winter): 19–23.

Kelly, Julie. 1990. Interview with author, September, New Bedford, Mass.

King, Charles R. 1993. "Calling Jane: The Life and Death of a Women's Illegal Abortion Service." *Women and Health* 20 (3): 75–93.

Kintch, Robert. 1974. Discussion of "The Challenge of the Women's Movement to American Gynecology." *American Journal of Obstetrics and Gynecology* 120 (5): 663–664.

Klawiter, Maren. 1999. "Racing for the Cure, Walking Women, and Toxic Touring: Mapping Cultures of Action within the Bay Area." *Social Problems* 46 (1): 104–127.

Kotelchuck, David. 1976. *Prognosis Negative: Crisis in the Health Care System.* New York: Vintage.

Krase, Kathryn. 1996. "Dr. Helen Rodriguez-Trias: A Warrior in the Struggle for Reproductive Rights." *Network News* (January/February): 4.

Krust, Lin, and Charon Asetoyer. 1993. *A Study of the Use of Depo-Provera and Norplant by the Indian Health Services (Revised).* Lake Andes, S.D.: NAWHERC.

Kushner, Rose. 1975. *Breast Cancer: A Personal History and Investigative Report.* New York: Harcourt, Brace, Jovanovitch.

Ladner, Joyce A. 1971. *Tomorrow's Tomorrow: The Black Woman.* Garden City, N.Y.: Doubleday.

Lamphere, Louise. 1987. *From Working Daughters to Working Mothers: Immigrant Women in a New England Industrial Community.* Ithaca, N.Y.: Cornell University Press.

Larson, Vicki. 1991. "Making Choices." *Hispanic* (March): 46.

La Rue, Linda. 1970. "The Black Movement and Women's Liberation." *Black Scholar* 1 (May): 32–42.

Latinas for Reproductive Choice. 1990–1991. "Latinas for Reproductive Choice." *Organizacion Nacional de la Salud de la Mujer Latina/National Latina Health Organization* 1 (1).

Laurence, Leslie, and Beth Weinhouse. 1997. *Outrageous Practices: How Gender Bias Threatens Women's Health.* New Brunswick, N.J.: Rutgers University Press.

Leavitt, Judith Walzer, and Ronald L. Numbers, eds. 1978. *Sickness and Health in America: Readings in the History of Medicine and Public Health.* Madison: University of Wisconsin Press.

Leigh, Wilhelmina A., and Malinda A. Lindquist. 1998. *Women of Color Health Data Book: Adolescents to Seniors.* [Bethesda, Md.]: Office of Research on Women's Health, Office of the Director, National Institutes of Health.

Leopold, Ellen. 1999. *A Darker Ribbon: Breast Cancer, Women, and Their Doctors in the Twentieth Century.* Boston: Beacon Press.

Leste, Judy et al. 1974. "Calling It Quits." *Off Our Backs* 4: 2.

Lewin, Tamar. 2001. "Women's Health Is No Longer a 'Man's World.'" *New York Times,* February 7, 1.

Lewry, Natasha, and Charon Asetoyer. 1992. *The Impact of Norplant in the Native American Community.* Lake Andes, S.D.: NAWHERC.

Looker, Patty. 1993. "Women's Health Centers: History and Evolution." *Women's Health Issues* 3 (2): 95–100.

Lorber, Judith. 1984. *Women Physicians: Careers, Status, and Power.* New York and London: Tavistock.

Lorde, Audre. 1980. *The Cancer Journals.* Argyle, N.Y.: Spinsters, Ink.

———. 1984. *Sister Outsider: Essays and Speeches.* Trumansburg, N.Y.: Crossing Press.

Luker, Kristen. 1984. *Abortion and the Politics of Motherhood.* Berkeley: University of California Press.

Lutz, Catherine. 1988. *Unnatural Emotions: Everyday Sentiments on a Micronesian Atoll & Their Challenge to Western Theory.* Chicago: University of Chicago Press.

———. 1990. "Engendered Emotion: Gender, Power and the Rhetoric of Emotional Control in American Discourse." In *Language and the Politics of Emotion,* edited by Catherine Lutz and Lila Abu-Lughod. Cambridge, U.K.: Cambridge University Press.

Lutz, Catherine, and Geoffrey White. 1986. "The Anthropology of Emotions." *Annual Review of Anthropology* 15: 405–436.

Lutz, Catherine A., and Lila Abu-Lughod. 1990. *Language and the Politics of Emotion.* New York: Cambridge University Press.

Malasky, Sandra. 1979. "Some Reminiscences." *Women Wise* 2, no. 3 (fall): 1–2.

Mansbridge, Jane. 1973. "Time, Emotion, and Inequality: Three Problems of Participatory Groups." *Journal of Applied Behavioral Science* 9 (2/3): 351–368.

———. 1979. "The Agony of Inequality." In *Coops, Communes, and Collectives: Experiments in Social Change in the 1960 and 1970s,* edited by John Case and Rosemary Taylor. New York: Pantheon.

———. 1980. *Beyond Adversary Democracy.* New York: Basic Books. Reprint, Chicago: University of Chicago Press, 1983.

———. 1982. "Fears of Conflict in Face-to-Face Democracies." In *Workplace Democracy and Social Change,* edited by Frank Lindfield and Joyce Rothschild-Whitt. Boston: Porter Sargent Publishers.

———. 1995. "What Is the Feminist Movement?" In *Feminist Organizations: Harvest of the Women's Movement,* edited by Myra Marx Ferree and Patricia Yancey Martin. Philadelphia: Temple University Press.

Marco, Gina, Robert Hollingworth, and William Durham, eds. 1987. *Silent Spring Revisited.* Washington, D.C.: American Chemical Society.

Marieskind, Helen. 1980. *Women in the Health System: Patients, Providers, Programs.* St. Louis, Mo.: C.V. Mosby.

Marieskind, Helen, and Barbara Ehrenreich. 1975. "Toward Socialist Medicine: The Women's Health Movement." *Social Policy* 6 (2): 34–42.

Martin, Patricia Yancey. 1990. "Rethinking Feminist Organizations." *Gender and Society* 4 (2): 182–206.

Martinez, Elizabeth. 1992. "Caramba, Our Anglo Sisters Just Didn't Get It." *Network News* (November/December): 1, 4–5.

Maskovsky, Jeff. 2000. "'Managing' the Poor: Neoliberalism, Medicaid HMOs and the Triumph of Consumerism among the Poor in Philadelphia." *Medical Anthropology* 19: 121–146.

Matthews, Nancy. 1994. *Confronting Rape: The Feminist Anti-Rape Movement and the State.* New York: Routledge.

————. 1995. "Feminist Clashes with the State: Tactical Choices by State Funded Rape Crisis Centers." In *Feminist Organizations: Harvest of the Women's Movement*, edited by Myra Marx Ferree and Patricia Yancey Martin. Philadelphia: Temple University Press.

McBride, Angela B., and W. McBride. 1994. "Women's Health Scholarship: From Critique to Assertion." *Journal of Women's Health* 2 (1): 43–47.

McIntosh, Mary. 1978. "The State and the Oppression of Women." In *Feminism and Materialism*, edited by Annette Kuhn and AnnMarie Wolpe. London: Routledge & Kegan Paul.

McKinney Barfoot, Julia. 1973. "Free Health Care for Women by Women: The Berkeley Women's Health Collective." In *Getting Clear: Body Work for Women*, by Anne Kent Rush. New York: Random House.

Mellow, Gail. 1989. "Sustaining Our Organizations: Feminist Health Activism in an Age of Technology." In *Healing Technology*, edited by Katherine Strother Ratcliff. Ann Arbor: University of Michigan Press.

Melosh, Barbara. 1982. *"The Physician's Hand": Work Culture and Conflict in American Nursing*. Philadelphia: Temple University Press.

Merrill, James. 1974. Discussion of "The Challenge of the Women's Movement to American Gynecology." *American Journal of Obstetrics and Gynecology* 120 (5): 663.

Merton, Robert. 1968. *Social Theory and Social Structure*. New York: Free Press.

Michels, Robert. [1959]. *Political Parties: A Sociological Study of the Oligarchical Tendencies of Modern Democracy*. Trans. by Eden and Cedar Paul. New York: Dover.

Mohanty, Chandra Talpade. 1992. "Feminist Encounters: Locating the Politics of Experience." *Destabilizing Theory: Contemporary Feminist Debates*, edited by Michele Barrett and Anne Phillips. Stanford, Calif.: Stanford University Press.

Moraga, Cherrie, and Gloria Anzaldua. 1981. *This Bridge Called My Back: Writings by Radical Women of Color*. Watertown, Mass.: Persephone Press.

Morantz-Sanchez, Regina Markell. 1985. *Sympathy and Science: Women Physicians in American Medicine*. New York: Oxford University Press.

Morgen, Sandra. 1982. *Ideology and Change in a Feminist Health Center: The Experience and Dynamics of Routinization*. Ph.D. Diss., University of South Carolina.

————. 1983. "Towards a Politics of Feelings: Beyond the Dialectic of Thought and Action." *Women's Studies* 10(2): 203–223.

————. 1986. "The Dynamics of Cooptation in a Feminist Health Clinic." *Social Science and Medicine* 23 (2): 201–210.

————. 1988a. "The Dream of Diversity, the Dilemmas of Difference: Race and Class Contradictions in a Feminist Health Clinic" In *Anthropology for the Nineties*, edited by Johnetta Cole. New York: Free Press.

————. 1988b. "It's the Whole Power of the City Against Us!": The Development of Political Consciousness in a Women's Health Care Coalition." In *Women and the Politics of Empowerment*, edited by Ann Bookman and Sandra Morgen. Philadelphia: Temple University Press.

————. 1990. "Two Faces of the State: Women, Social Control and Empowerment." In *Uncertain Terms: Negotiating Gender in America*, edited by Faye Ginsburg and Anna Tsung. Boston: Beacon Press.

————. 1995. "It Was the Best of Times, It Was the Worst of Times: Emotional Discourse in the Work Culture of Feminist Clinics." In *Feminist Organizations: Harvest of the*

Women's Movement, edited by Myra Marx Ferree and Patricia Yancey Martin. Philadelphia: Temple University Press.

———. 1997. "Class Experience and Conflict in a Feminist Workplace: A Case Study." In *Women and Work: Exploring Race, Ethnicity, and Class*, edited by Elizabeth Higginbotham and Mary Romero. Thousand Oaks, Calif.: Sage Publishers.

Morgen, Sandra, and Alice Julier. 1991. "Women's Health Movement Organizations: Two Decades of Struggle and Change." Unpublished report.

Morgen, Sandra, and Jill Weigt. 2001. "Poor Women, Fair Work and Welfare-to-Work That Works." In *New Poverty Studies: The Ethnography of Politics, Policy and Impoverished People in the U.S*, edited by Judith Goode and Jeff Maskovsky. New York: New York University Press.

Ms. 1995. "Special Report: Abortion." 5(6): 42–66.

Mumby, Dennis, and Linda Putnam. 1992. "The Politics of Emotion: A Feminist Reading of Bounded Rationality." *Academy of Management Review* 17 (3): 465–486.

Narrigan, Deborah, et al. 1997. "Research to Improve Women's Health: *An Agenda for Equity.*" In *Women's Health: Complexities and Differences*, edited by Sheryl Burt Ruzek, Virginia L. Olesen, and Adele E. Clarke. Columbus: Ohio State University Press.

Nathan, Richard P., Fred C. Doolittle, and Associates. 1983. *The Consequences of Cuts: The Effects of the Reagan Domestic Program on State and Local Governments.* Princeton, N.J.: Princeton Urban and Regional Research Center; distributed by Princeton University Press.

———. 1987. *Reagan and the States.* Princeton, N.J.: Princeton University Press.

National Abortion Federation. 1987. *Network News* (May/June).

———. 1997. "Fact Sheet: Economics of Abortion." Retrieved June 27 from http://www.cais.com/naf/facts/econ.htm.

National Abortion Rights Action League (NARAL). 2000. NARAL web site. Retrieved from http://www.naral.org/index.html.

National Asian Women's Health Organization (NAWHO). 1993–1994. *Report.* NAWHO.

———. 1995. *Perceptions of Risk: An assessment of the Factors Influencing Use of Reproductive and Sexual Health Services by Asian American Women.* NAWHO.

———. 1996. "On the Issues: Breast Cancer in the Asian Community." *NAWHO Quarterly Newsletter* 2 (2): 1.

———. 1999. "New Study Reveals Startling Trends in Health Habits of Asian American Men." *NAWHO Press Release* (May 10).

———. 2000. *National Asian Women's Health Organization.* Retrieved June 16 from http://www.nawho.org/.

National Black Women's Health Project (NBWHP). 1985. *Vital Signs* 2, no. 1 (April).

———. 1994a. *Tenth Anniversary Conference and Homecoming Celebration Program.* June 30–July 3, Atlanta, Ga.

———. 1994b. *Vital Signs.* Tenth Anniversary Issue.

———. 2001. "Eliminating Racial and Ethnic Disparities in Health." Retrieved from the NBWHP web site: http://www.nationalblackwomenshealthproject.org.

National Latina Health Organization (NLHO). n.d. Organización Nacional de la Salud de la Mujer Latina/National Health Organization Brochure.

———. 1988a "New Latina Health Organization." Coalition to Fight Infant Mortality Newsletter, 6, 8.

————. 1988b. "Raising Health Issues for Latinas by Latinas." *Organizers Notes: Newsletter of the Reproductive Rights Access Project* 3, no. 4 (November–January): 1, 5.

————. 1995. "Don't Panic." *Organización Nacional de la Salud de la Mujer Latina/National Health Organization* (winter): 1.

National Latina Institute for Reproductive Health (NLIRH). 1999. "National Latina Institute for Reproductive Health (NLIRH)." *Pro-Choice Public Education Project.* Retrieved May 28 from http://www.protectchoice.org/partnerNLIRH.html.

National Women's Health Network (NWHN). 1976. *Network News* (October): 1–2.

————. 1994. *Network News* (September/October).

Native American Women's Health Education Resource Center (NAWHERC). 2000. "Indigenous Women's Reproductive Rights and Pro-Choice." Retrieved June 15 from http://www.nativeshop.org/pro-choice.html.

————. 1994a. "Native Women Gather for Third Annual Reproductive Rights Conference." *Wicozanni Wowapi: Good Health Newsletter* (spring): 1, 3.

————. 1994b. *Wicozanni Wowapi: Good Health Newsletter* (summer): 1, 4.

New Hampshire Feminist Health Center (NHFHC). 1982. "NHFHC Cervical Cap Study: First Year Results Compiled." *Women Wise* (summer): 1.

Newman, Katherine. 1980. "Incipient Bureaucracy: The Development of Hierarchies in Egalitarian Organizations." In *Hierarchy and Society: Anthropological Perspectives on Bureaucracy,* edited by Gerald Britain and Ronald Cohen. Philadelphia: Institute for the Study of Human Issues.

Nicholson, Linda, ed. 1990. *Feminism/Postmodernism.* New York and London: Routledge.

Norsigian, Judy. 1994. "Women and National Health Care Reform: A Progressive Feminist Agenda." In *Reframing Women's Health: Multidisciplinary Research and Practice,* edited by Alice Dan. Thousand Oaks, Calif.: Sage.

————. 1996. "The Women's Health Movement in the U.S." In *Man-Made Medicine: Women's Health, Public Policy, and Reform,* edited by Kary Moss. Durham, N.C.: Duke University Press.

Norsigian, Judy, and Wendy Coppedge Sanford. 1987. "Ten Years in the 'Our Bodies, Ourselves' Collective." *Women and Therapy* 6 (1/2): 287–292.

Nowrojee, Sia, and Jael Silliman. 1997. "Asian Women's Health: Organizing a Movement." In *Dragon Ladies: Asian American Feminist Breathe Fire,* edited by Sonia Shah. Boston: South End Press.

Nye, Alice, et al. 1994. "New Hampshire Feminist Health Center Is Twenty Years Old." *Women Wise* (fall): 1, 10.

O'Connor, James. 1973. *The Fiscal Crisis of the State.* New York: St. Martin's Press.

O'Connor, Julia, Ann Orloff, and Sheila Shaver. 1999. *States, Markets, Families: Gender, Liberalism and Social Policy in Australia, Canada, Great Britain and the U.S.* New York: Cambridge University Press.

Olesen, Virginia. 1997. "Who Cares? Women as Informal and Formal Caregivers." In *Women's Health: Complexities and Differences,* edited by Sheryl Burt Ruzek, Virginia L. Olesen and Adele E. Clarke. Columbus: Ohio State University Press.

Oppenheimer, Amy. 1976. Personal unpublished document.

Organization for Economic Co-operation and Development. 1992. "The Reform of Health Care: A Comparative Study of Seven OECD Countries." *OECD Health Policy Studies* No. 2. Paris: OECD

Palmer John L., and Isabel Sawhill. 1982. *The Reagan Experiment: An Examination of*

Economic and Social Policies under the Reagan Administration. Washington, D.C.: Urban Institute Press.

——, eds. 1984. *The Reagan Record: An Assessment of America's Changing Domestic Priorities.* Cambridge, Mass.: Ballinger Publishing Co.

Payne, Charles. 1995. *I've Got the Light of Freedom: The Organizing Tradition and the Mississippi Freedom Struggle.* Berkeley: University of California Press.

Pearson, Cindy. 1996. "Self Help Clinic Celebrates 25 Years." *Network News* (March/April): 1, 2–4.

——. 1987. "Women's Clinic Directors Harassed." *Network News* (May/June):5.

Petchesky, Rosalind P. 1984. *Abortion and Woman's Choice: The State, Sexuality, and Reproductive Freedom.* New York: Longman.

——. 1990. *Abortion and Women's Choice: The State, Sexuality, and Reproductive Freedom.* Boston: Northeastern University Press.

Piven, Frances Fox. 1985. "Women and the State: Ideology, Power, and the Welfare State." In *Gender and the Life Course*, edited by Alice Rossi. New York: Aldine de Gruytar Publishers.

Piven, Frances Fox, and Richard Cloward. 1971. *Regulating the Poor: The Functions of Public Welfare.* New York: Pantheon Books.

——. 1974. *The Politics of Turmoil: Essays on Poverty, Race, and Urban Crisis.* New York: Pantheon.

——. 1977. *Poor People's Movements.* New York: Pantheon.

Podell, Jane, ed. 1990. *Abortion.* New York: Wilson Co.

Pollner, Fran. 1975. "Feminist Movement's Impact on Obstetrics and Gynecological Care Is Not Debatable." *Obstetrics/Gynecology News* (June 15): 13, 34.

Ponge, Lori, and Judith Stein. 1981. Letter. July 22.

Portland Feminist Women's Health Center (PFWHC). 1995a. *FWHC News* (winter): 1, 7.

——. 1995b. *FWHC News* (spring): 2.

Pringle, Rosemary. 1998. *Sex and Medicine: Gender, Power and Authority in the Medical Profession.* New York: Cambridge University Press.

Putnam, Linda, and Dennis Mumby. 1993. "Organizations, Emotion and the Myth of Rationality." In *Emotion in Organizations*, edited by Stephen Fineman. London: Sage Publications.

Reinelt, Claire. 1995. "Moving onto the Terrain of the State: The Battered Women's Movement and the Politics of Engagement." In *Feminist Organizations: Harvest of the Women's Movement*, edited by Myra Marx Ferree and Patricia Yancey Martin. Philadelphia: Temple University Press.

Reverby, Susan, and David Rosner. 1979. *Health Care in America: Essays in Social History.* Philadelphia: Temple University Press.

Rich, Adrienne. 1976. *Of Woman Born.* New York: W. W. Norton.

Ricoeur, Paul. 1978. *Main Trends in Philosophy.* New York: Holmes and Meier.

Rix, Sara, and Anne Stone. 1983. *Reductions and Realities: How the Federal Budget Affects Women.* Washington, D.C.: Women's Research and Education Institute.

Robb, Christina. 1979. "Take Good Care of Yourself." *New England Boston Sunday Globe*, February 18, 8–10, 21, 24, 33.

Roberts, Dorothy. 1997. *Killing the Black Body: Race, Reproduction, and the Meaning of Liberty.* New York: Pantheon Books.

Rodriguez-Trias, Helen 1997a. Interview with author, February 8, Eugene, Oreg.

———. 1997b. Foreword to *Women's Health: Complexities and Differences*, edited by Sheryl Ruzek, Virginia L. Olesen and Adele E. Clarke. Columbus: Ohio State University Press.

Rodriguez-Trias, Helen, and Carola Marte. 1995. "Challenges and Possibilities: Women, HIV, and the Health Care System in the 1990s." In *Women Resisting AIDS: Feminist Strategies of Empowerment*, edited by Beth Schneider and Nancy Stoller. Philadelphia: Temple University Press.

Ropes, Linda Brubaker. 1991. *Health Care Crisis in America: A Reference Handbook*. Santa Barbara, Calif.: ABC-CLIO.

Rose, Liz. 1975. Unpublished Document.

———. 1991. Interview with the author.

Ross, Loretta. 1998. "African-American Women and Abortion." In *Abortion Wars: A Half Century of Struggle, 1950–2000*, edited by Rickie Solinger. Berkeley: University of California Press.

Rothschild-Whitt, Joyce. 1976. "Conditions Facilitating Participatory Democratic Organizations." *Sociological Inquiry* 46 (2): 75–86.

———. 1979. "The Collectivist Organization: An Alternative to Rational-Bureaucratic Models." *American Sociological Review* 44 (4): 509–527.

———. 1986. *The Cooperative Workplace*. Cambridge, U.K.: Cambridge University Press.

Ruzek, Sheryl B. 1978. *The Women's Health Movement*. New York: Praeger.

———.1999. "Rethinking Feminist Ideologies and Actions: Thoughts on the Past and Future of Health Reform." In *Revisioning Women, Health and Healing: Feminist, Cultural and Technoscience Perspectives*, edited by Adele E. Clarke and Virginia L. Olesen. New York: Routledge.

Ruzek, Sheryl B., and Julie Becker. 1999. "The Women's Health Movement in the U.S.: From Grassroots Activism to Professional Agendas." *Journal of the American Medical Women's Association* 54 (1): 4–8, 40.

Ruzek, Sheryl Burt, Virginia L. Olesen, and Adele E. Clarke. 1997. *Women's Health : Complexities and Differences*. Columbus: Ohio State University Press.

Ryan, Barbara. 1992. *Feminism and the Women's Movement: Dynamics of Change in Social Movement, Ideology, and Activism*. New York: Routledge.

Rynne, Sally. 1989."The Women's Center: A Bold Strategy." *Health Management Quarterly* (fall/winter).

Sacks, Karen Brodkin. 1988. *Caring by the Hour: Women, Work, and Organizing at Duke Medical Center*. Urbana: University of Illinois Press.

Salaman, Graeme. 1986. *Working*. Chichester, U.K.: E. Horwood.

Santa Cruz Women's Health Center (SCWHC). 1988. "Statement of Purpose." Unpublished document.

Schechter, Susan. 1981. "Speaking to the Battered Women's Movement." *Aegis* 32.

———. 1982. *Women and Male Violence: The Visions and Struggles of the Battered Women's Movement*. Boston: South End Press.

Scherzer, Martha. 1995. "Byllye Avery and the National Black Women's Health Project." *Network News* (May/June): 1, 4, 6.

Schneider, Beth, and Nancy Stoller, eds. 1995. *Women Resisting AIDS: Feminist Strategies of Empowerment*. Philadelphia: Temple University Press.

Schnitger, Eileen. 1981. "Feminist Women's Health Center Attacked." *Women's Health Movement Papers*, compiled by the Federation of Feminist Women's Health Centers. Los Angeles, Calif.: FFWHC.

Scott, Ellen K. 1998. "Creating Partnerships for Change." *Gender and Society* 12 (4): 400–424.

———. 2000. "Everyone against Racism: Agency and the Production of Meaning in the Anti-racism Practices of Two Feminist Organizations." *Theory and Society* 29 (6): 785–819.

Scott, Julia. 1991. Interview with author, June, Washington, D.C.

Seaman, Barbara. 1969. *The Doctor's Case against the Pill*. New York: Wyden Books.

———. 1975. "The New 'Pill' Scare—Important Research from England." *Ms.* 3 (June): 61–64, 98–102.

———. 1977. "The Dangers of Sex Hormones." In *Seizing Our Bodies: The Politics of Women's Health*, edited by Claudia Dreifus. New York: Vintage.

Seaman, Barbara, and Susan Wood. 2000. "Role of Advocacy Groups in Research on Women's Health." In *Women and Health*, edited by Marlene B. Goldman and Maureen C. Hatch. San Diego, Calif.: Academic Press.

Selznick, Phillip. 1966. *TVA and the Grassroots: A Study in the Sociology of Formal Organizations*. New York: Harper Torchbooks.

Shapiro, Thomas. 1985. *Population Control Politics: Women, Sterilization and Reproductive Choice*. Philadelphia: Temple University Press.

Sheklow, Sally. 1994. Clinic Newsletter, Feminist Women's Health Center.

Shorter, Edward. 1982. *A History of Women's Bodies*. New York: Basic Books.

———. 1985. *Bedside Manners: The Troubled History of Doctors and Patients*. New York: Simon and Schuster.

Simmons, Judy Dothard. 1995. "Heroes at Work in an Alabama Clinic." *Ms.* 5 (6): 48–53.

Simmons, Ruth, Bonnie Kay, and Carol Regan. 1984. "Women's Health Groups: Alternatives to the Health Care System." *International Journal of Health and Services* 14 (4): 619–634.

Simonds, Wendy. 1995. "Feminism on the Job: Confronting Opposition in Abortion Work." In *Feminist Organizations: Harvest of the Women's Movement*, edited by Myra Marx Ferree and Patricia Yancey Martin. Philadelphia: Temple University Press.

———. 1996. *Abortion at Work: Ideology and Practice in a Feminist Clinic*. New Brunswick, N.J.: Rutgers University Press.

SisteReach. n.d. SisteReach: International Program of the National Black Women's Health Project Brochure.

Smith, Barbara. 1993. "Some Home Truths on the Contemporary Black Feminist Movement." In *Words of Fire: An Anthology of Movement*, edited by Beverly Guy-Sheftall. New York: New Press.

Smith, Steven, and Michael Lipsky. 1993. *Nonprofits for Hire: The Welfare State in the Age of Contracting*. Cambridge, Mass.: Harvard University Press.

Smith, Susan L. 1995. *Sick and Tired of Being Sick and Tired: Black Women's Health Activism in America, 1890–1950*. Philadelphia: University of Pennsylvania Press.

Solarz, Andrea L., ed. 1999. *Lesbian Health: Current Assessment and Directions for the Future*. Washington, D.C.: National Academy Press.

Solinger, Rickie. 1992. *Wake up Little Suzie: Single Pregnancy and Race before* Roe ver-
sus Wade. New York: Routledge.
———, ed. 1998. *Abortion Wars: A Half Century of Struggle, 1950–2000.* Berkeley: Uni-
versity of California Press.
Sommers, Elizabeth, et al. 1977. "A Report from Women's Community Health Center."
Quest 4, 1 (summer): 13–21.
Source Collective. 1974. *Source Catalog 3. Organizing for Health Care: A Tool for Change.*
Boston: Beacon Press.
Spangler, Luita. 1992. "Diary of a Mad Health Worker." *Women Wise* (spring): 7, 9.
Starr, Paul. 1982. *The Social Transformation of American Medicine: The Rise of a Sover-
eign Profession and the Making of a Vast Industry.* New York: Bantam Books.
Strobel, Margaret. 1995. "Organizational Learning in the Chicago Women's Liberation
Union." In *Feminist Organizations: Harvest of the Women's Movement,* edited by Myra
Marx Ferree and Patricia Yancey Martin. Philadelphia: Temple University Press.
Sullivan, Deborah, and Rose Weitz. 1988. *Labor Pains: Modern Midwives and Home Birth.*
New Haven, Conn.: Yale University Press.
Swartz, Donald. 1974. Discussion of "The Challenge of the Women's Movement to Ameri-
can Gynecology." *American Journal of Obstetrics and Gynecology* 120 (5): 661–663.
Taylor, Carol. 1994. "Gender Equity in Research." *Journal of Women's Health* 3 (3): 143–
153.
Taylor, Rosemary. 1979. "Free Medicine." In *Cooperatives, Communes, and Collectives:
Experiments in Social Change in the 1960s and 1970s,* edited by John Case and Rose-
mary Taylor. New York: Pantheon.
Taylor, Verta. 1983. "The Future of Feminism in the 1980's: A Social Movement Analy-
sis." In *Feminist Frontiers: Rethinking Sex, Gender and Society,* edited by Laura
Richardson and Verta Taylor. Reading, Mass.: Addison-Wesley.
———. 1995. "Watching for Vibes: Bringing Emotions into the Study of Feminist Orga-
nizations." In *Feminist Organizations: Harvest of the Women's Movement,* edited by
Myra Marx Ferree and Patricia Yancey Martin. Philadelphia: Temple University
Press.
Taylor, Verta, and Nancy Whittier. 1995. "Frameworks for the Analysis of Social Move-
ment Culture: The Culture of the Women's Movement." In *Culture and Social Move-
ments,* edited by Hank Johnson and Kent Klanderman. Minneapolis: University of
Minnesota Press.
Thomas, Jan E. 1999. "'Everything about Us Is Feminist': The Significance of Ideology
in Organizational Change." *Gender and Society* 13 (1): 101–119.
Touraine, Alain. 1981. *The Voice and the Eye: An Analysis of Social Movements.* New York:
Cambridge University Press.
Ulstad, Valerie K. 1993. "How Women Are Changing Medicine." *Journal of the Ameri-
can Medical Women's Association* 48, no. 3 (May/June): 75–78.
U.S. Women of Color Delegation to the International Conference on Population and De-
velopment. 1994. *Executive Summary: Statement on Poverty, Development and Popu-
lation.*
Van Gelder, Lindsy. 1991. "The Jane Collective: Seizing Control." *Ms.* 2, 2: 83–86.
Vaughn, Susan. 1987. "A Healthy Interest." *The Tab* (December 8).
Viguerie, Richard. 1982. "Defund the Left." *New York Times,* August 11, A23.
Villarosa, Linda, ed. 1994. *Body and Soul: The Black Women's Guide to Physical Health
and Emotional Well-Being.* New York: HarperPerennial.

Wallis, Lila A., Glenda D. Donoghue, and Jean L. Fourcroy. 1994. "Feminists and Women Physicians." *Journal of Women's Health* 3 (6).

Weber, Max. 1947. *The Theory of Social and Economic Organization*. London: William Hodge.

————. 1978. *Economy and Society*, edited by Guenther Roth and Klaus Wittich. Berkeley: University of California Press.

Weideger, Paula. 1975. *Menstruation and Menopause*. New York: Knopf.

Weisman, Carol. 1998. *Women's Health Care: Activist Traditions and Institutional Change*. Baltimore: Johns Hopkins University Press.

Weisman, Carol et al. 1995. "The National Survey of Women's Health Centers: Current Models of Women-Centered Care." *Women's Health Issues* 5 (3): 103–117.

Wentz, Anne Colston. 1994. Editorial. *Journal of Women's Health* 3 (4): 249–250.

White, Evelyn. 1990. *The Black Women's Health Book: Speaking for Ourselves*. Seattle, Wash.: Seal Press.

Williams, Patricia. 1991. *The Alchemy of Race and Rights*. Cambridge, Mass.: Harvard University Press.

Wolfson, Alice. 1998. "Clenched Fist, Open Heart." In *The Feminist Memoir Project: Voices from Women's Liberation*, edited by Rachel DuPlessis Blau and Ann Snitow. New York: Three Rivers Press.

Women's Community Health Center (WCHC). 1975. *First Annual Report* (August).

————. 1976a. "Experience of a Pelvic Teaching Group." *Women and Health* 1 (July/August): 19–20.

————. 1976b. Second Annual Report [August].

————. 1977a. Third Annual Report (September).

————. 1977b. Letter, May 10.

————. 1979. Fifth Annual Report.

————. 1981. Letter, July 22.

Worcester, Nancy, and Mariamne Whatley. 1988. "The Response of the Health Care System to the Women's Health Movement: The Selling of Women's Health Centers." In *Feminism within the Science and Health Care Profession: Overcoming Resistance*, edited by Sue Rosser. Oxford, U. K.: Pergamon Press.

Wright, Erik. 1975. "Alternative Perspectives in the Marxist Theory of Accumulation and Crisis." *Insurgent Sociologist* 6 (1): 5–39.

Yallof, Barrie E. 1994. "Feminism and Health Care: The Boston Women's Health Book Collective." Honor's thesis, Amherst College.

Zald, Mayer, and Roberta Ash. 1966. "Social Movement Organizations: Growth, Decay, and Change." *Social Forces* 44 (3): 327–341.

Zavella, Patricia. 1987. *Women's Work and Chicano Families: Cannery Workers of the Santa Clara Valley*. Ithaca, N.Y.: Cornell University Press.

Ziegler, Vicki, and Elizabeth Campbell, eds. 1973. *Circle One Self Health Handbook*. Colorado Springs, Colo.: Colorado Springs Women's Health.

Zimmerman, Mary K. 1987. "The Women's Health Movement: A Critique of Medical Enterprise and the Position of Women." In *Analyzing Gender: A Handbook of Social Science Research*, edited by Beth B. Hess and Myra Marx Ferree. Beverly Hills: Sage.

Index

abortion: feminist health clinic services, 43, 70–71, 74, 85, 150–151, 188, 245n1; Hyde Amendment and, 51, 58, 172–173, 181, 199, 234, 248–249n4; Janes' role in illegal abortion, 5–7, 31–35; laws, 4, 7, 155, 182, 249n1; for low-income women, 41, 51; Planned Parenthood clinics, 150–151; referral collective for illegal abortion, 90; Supreme Court rulings on, 201, 245n2. *See also* antiabortion movement; reproductive rights

Abortion Counseling Service of Women's Liberation, 5, 32

Abramovitz, Mimi, 154

Abramson, Alan, 184

Abramson, Hilary, 129, 202, 203

Acker, Joan, 119

advocacy groups, 30–31; AIDS and, 203–205, 235; breast cancer and, 143–145, 235; for women's health research, 141–142, 234. *See also* National Asian Women's Health Organization; National Black Women's Health Project; National Latina Health Organization; National Women's Health Network

Advocates for Life (AFL), 193, 196

Advocates for Medical Information (AMI), 10, 27

affirmative action, 224. *See also* race conflicts/differences

African American women. *See* Black women's health movement; National Black Women's Health Project; racial/ethnic diversity, staff

Ahrens, Lois, 111, 112

Ahron, Jonina, 49

AIDS, 13, 203–205, 235

Akron Center for Reproductive Health vs. The City of Akron, 201

Allen, Lillie, 49

Allen, Robert, 167

Alonso, Ana, 12

Alvarez Martinez, Luz, 55–58, 59, 60, 61, 68

Amaro, Hortensia, 204

American College of Obstetricians and Gynecologists, 126, 135

American Gynecological Association, 124–125

American Medical Association (AMA), 121, 122, 127, 129

American Medical Women's Association (AMWA), 141

About the Author

Sandra Morgen is director of the Center for the Study of Women in Society and a professor in the department of sociology at the University of Oregon. She is an anthropologist whose research has focused on women's health, social welfare policy, and women's political activism. Her publications include *Women and the Politics of Empowerment* (1988, edited with Ann Bookman), *Gender and Anthropology: Critical Reviews for Research and Teaching* (1989), and *EnGendering Rationalities* (2001, edited with Nancy Tuana), as well as a host of articles in professional journals and anthologies. She lives in Eugene, Oregon, with her husband and two children.